Cardiac Valvular Medicine

Nalini M. Rajamannan
Editor

Cardiac Valvular Medicine

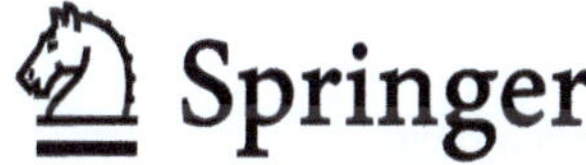

Editor
Nalini M. Rajamannan, M.D.
Mayo Clinic
Rochester, MN
USA

ISBN 978-1-4471-4131-0 ISBN 978-1-4471-4132-7 (eBook)
DOI 10.1007/978-1-4471-4132-7
Springer Dordrecht Heidelberg New York London

Library of Congress Control Number: 2012945531

Printed on acid-free paper

Springer is part of Springer Science+Business Media (www.springer.com)

This textbook is dedicated to my Roman Catholic Faith, to my dear Mother Concie Armstrong Rajamannan who dedicated her life to her Roman Catholic Faith, and to her family, to my extended family, and to my Godchildren Hugh, Hazen and Sophia, to all my patients past, present and future, and finally to my educators at Immaculate Conception School, Totino Grace High School, the University of Notre Dame, and the Institute of Christ the King Sovereign Priest.

Preface

Valvular Medicine is a textbook which represents an overview of recent discoveries and scientific contributions in the field of valvular heart disease. The book is designed to update cardiologists, internists, family practice physicians, cardiac surgeons, and basic scientists regarding the most recent science, clinical trials, and new discoveries in the field of valvular heart disease. For decades, cardiac valve lesions have been thought to be due to a degenerative process, which has been for years described as "a wear and tear phenomena"; however experimental studies in the field of cardiac valve biology have demonstrated that this disease process is an active biology.

Since 1968, the only therapy for calcific aortic valve disease has been careful observation until the time of the classic triad of symptoms, which includes chest pain, shortness of breath, and lightheadedness. When these symptoms develop, the timing to surgical valve replacement is critical to avoid the increase in morbidity and mortality for the patient. Across the world, percutaneous intervention for aortic stenosis is soon becoming the next option for therapies for patients.

Over the past 15 years, epidemiologists have discovered that valvular risk factors are similar to vascular risk factors. These vascular risk factors an atherosclerotic valve lesion which is similar to the vasculature lesion in experimental models. The final common pathway for the disease phenotype is bone formation in the valve. These studies will help to further understand not only the cellular mechanisms, but also the potential to target this disease with medical therapies.

Similar discoveries in the field of mitral valve biology and risk factors are also evolving rapidly, to will give physicians and scientists insight into the cellular mechanisms, and the possibility of treating this valve lesions with other options besides surgical valve repair. The future results of the randomized surgical trial for mitral regurgitation will provide the template for the timing of intervention.

Our understanding of right sided valve lesions is also rapidly becoming important in the field of valvular medicine. Not only is the pathology different from the left sided valve lesion, but the hemodynamic compromise is more complex and difficult to treat in patients who develop tricuspid or pulmonic valve disease. Early diagnosis and careful management of this patient population is critical for long term outcomes in this patient population.

The most important lesson in the care of the patient is a careful history and physical exam. The stethoscope and the art of auscultation will continue to be important in screening for cardiac and pulmonary disease, but a future window to diagnose early atherosclerosis in patients who have aortic valve sclerosis. The authors and I hope that this textbook will bring the most recent developments in the field of valvular heart disease to the reader and provide a translational understanding from bench to bedside for the future treatments for this patient population.

Nalini Marie Rajamannan, M.D.
Editor Valvular Medicine

Contents

Contributors

Elena Aikawa Department of Medicine, Cardiovascular Medicine, Brigham and Women's Hospital, Harvard Medical School, Boston, MA, USA

Francesco Antonini-Canterin Department of Cardiology, Cardiologia, ARC, Azienda Ospedaliera S. Maria degli Angeli, Pordenone, Italy

Luigi P. Badano, M.D. Department of Cardiac, Thoracic and Vascular Sciences, University of Padua, Padua, Italy

Cristina Basso, M.D., Ph.D. Department of Cardiac, Thoracic and Vascular Sciences, University of Padua, Padua, Italy

M. Chrissoheris, M.D. Transcatheter Heart Valve Department, HYGEIA Hospital, N. Attikis, Greece

José Juan GómezdeDiego, M.D. Cardiac Imaging Laboratory, La Paz Hospital, Madrid, Spain

Jean G. Dumesnil, M.D., FRCP(C) Department of Medicine, Laval University, Ottawa, ON, Canada

Sammy Elmariah, M.D., MPH Interventional and Structural Heart Disease, Division of Cardiology, Massachusetts General, Hospital, Harvard Medical School, Boston, MA, USA

Alexandra Gonçalves, M.D. Cardiology Department, University Hospital Ramón y Cajal, Madrid, Spain

Hospital S. João/University of Porto Medical School, Porto, Portugal

K. Jane Grande-Allen Department of Bioengineering, Rice University, Houston, TX, USA

Anders M. Greve, M.D. Department of Cardiology, The Heart Center, Rigshospitalet, Copenhagen, Denmark

Department of Cardiology, Gentofte Hospital, Hellerup, Denmark

Gilbert Habib Department of Cardiology, La Timone Hospital, Marseille, France

Helena J. Heuvelman Department of Cardio-Thoracic Surgery, Erasmus University Medical Center, Rotterdam, The Netherlands

Patrizio Lancellotti, M.D., Ph.D Department of Cardiology, Heart Valve Clinic, University Hospital Sart Tilman, University of Liège, Liège, Belgium

Margaret A. Lloyd, M.D. Department of Cardiology, Mayo Clinic, Rochester, MN, USA

Chaim Lotan Department of Cardiology, Heart Institute Hadassah Hebrew University Medical Center, Jerusalem, Israel

Julien Magne, Ph.D Department of Cardiology, Heart Valve Clinic, University Hospital Sart Tilman, University of Liège, Liège, Belgium

Antonia Delgado Montero, M.D. Cardiology Department, University Hospital Ramón y Cajal, Madrid, Spain

Luis Moura Department of Cardiology, Hospital S. João/University of Porto Medical School, Porto, Portugal

Denisa Muraru, M.D. Department of Cardiac, Thoracic and Vascular Sciences, University of Padua, Padua, Italy

Philippe Pibarot, DVM, Ph.D. Canada Research Chair in Valvular Hear Disease, Canadian Institutes of Health research, Ottawa, Canada

Department of Medicine, Laval University, Ottawa, ON, Canada

Nalini Marie Rajamannan, M.D. Department of Molecular Biology and Biochemistry, Mayo Clinic, Rochester, MN, USA

Department of Aerospace Engineering, University of Notre Dame, South Bend, IN, USA

Charanjit S. Rihal, M.D. Division of Cardiovascular Diseases, Mayo Clinic, Rochester, MN, USA

Mony Shuvy Department of Cardiology, Heart Institute Hadassah Hebrew University Medical Center, Jerusalem, Israel

K. Spargias, M.D. Transcatheter Heart Valve Department, HYGEIA Hospital, N. Attikis, Greece

Thomas C. Spelsberg, Ph.D. Department of Molecular Biology and Biochemistry, Mayo Clinic, Rochester, MN, USA

Malayannan Subramaniam, Ph.D. Department of Molecular Biology and Biochemistry, Mayo Clinic, Rochester, MN, USA

Philippe Sucosky, Ph.D. Department of Molecular Biology and Biochemistry, Mayo Clinic, Rochester, MN, USA

M.J. Swaans, M.D. Department of Cardiology, St. Antonius Hospital, Nieuwegein, the Netherlands

Johanna J.M. Takkenberg Department of Cardio-Thoracic Surgery, Erasmus University Medical Center, Rotterdam, The Netherlands

Gaetano Thiene, M.D., FRCP Department of Cardiac, Thoracic and Vascular Sciences, University of Padua, Padua, Italy

Franck Thuny Department of Cardiology, La Timone Hospital, Marseille, France

Kristian Wachtell, M.D., Ph.D., DrMedSci Department of Cardiology, The Heart Center, Rigshospitalet, Copenhagen, Denmark

Department of Cardiology, Gentofte Hospital, Hellerup, Denmark

University of Copenhagen, Copenhagen, Denmark

José Luis Zamorano, M.D., Ph.D., FESC Cardiology Department, University Hospital Ramón y Cajal, Madrid, Spain

1 Modifying the Natural History of Aortic Valve Stenosis

Helena J. Heuvelman, Nalini Marie Rajamannan, and Johanna J.M. Takkenberg

Introduction

Aortic valve stenosis (AS) is the most common heart valve disease in the world, with a prevalence up to 3% of adults over the age of 75 years (Nkomo et al. 2006). One-third of US adults ≥65 years has aortic valve sclerosis and of these at least one-third will develop some degree of AS within 5 years (Faggiano et al. 2003; Otto et al. 1999). The natural history, diagnosis, and cellular mechanisms of this disease process have evolved over the past several decades. Over the last 10 years, the scientific progress in the field of calcific aortic valve stenosis has increased exponentially. A critical discovery in our understanding of calcification as the end-stage pathogenesis of a congenital bicuspid or tricuspid aortic valve is the osteogenic process (Rajamannan et al. 2003; Otto 2006; Rosenhek et al. 2000a). Progressive calcification of the leaflets usually leads to severe narrowing of the aortic valve orifice and fibrosis of the left ventricular wall, finally resulting in left ventricular outflow tract obstruction and severe aortic stenosis. After a prolonged asymptomatic period with low morbidity and mortality, the development of the classic triad of symptoms including: angina, syncope, or heart failure marks the critical point in the natural history of aortic valve disease. AS is a progressive disease and without intervening treatment associated with high morbidity and mortality rates within a few years of diagnosis (Horstkotte and Loogen 1988). Survival declines when a patient with AS develops angina or syncope, and is even more limited when the patient develops congestive heart failure. Because AS is a disease of the elderly, it can be difficult to distinguish the gradual decrease in physical functioning attributed to advanced age and multiple co-morbidities such as frailty, lung disease, neurological disease, and symptoms from the worsening AS disease. It is not uncommon that patients will lower their activity level below their symptom threshold, to accommodate to the progressive left ventricular outflow tract obstruction. This chapter will outline the studies in the field of diagnosis and the impact of the evolving science of clinical risk factors for calcific aortic valve disease. Traditional Timing to Intervention.

Patients with mild to severe asymptomatic AS are monitored until the development of symptoms. Sudden death is a rare event with an occurrence of 1% per year without preceding symptoms (Pellikka

H.J. Heuvelman, M.D. (✉) •
J.J.M. Takkenberg, M.D., Ph.D.
Department of Cardio-Thoracic Surgery,
Erasmus University Medical Center,
Rotterdam, The Netherlands
e-mail: h.heuvelman@erasmusmc.nl

N.M. Rajamannan, M.D.
Department of Molecular Biology
and Biochemistry, Mayo Clinic,
Rochester, MN, USA

Department of Aerospace Engineering,
University of Notre Dame,
South Bend, IN, USA
e-mail: nrajamannan@gmail.com

N.M. Rajamannan (ed.), *Cardiac Valvular Medicine*,
DOI 10.1007/978-1-4471-4132-7_1, © Springer-Verlag London 2013

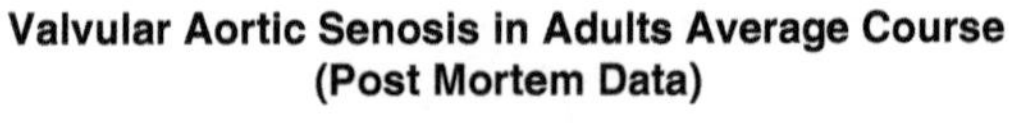

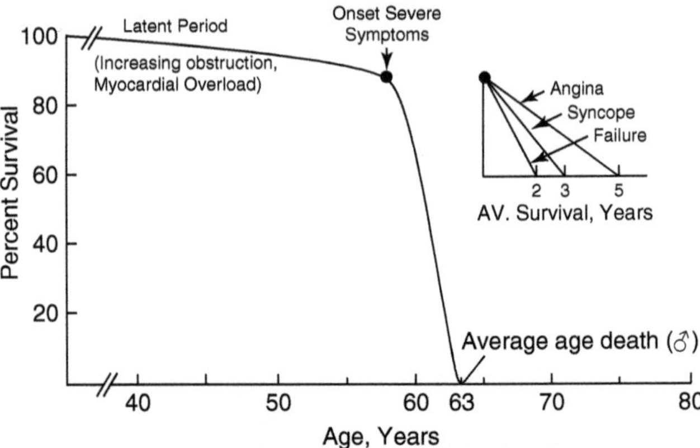

Fig. 1.1 Average course of valvular aortic stenosis in adults. Data assembled from post-mortem studies (Reprinted with permission)

et al. 2005). If symptomatic severe AS is present, according to the present ACC/AHA and ESC guidelines, aortic valve replacement is indicated (Bonow et al. 2006; Vahanian et al. 2007). An evolving option in the twenty-first century for patients who are not candidates for surgery, is the transcatheter aortic valve implantation which is performed in specific patient populations in Europe and US. In an effort to assess AS severity and progression for the individual adult patient, it is important to consider the changing basic concept of AS disease, current knowledge about AS progression, and insight in the factors associated with AS progression. These topics will be described in the following paragraphs of this chapter.

Historical Perspective of AS Disease

Early reports on the natural history of AS are based on post-mortem studies, invasive cardiac catheterization studies, and Doppler echocardiography. Historically, symptomatic AS was seen as a passive degenerative disease and associated with a significant risk (>15%) of sudden death while asymptomatic AS reportedly had a risk of sudden death of 3–5% (Ross and Braunwald 1968). According to the post mortem studies from the period 1930–1950, the time from symptom onset until death was on average less than 5 years for patients with angina and only 2 years for patients with heart failure as shown in Fig. 1.1. With the development of cardiac catheterization in the 1930s, hemodynamic assessment of AS severity became possible. Although the published catheterization studies in patients with AS often consist of small study populations, they provide the first quantitative data of AS progression over time (Lester et al. 1998). In the late 1980s, the non-invasive Doppler echocardiography technique became available and offered an opportunity for longitudinal studies regarding AS disease and progression. These studies provide further information for the understanding of this complex disease process via non-invasive imaging.

On July 13, 1912, Theodore Tuffier, a French surgeon, performed the first successful closed heart surgery in a young patient with severe AS by digitally invaginating the aortic wall into the aortic valve orifice to dilate the stenosed valve (Lichtenstein 2006). Several different invasive approaches to palliate severe AS followed with poor outcomes (Shumacker 1992). The first aortic valve replacements were performed with an caged-ball valve prosthesis in the 1960s and were accompanied by mortality rates ranging from 25% to 50%, but over time, mortality rates decreased considerably, even for complex aortic valve procedures (Harken 1958). The introduction of cardiopulmonary bypass in the 1950s and cardioplegia in the mid 1960s was associated with the continuous improvements in operative techniques and postoperative care. The development of new valve substitutes, such as bioprosthetic valves, are important developments which have resulted in the extremely low morbidity and mortality that is observed in contemporary clinical practice.

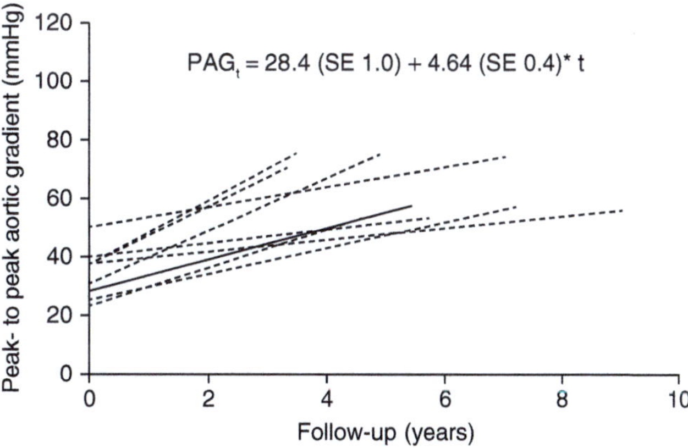

Fig. 1.2 AS progression in cardiac catheterization studies. *AS* aortic valve stenosis, *PAG$_t$* peak-to-peak aortic gradient at time t, *SE* standard error, *t* time. *Interrupted lines* individual study estimates, *solid line* pooled estimate (Heuvelman et al. 2012) (Reprinted with permission)

In more recent years, the concept that AS is passive and degenerative is not valid anymore. It is now proven that AS represents a more active regulated disease process characterized by lipoprotein deposition, active leaflet calcification, and chronic inflammation for which medical treatment possibly could play a role (Rajamannan et al. 2011; Freeman and Otto 2005; Mohler 2000). The understanding of this biologic process may offer an opportunity to treat AS with medications, in order to prevent, reverse or slow down the disease as more scientific studies in this field are performed.

What Is Known About AS Progression?

There are several studies investigating AS progression and its potential determinants, however, due to small sample size, non-randomized retrospective study design, heterogenic study populations, large variability in AS progression estimates, and limited follow-up duration, it has been difficult in the past to draw general conclusions. A meta-analysis on the diagnostic studies in cardiac catheterization and echocardiography demonstrates the differences in these diagnostic approaches, and the challenges that are present in following the natural history of this disease by echo and cardiac catheterization data.

Figure 1.2 shows progression of AS measured by cardiac catheterization according to nine published reports from the 1970s and 1980s, describing the course of AS disease over time in patients with a mean age of 55 years (range 37–61 years) of whom 75% males (Bogart et al. 1979; Cheitlin et al. 1979; Wagner and Selzer 1982; Jonasson et al. 1983; Nestico et al. 1983; Larsen and Jensen 1985; Ng et al. 1986; Nitta et al. 1988; Turina et al. 1987). The studies include predominantly male patients with ages ranging from 40 to 60 years with mostly non-severe AS who underwent serial measurements for clinical reasons, for example for the evaluation of a systolic murmur. Progression of AS disease, as measured by the aortic valve area calculated with the Gorlin formula and the peak-to-peak aortic gradient, shows a large variability in the progression rates between studies. Annual reductions of the aortic valve area vary from 0.03 to 0.24 cm^2/year and annual increase in aortic peak-to-peak gradients ranging from 2 to 11 mmHg/year.

Figure 1.3 displays echocardiographic AS progression from a systematic review and meta-analysis of observational reports published between 1989 and 2009 (Heuvelman et al. 2012). The results of this analysis demonstrate a similar large variability in AS progression rates compared to cardiac catheterization studies. Annual reductions in aortic valve area vary from 0.04 to 0.22 cm^2/year. There is an annual increase in maximum aortic jet velocity ranging from 0.06 to 0.40 m/s/year. The annual increase in peak and mean aortic gradient varying from 2 to 15 and from 2 to 8 mmHg respectively (Heuvelman et al. 2012). This meta-analysis for catheterization and echo variability demonstrates further understanding into the complex assessment of the hemodynamic parameters, which reflects most probably

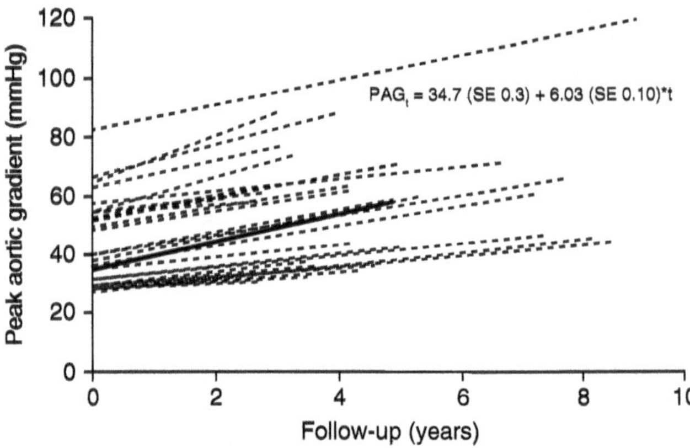

Fig. 1.3 AS progression in observational studies. *AS* aortic valve stenosis, *PAG$_t$* peak aortic gradient at time t, *SE* standard error, *t* time. *Interrupted lines* individual study estimates, *solid line* pooled estimate (Heuvelman et al. 2012) (Reprinted with permission)

institutional variability in measurements and differences in patients' clinical risk factors. Assessing the degree of stenosis, hemodynamic severity, and anatomic criteria for TAVI is also evolving quickly and the results of this meta-analysis will help to further understand this process.

In addition to the measures above, assessing the amount of aortic valve calcification can also be used to monitor AS severity and progression. This has been measured in a few studies in which different methods were employed to assess aortic calcification, often without a reference test to quantify the extent of aortic valve calcification and the timing to progression (Rubler et al. 1985; Rosenhek et al. 2004; Cowell et al. 2003; Dichtl et al. 2008). This textbook will provide an overview for why these differences may exist which include risk factors, diagnostic techniques, and understanding the variable stages of this disease by assessing the calcification in the overall outcome of this patient population.

Factors Associated with AS Progression and Clinical Outcome

Many factors are reportedly potentially associated with faster AS progression and/or impaired clinical outcome of AS disease: advanced patient age, male gender, obesity, smoking, hypertension, diabetes, coronary artery disease, chronic obstructive lung disease, severe pulmonary hypertension, significant aortic valve calcification, a higher maximum aortic jet velocity at baseline and faster progression rate, decreased aortic valve area, left ventricular dysfunction, aortic regurgitation, impaired functional status, abnormal exercise response on exercise testing, inactivity, elevated levels of serum cholesterol, calcium, creatinine, C-reactive protein, and natriuretic peptides, osteoporosis treatment, chronic renal failure, and hemodialysis (Pellikka et al. 2005; Rosenhek et al. 2000b, 2004, 2010; Otto et al. 1997; Avakian et al. 2008; Brener et al. 1995; Peter et al. 1993; Bahler et al. 1999; Palta et al. 2000; Ngo et al. 2001; Wongpraparut et al. 2002; Davies et al. 1991; Sanchez et al. 2006; Antonini-Canterin et al. 2003; Faggiano et al. 1996; Bergler-Klein et al. 2004; Skolnick et al. 2009; Lafitte et al. 2009; Varadarajan et al. 2006; Ohara et al. 2005).

As the basic concept of AS disease as a passive degenerative disease is now a concept of the past, and we are moving to the notion that it represents an active disease process with many similarities to atherosclerosis, the interest in potential medical treatments of AS disease is growing. The recent Working group of the National Heart Lung and Blood Institute/NIH, has defined the concept that CAVD is not a passive degenerative process but an active biology (Rajamannan et al. 2011). In this respect, five randomized controlled trials on AS progression were developed to determine whether statins could reduce AS progression in adult patients with AS (Dichtl et al. 2008; Chan et al. 2010; Rossebo et al. 2008; Cowell et al. 2005; van der Linde et al. 2011). These statin trials provide invaluable information into future trial design and also the effects of statins on the

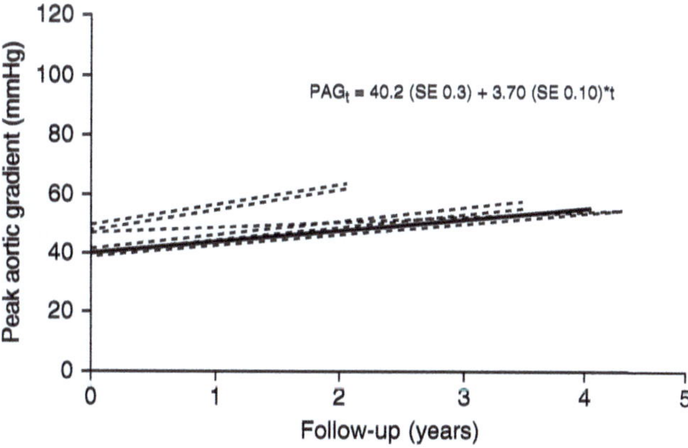

Fig. 1.4 AS progression in randomized controlled trials. *AS* aortic valve stenosis, *PAG$_t$* peak aortic gradient at time t, *SE* standard error, *t* time. *Interrupted lines* individual study estimates, *solid line* pooled estimate (Heuvelman et al. 2012) (Reprinted with permission)

progression of AS in vastly different patient populations. The TASS trial, the SALTIRE trial, the large SEAS trial, and the ASTRONOMER trial included patients with mild to severe AS, a mean age varying from 54 to 70 years with predominantly male patients and show an annual decrease in aortic valve area ranging from 0.03 to 0.08 cm^2/year, an annual increase in maximum aortic jet velocity of 0.15–0.20 m/s/year, an annual increase in peak aortic gradient of 2–7 mmHg/year, and an annual increase in mean aortic gradient of 1–4 mmHg/year and showed no significantly reduction in AS progression in patients receiving lipid-lowering therapy, in this range of patient population (Heuvelman et al. 2012; Dichtl et al. 2008; Chan et al. 2010; Rossebo et al. 2008; Cowell et al. 2005). Figure 1.4 displays the echocardiographic AS progression from a systematic review and meta-analysis of these published randomized controlled statin trials between 2005 and 2010 (Heuvelman et al. 2012). Again there is some variability in the echo results as shown in Fig. 1.4, but not as significant as the progression study analysis in Figs. 1.2 and 1.3. Recently, the hypothesis of lipid-lowering therapy on AS progression was tested in congenital AS patient population, entitled the PROCAS trial. This trial included 63 patients with an age range of 18–45 years and no decrease in AS progression in patients randomized to rosuvastatin 10 mg for the duration of the trial (van der Linde et al. 2011). The results of these randomized trials can be possibly attributed to trial design, timing of treatment, and level of LDL lowering. Earlier initiation of therapy may be the key to success in the future clinical trials to treat this disease. The only study to demonstrate the positive effects of a statin in the treatment of calcific aortic valve disease is the RAAVE trial, Rosuvastatin Affecting Aortic Valve Endothelium in aortic stenosis (Moura et al. 2007). This open label hypothesis driven study demonstrating slowing of progression of AS using Rosuvastatin 10 mg a day by measuring aortic valve area, mean gradient, and peak jet velocity. The retrospective, prospective and animal models are providing the foundation for the treatment of this disease in the future.

Several observational studies suggest that in particular age, baseline severity of AS disease, and aortic valve morphology like calcification and the presence of a bicuspid valve, may affect AS progression rate (Pellikka et al. 2005; Otto et al. 1997; Rosenhek et al. 2000b). The ASTRONOMER trial sub-study identified aortic valve calcification as an independent factor associated with a faster AS progression after correcting for age, baseline AS severity, and tricuspid aortic valve morphology (Chan et al. 2010). It represents more severe and aggressive disease in bicuspid patients as compared to tricuspid patients, and therefore alerts the physician to careful clinical decision making for patients with bicuspid aortic valve disease.

These studies illustrate a wide variation in the observed progression of AS over time. As compared to observational studies, randomized controlled trials show smaller AS progression estimates which may be explained by selection bias and different echocardiographic methods employed to monitor AS disease. Our observations of AS progression are biased in many ways. Another recent report shows that the hemodynamic criteria for AS severity are applied inconsistently for grading AS, even in patients with normal left ventricular function (Minners et al. 2008). If AS severity is assessed using the aortic valve area method, more patients are classified as having severe AS compared to AS assessment with the mean aortic pressure or maximum aortic jet velocity method. These observations call for a universal classification of AS severity, in order to optimize uniformity in assessment of AS disease. This textbook of valvular medicine provides further understanding into establishing criteria to include these novel findings and clinical risk factors for this disease process.

Conclusions

This chapter aimed to provide insight in the natural history of AS over time and the complex nature of AS disease, especially to identify factors associated with AS progression and clinical outcome of AS disease in the aging population. We are only starting to understand the mechanisms underlying AS disease, and its complexity. From basic science to applied clinical studies, there are so many aspects of AS disease, which are under intense investigation. For example, there is increasing evidence that genetics may play a role in bicuspid valve disease and the calcification of the tricuspid aortic valve (Rajamannan et al. 2011). Improved insights into genetic factors associated with AS disease may help clinicians to better diagnose and treat our patients. On a more general note, the emerging knowledge of the mechanisms underlying AS disease may provide us with drugs that prevent, reverse or slow down AS disease. Also, the tremendous development of different non-invasive imaging techniques will help clinicians better diagnose disease severity, provided that a universal classification of AS severity is achieved. Biomarkers that are at the horizon may also help prognostication. Using the information obtained from emerging knowledge, the next step is to integrate this knowledge into clinical decision tools that can provide evidence-based estimates of outcome for individual patients, allowing optimal individualized treatment and improvement in the natural history of AS.

References

Antonini-Canterin F, Huang G, Cervesato E, Faggiano P, Pavan D, Piazza R, Nicolosi GL. Symptomatic aortic stenosis: does systemic hypertension play an additional role? Hypertension. 2003;41(6):1268–72.

Avakian SD, Grinberg M, Ramires JA, Mansur AP. Outcome of adults with asymptomatic severe aortic stenosis. Int J Cardiol. 2008;123(3):322–7.

Bahler RC, Desser DR, Finkelhor RS, Brener SJ, Youssefi M. Factors leading to progression of valvular aortic stenosis. Am J Cardiol. 1999;84(9):1044–8.

Bergler-Klein J, Klaar U, Heger M, Rosenhek R, Mundigler G, Gabriel H, Binder T, Pacher R, Maurer G, Baumgartner H. Natriuretic peptides predict symptom-free survival and postoperative outcome in severe aortic stenosis. Circulation. 2004;109(19):2302–8.

Bogart DB, Murphy BL, Wong BY, Pugh DM, Dunn MI. Progression of aortic stenosis. Chest. 1979;76(4):391–6.

Bonow RO, Carabello BA, Chatterjee K, de Leon Jr AC, Faxon DP, Freed MD, Gaasch WH, Lytle BW, Nishimura RA, O'Gara PT, O'Rourke RA, Otto CM, Shah PM, Shanewise JS, Smith Jr SC, Jacobs AK, Adams CD, Anderson JL, Antman EM, Fuster V, Halperin JL, Hiratzka LF, Hunt SA, Lytle BW, Nishimura R, Page RL, Riegel B. ACC/AHA 2006 guidelines for the management of patients with valvular heart disease: a report of the American College of Cardiology/American Heart Association Task Force on Practice Guidelines (writing Committee to Revise the 1998 guidelines for the management of patients with valvular heart disease) developed in collaboration with the Society of Cardiovascular Anesthesiologists endorsed by the Society for Cardiovascular Angiography and Interventions and the Society of Thoracic Surgeons. J Am Coll Cardiol. 2006;48(3):e1–148.

Brener SJ, Duffy CI, Thomas JD, Stewart WJ. Progression of aortic stenosis in 394 patients: relation to changes in myocardial and mitral valve dysfunction. J Am Coll Cardiol. 1995;25(2):305–10.

Chan KL, Teo K, Dumesnil JG, Ni A, Tam J. Effect of lipid lowering with rosuvastatin on progression of aortic stenosis: results of the aortic stenosis progression observation: measuring effects of rosuvastatin (ASTRONOMER) trial. Circulation. 2010;121(2):306–14.

Cheitlin MD, Gertz EW, Brundage BH, Carlson CJ, Quash JA, Bode Jr RS. Rate of progression of severity of valvular aortic stenosis in the adult. Am Heart J. 1979;98(6):689–700.

Cowell SJ, Newby DE, Burton J, White A, Northridge DB, Boon NA, Reid J. Aortic valve calcification on computed tomography predicts the severity of aortic stenosis. Clin Radiol. 2003;58(9):712–6.

Cowell SJ, Newby DE, Prescott RJ, Bloomfield P, Reid J, Northridge DB, Boon NA. A randomized trial of intensive lipid-lowering therapy in calcific aortic stenosis. N Engl J Med. 2005;352(23):2389–97.

Davies SW, Gershlick AH, Balcon R. Progression of valvar aortic stenosis: a long-term retrospective study. Eur Heart J. 1991;12(1):10–4.

Dichtl W, Alber HF, Feuchtner GM, Hintringer F, Reinthaler M, Bartel T, Sussenbacher A, Grander W, Ulmer H, Pachinger O, Muller S. Prognosis and risk factors in patients with asymptomatic aortic stenosis and their modulation by atorvastatin (20 mg). Am J Cardiol. 2008;102(6):743–8.

Faggiano P, Aurigemma GP, Rusconi C, Gaasch WH. Progression of valvular aortic stenosis in adults: literature review and clinical implications. Am Heart J. 1996;132(2 Pt 1):408–17.

Faggiano P, Antonini-Canterin F, Erlicher A, Romeo C, Cervesato E, Pavan D, Piazza R, Huang G, Nicolosi GL. Progression of aortic valve sclerosis to aortic stenosis. Am J Cardiol. 2003;91(1):99–101.

Freeman RV, Otto CM. Spectrum of calcific aortic valve disease: pathogenesis, disease progression, and treatment strategies. Circulation. 2005;111(24):3316–26.

Harken DE. The surgical treatment of acquired valvular disease. Circulation. 1958;18(1):1–6.

Heuvelman HJ, Van Geldorp MWA, Eijkemans MJC, Rajamannan NM, Bogers AJJC, Roos-Hesselink JW, Takkenberg JJM. Progression of aortic valve stenosis is adults: a systematic review. J Heart Valve Dis. 2012; 21:454–462.

Horstkotte D, Loogen F. The natural history of aortic valve stenosis. Eur Heart J. 1988;9(Suppl E):57–64.

Jonasson R, Jonsson B, Nordlander R, Orinius E, Szamosi A. Rate of progression of severity of valvular aortic stenosis. Acta Med Scand. 1983;213(1):51–4.

Lafitte S, Perlant M, Reant P, Serri K, Douard H, Demaria A, Roudaut R. Impact of impaired myocardial deformations on exercise tolerance and prognosis in patients with asymptomatic aortic stenosis. Eur J Echocardiogr. 2009;10(3):414–9.

Larsen VH, Jensen BS. Spontaneous progression of valvular aortic stenosis. Dan Med Bull. 1985;32(1):69–72.

Lester SJ, Heilbron B, Gin K, Dodek A, Jue J. The natural history and rate of progression of aortic stenosis. Chest. 1998;113(4):1109–14.

Lichtenstein SV. Closed heart surgery: back to the future. J Thorac Cardiovasc Surg. 2006;131(5):941–3.

Minners J, Allgeier M, Gohlke-Baerwolf C, Kienzle RP, Neumann FJ, Jander N. Inconsistencies of echocardiographic criteria for the grading of aortic valve stenosis. Eur Heart J. 2008;29(8):1043–8.

Mohler 3rd ER. Are atherosclerotic processes involved in aortic-valve calcification? Lancet. 2000;356(9229): 524–5.

Moura LM, Ramos SF, Zamorano JL, Barros IM, Azevedo LF, Rocha-Goncalves F, Rajamannan NM. Rosuvastatin affecting aortic valve endothelium to slow the progression of aortic stenosis. J Am Coll Cardiol. 2007;49(5):554–61.

Nestico PF, DePace NL, Kimbiris D. Progression of isolated aortic stenosis: analysis of 29 patients having more than 1 cardiac catheterization. Am J Cardiol. 1983;52(8):1054–8.

Ng AS, Holmes Jr DR, Smith HC, Connolly DC, Hynes JK, Ilstrup DM, Danielson GK. Hemodynamic progression of adult valvular aortic stenosis. Cathet Cardiovasc Diagn. 1986;12(3):145–50.

Ngo MV, Gottdiener JS, Fletcher RD, Fernicola DJ, Gersh BJ. Smoking and obesity are associated with the progression of aortic stenosis. Am J Geriatr Cardiol. 2001;10(2):86–90.

Nitta M, Takamoto T, Taniguchi K. Progression of aortic stenosis in the elderly detected by noninvasive methods. Bull Tokyo Med Dent Univ. 1988;35(1–2):19–24.

Nkomo VT, Gardin JM, Skelton TN, Gottdiener JS, Scott CG, Enriquez-Sarano M. Burden of valvular heart diseases: a population-based study. Lancet. 2006;368(9540): 1005–11.

Ohara T, Hashimoto Y, Matsumura A, Suzuki M, Isobe M. Accelerated progression and morbidity in patients with aortic stenosis on chronic dialysis. Circ J. 2005; 69(12):1535–9.

Otto CM. Valvular aortic stenosis. Disease severity and timing of intervention. J Am Coll Cardiol. 2006;47(11):2141–51.

Otto CM, Burwash IG, Legget ME, Munt BI, Fujioka M, Healy NL, Kraft CD, Miyake-Hull CY, Schwaegler RG. Prospective study of asymptomatic valvular aortic stenosis. Clinical, echocardiographic, and exercise predictors of outcome. Circulation. 1997;95(9):2262–70.

Otto CM, Lind BK, Kitzman DW, Gersh BJ, Siscovick DS. Association of aortic-valve sclerosis with cardiovascular mortality and morbidity in the elderly. N Engl J Med. 1999;341(3):142–7.

Palta S, Pai AM, Gill KS, Pai RG. New insights into the progression of aortic stenosis: implications for secondary prevention. Circulation. 2000;101(21):2497–502.

Pellikka PA, Sarano ME, Nishimura RA, Malouf JF, Bailey KR, Scott CG, Barnes ME, Tajik AJ. Outcome of 622 adults with asymptomatic, hemodynamically significant aortic stenosis during prolonged follow-up. Circulation. 2005;111(24):3290–5.

Peter M, Hoffmann A, Parker C, Luscher T, Burckhardt D. Progression of aortic stenosis. Role of age and concomitant coronary artery disease. Chest. 1993;103(6): 1715–9.

Rajamannan NM, Subramaniam M, Rickard D, Stock SR, Donovan J, Springett M, Orszulak T, Fullerton DA, Tajik AJ, Bonow RO, Spelsberg T. Human aortic valve calcification is associated with an osteoblast phenotype. Circulation. 2003;107(17):2181–4.

Rajamannan NM, Evans FJ, Aikawa E, Grande-Allen KJ, Demer LL, Heistad DD, Simmons CA, Masters KS, Mathieu P, O'Brien KD, Schoen FJ, Towler DA, Yoganathan AP, Otto CM. Calcific aortic valve disease: not simply a degenerative process: a review and agenda for research from the National Heart and Lung and Blood Institute Aortic Stenosis Working Group. Executive summary: calcific aortic valve disease-2011 update. Circulation. 2011;124(16):1783–91.

Rosenhek R, Binder T, Porenta G, et al. Predictors of outcome in severe asymptomatic aortic stenosis. N Engl J Med. 2000a;343:611–7.

Rosenhek R, Binder T, Porenta G, Lang I, Christ G, Schemper M, Maurer G, Baumgartner H. Predictors of outcome in severe, asymptomatic aortic stenosis. N Engl J Med. 2000b;343(9):611–7.

Rosenhek R, Klaar U, Schemper M, Scholten C, Heger M, Gabriel H, Binder T, Maurer G, Baumgartner H. Mild and moderate aortic stenosis. Natural history and risk stratification by echocardiography. Eur Heart J. 2004; 25(3):199–205.

Rosenhek R, Zilberszac R, Schemper M, Czerny M, Mundigler G, Graf S, Bergler-Klein J, Grimm M, Gabriel H, Maurer G. Natural history of very severe aortic stenosis. Circulation. 2010;121(1):151–6.

Ross Jr J, Braunwald E. Aortic stenosis. Circulation. 1968;38(1 Suppl):61–7.

Rossebo AB, Pedersen TR, Boman K, Brudi P, Chambers JB, Egstrup K, Gerdts E, Gohlke-Barwolf C, Holme I, Kesaniemi YA, Malbecq W, Nienaber CA, Ray S, Skjaerpe T, Wachtell K, Willenheimer R. Intensive lipid lowering with simvastatin and ezetimibe in aortic stenosis. N Engl J Med. 2008;359(13):1343–56.

Rubler S, King ML, Tarkoff DM, Dolgin M, Reitano J, Schreiber J. The role of aortic valve calcium in the detection of aortic stenosis: an echocardiographic study. Am Heart J. 1985;109(5 Pt 1):1049–58.

Sanchez PL, Santos JL, Kaski JC, Cruz I, Arribas A, Villacorta E, Cascon M, Palacios IF, Martin-Luengo C. Relation of circulating C-reactive protein to progression of aortic valve stenosis. Am J Cardiol. 2006; 97(1):90–3.

Shumacker Jr HB. The evolution of cardiac surgery. Bloomington: Indiana University Press; 1992.

Skolnick AH, Osranek M, Formica P, Kronzon I. Osteoporosis treatment and progression of aortic stenosis. Am J Cardiol. 2009;104(1):122–4.

Turina J, Hess O, Sepulcri F, Krayenbuehl HP. Spontaneous course of aortic valve disease. Eur Heart J. 1987;8(5): 471–83.

Vahanian A, Baumgartner H, Bax J, Butchart E, Dion R, Filippatos G, Flachskampf F, Hall R, Iung B, Kasprzak J, Nataf P, Tornos P, Torracca L, Wenink A. Guidelines on the management of valvular heart disease: the task force on the management of valvular heart disease of the European Society of Cardiology. Eur Heart J. 2007;28(2):230–68.

van der Linde D, Yap SC, van Dijk AP, Budts W, Pieper PG, van der Burgh PH, Mulder BJ, Witsenburg M, Cuypers JA, Lindemans J, Takkenberg JJ, Roos-Hesselink JW. Effects of rosuvastatin on progression of stenosis in adult patients with congenital aortic stenosis (PROCAS Trial). Am J Cardiol. 2011;108(2):265–71.

Varadarajan P, Kapoor N, Bansal RC, Pai RG. Clinical profile and natural history of 453 nonsurgically managed patients with severe aortic stenosis. Ann Thorac Surg. 2006;82(6):2111–5.

Wagner S, Selzer A. Patterns of progression of aortic stenosis: a longitudinal hemodynamic study. Circulation. 1982;65(4):709–12.

Wongpraparut N, Apiyasawat S, Crespo G, Yazdani K, Jacobs LE, Kotler MN. Determinants of progression of aortic stenosis in patients aged > or =40 years. Am J Cardiol. 2002;89(3):350–2.

Cardiovascular Risk Factors for Calcific Aortic Valve Disease

2

Mony Shuvy, Chaim Lotan, and Nalini Marie Rajamannan

Introduction

Over the past decade epidemiological studies have revealed the risk factors associated for vascular atherosclerosis, including male gender, smoking, hypertension and elevated serum cholesterol, are similar to the risk factors associated with development of aortic valve stenosis. There is also growing evidence that renal failure (RF) is responsible for accelerated vascular calcification. These clinical studies demonstrate that defining these risk factors for this disease may delineate preventive strategies to slow progression and to possibly modify the disease process. In summary, these findings suggest that medical therapies may have a potential role in patients in the early stages of this disease process to slow the progression to severe calcific aortic valve disease and delay the timing to intervention.

M. Shuvy, M.D. (✉) • C. Lotan, M.D.
Department of Cardiology, Heart Institute Hadassah Hebrew University Medical Center, Jerusalem, Israel
e-mail: monysh@gmail.com

N.M. Rajamannan, M.D.
Department of Molecular Biology and Biochemistry, Mayo Clinic, 200 First St SW, Rochester, MN 55905, USA
Department of Aerospace Engineering, University of Notre Dame, South Bend, IN, USA
e-mail: nrajamannan@gmail.com

With the decline incidence of rheumatic carditis, calcific aortic stenosis (AS) has become the most common indication for surgical valve replacement in the US. Numerous epidemiologic studies identified risk factors for AS disease development, which are similar to those of vascular atherosclerosis, including smoking, male gender, body mass index, hypertension, elevated lipid and inflammatory markers, metabolic syndrome and renal failure (Deutscher et al. 1984; Hoagland et al. 1985; Aronow et al. 2001; Mohler et al. 1991; Lindroos et al. 1994; Boon et al. 1997; Chui et al. 2001; Wilmshurst et al. 1997; Chan et al. 2001; Briand et al. 2006; Palta et al. 2000; Peltier et al. 2003; Stewart et al. 1997; Otto et al. 1999; Faggiano et al. 2006; Pohle et al. 2001).

Aortic Valve Cardiovascular Risk Factors

Stewart et al. (1997, 1999), described the risk factors for calcific AS identified in the Cardiovascular Health Study. The investigators examined 5,621 patients older than the age of 65 years found by Doppler Echocardiography that the prevalence of aortic valve sclerosis was 29% and AS was 2% in this population. The investigators demonstrated that the clinical risk factors important for the development of atherosclerosis are also the independent risk factors for AS including age, male gender, height (inverse relationship), history of hypertension, smoking and elevated serum levels of lipoprotein(a) and LDL levels (Stewart et al. 1997).

N.M. Rajamannan (ed.), *Cardiac Valvular Medicine*,
DOI 10.1007/978-1-4471-4132-7_2, © Springer-Verlag London 2013

Data from several studies have confirmed that all of these traditional risk factors including metabolic syndrome (Briand et al. 2006), and RF (Palta et al. 2000), which are important in the development of vascular atherosclerosis, are also implicated in the development of calcific AS. These findings provide the foundation to study targeted strategies for medical therapy, including for example, medications for hyperlipidemia, hypertension and diabetes. There are a growing number of experimental in vivo models of calcific AS which demonstrate primarily that lipids (Rajamannan et al. 2001, 2002; Drolet et al. 2003, 2006; Weiss et al. 2006; Aikawa et al. 2007; Shao et al. 2005), diabetes (Shao et al. 2005) and RF (Shuvy et al. 2008) are important in the development of this disease. Early studies have demonstrated that cholesterol (Ortlepp et al. 2006), and Vitamin D (Drolet et al. 2003), can induce early stenosis of the valve (Drolet et al. 2003) as documented by echocardiographic measurements.

Lipids and other cardiovascular risk factors induce oxidative stress (Weiss et al. 2006; Rajamannan et al. 2005a; Miller et al. 2008) in the aortic valve endothelium similar to vascular endothelium (Wilcox et al. 1997) which in turn activates the secretion of cytokines and growth factors important in cell signaling. The early atherosclerotic and abnormal oxidative stress environment also plays a role in the activation of the calcification process in the myofibroblast cell. The signaling molecules important in the development of vascular atherosclerosis are also important in the development of valve calcification including: MMP (Kaden et al. 2004a; Jian et al. 2001), Interleukin 1 (Kaden et al. 2003), transforming growth factor-beta(TGF-beta) (Jian et al. 2003), purine nucleotides (Osman et al. 2006a, b), RANK (Kaden et al. 2004b), osteoprotegrin(OPG) (Kaden et al. 2004b), elastolytic cathepsins S, K, and V and their inhibitor Cystatin C in stenotic aortic valves (Helske et al. 2006) Toll-like receptors (Yang et al. 2009), TNF alpha (Kaden et al. 2005), MAP Kinase (Gu and Masters 2009) and the canonical Wnt pathway (Shao et al. 2005; Rajamannan et al. 2005b; Caira et al. 2006). Similar to vascular atherosclerosis these events are potential cellular targets for pharmacologic agents to slow this disease process.

Renal Failure as a Risk Factor Associated with Calcific Aortic Valve Disease

Cardiovascular disease is the leading cause of mortality in patients with renal disease and is attributed to both traditional and non-traditional cardiovascular risk factors. One of the most devastating complications in this population is ectopic calcification. Ectopic calcification is defined as inappropriate biomineralization occurring in soft tissues as a result of systemic mineral and hormonal imbalance (Giachelli 2004; Goodman 2001). Aortic valve is one of the most important tissues which are involved in the calcification process.

The prevalence and extent of AS in this population of patients is poorly explained by traditional cardiovascular risk factors (Moe 2004; Yao et al. 2004) abnormalities of mineral metabolism are likely to contribute to AS development and progression. Contrary to "senile AS", patients with RF associated AS are characterized by significant mineral disturbances especially involving phosphate and calcium metabolism (Kalpakian and Mehrotra 2007; Tomson 2003). Most of these patients develop hyperphosphatemia as well as an increased Ca – phosphate product levels (Verberckmoes et al. 2007). Calcium-phosphorus product is associated with increased ectopic calcification and cardiovascular morbidity and mortality (Cozzolino et al. 2001).

Phosphorus excess is an independent cardiovascular risk factor for morbidity and mortality in patients with advanced RF (Kestenbaum et al. 2005; Menon et al. 2005) as well as in normal subjects. In addition to the effects of phosphate during passive mineralization, recent data suggest that phosphate induces calcification by activating osteoblast transformation in vascular smooth muscle cells (VSMC) (Giachelli 2003). Elevated phosphate level is a key element in activation of osteoblast specific maturation factors. Although the exact mechanism is still unknown, this effect seems to be mediated by a sodium-dependent phosphate cotransporter, Pit-1 (Glvr-1) (Giachelli 2003). In vitro studies in VSMC cells demonstrated that inhibition of phosphate uptake abolished calcification. The specific role of phosphate in RF associated AS is still under investigation, data obtained from animal study suggest that hyperphosphatemia and elevated parathyroid hormone (PTH) rather than uremia itself are the mediator of AS (Shuvy et al. 2008).

Parathyroid hormone is the most important regulator of calcium and phosphate metabolism (Goodman 2005). It is essential for both bone formation and osteoblast activity, and increases the conversion of vitamin D to its active metabolite (Murray et al. 2005). Hyperparathyroidism is often accompanied with hyperphosphatemia making the evaluation of the specific effect of PTH on calcification difficult. Nevertheless animal studies find the PTH induces ectopic calcification, which is unrelated to the serum levels of calcium and phosphate. The mechanism of this phenomenon is unclear and it may be related to elevated bone turnover (Neves et al. 2007). The role of calcium in the pathogenesis of AS is less established, and no significant increased progression of AS was found in women taking oral calcium supplementation (Bhakta et al. 2009).

Apart of mineral and hormonal disturbances numerous additional factors as oxidative stress, malnutrition, endothelial dysfunction and constant low-grade inflammation are common in that population (Pecoits-Filho et al. 2002). Available data suggest that pro-inflammatory cytokines play a central role in the genesis of both malnutrition and vascular disease in RF (Stenvinkel et al. 2005). Strong associations between malnutrition, inflammation and atherosclerosis suggest the presence of a syndrome malnutrition, inflammation, and atherosclerosis (MIA), which is associated cardiovascular morbidity.

Calcification Inhibitors

Although the majority of patients with significant RF develop ectopic calcification, not all of them have vascular calcification, naturally occurring inhibitors of calcification may be involved in this phenomenon. Fetuin-A (alpha-Heremans–Schmid glycoprotein), a 59 kDa glycoprotein, consisting of two cystatin-like domains and a smaller unrelated domain, is predominantly synthesized in liver (Westenfeld et al. 2009). It is secreted into the blood stream and deposited as a noncollagenous protein in mineralized bones. Fetuin-A binds calcium phosphate (Heiss et al. 2003), and thus directly prevents calcium-phosphate to cause ectopic calcification (Westenfeld et al. 2009). Dialysis patients have significantly reduced serum fetuin-A levels compared with control subjects (Ketteler et al. 2003). Interestingly, Ketteler et al. reported an inverse relationship between serum fetuin-A and C-reactive protein serum in dialysis patients, implying that inflammation decreases fetuin-A level, furthermore, its level is significantly decreased in patients with major components of the MIA syndrome (Wang et al. 2005). The role of futin A in preventing AS was demonstrated in RF population. This study demonstrates in patients with low serum fetuin-A have the greatest prevalence of valvular calcification and 0.01 g/l increase in serum fetuin-A is associated with a 6% decrease in the risk of valvular calcification (Wang et al. 2005). Recently low fetuin A level were found in patients with senile AS (Koos et al. 2009).

Matrix Gla protein (MGP) is one of three vitamin-K dependent proteins have been isolated in bones. MGP inhibit calcification via modulation of bone morphogenic protein-2 (BMP-2) activity, which is known to induce calcification. Warfarin treatment decreases MGP levels and may increase calcification, actually several clinical and experimental (Price et al. 1998) studies support this hypothesis. In patients undergoing valvular replacement or in patients with renal failure, warfarin treatment was associated with greater valvular calcification (Zebboudj et al. 2003). An addition protein that requires vitamin k and decreased during warfarin treatment, is the product of the gene growth arrest specific 6 (GAS6) (Nagata et al. 1996) which prevents apoptosis and calcification in VSMC. Phosphate is a negative modulator of GAS6, therefore hyperphosphatemia promotes apoptosis and calcification (Son et al. 2006).

Osteoprotegerin (OPG), a member of the tumor necrosis factor (TNF) superfamily of proteins, is involved in bone remodeling as well as ecotpic calcification, through its action as a decoy receptor for RANKL (Bennett et al. 2006). The exact role of the RANK-RANKL complex in the calcification process is not clear. It was shown to trigger and osteoclast differentiation and which are highly important in the calcification process. The importance of this pathway is demonstrated in OPG-deficient mice which develop severe osteoporosis, as well as ectopic calcification; administration of OPG reduces this calcification (Bucay et al. 1998). The role of RANK-RANKL-OPG was shown both in vitro and in vivo, especially in the pathogenesis of renal failure associated calcification. As opposed to fetuin-A, OPG plasma levels are increased in patients with significant calcification, furthermore high level of OPG may predict cardiovascular calcification in RF population (Morena et al. 2009). This unique observation may be explained that OPG is protective and its elevation in a compensation in patients with extensive disease (Schoppet et al. 2002). The specific role RANK-RANKL-OPG was demonstrated in a recent study showing high expression of RANKL in human calcified aortic valves (Kaden et al. 2004b), and in animal model of RF associated valve calcification (Shuvy et al. 2008).

Pathogenesis of Renal Failure Associated Valve Calcification

Vascular and valve calcification is considered to be an organized, regulated process comparable to bone mineralization which involves trans-differentiation of valvular myofibroblasts into osteoblasts. The presence of various components associated with bone mineralization such as bone specific proteins in valvular lesions supports this concept. There are three phases necessary for the myofibroblast cell to differentiate to form bone. These phases include first: activation of cell proliferation, second: extracellular matrix synthesis, third: mineralization of the bone formation. Several RF associated mediators are involved in this process: Activation of PTH receptor induces several osteoblast transcription factors (e.g. Runx-2) and proteins (e.g. osteopontin and osteocalcin) that stimulate osteoblast maturation. Runx-2 is crucial in the differentiation of mesenchymal cells to an osteoblastic phenotype, a process that may contribute to AS. Osteopontin and osteocalcin are the most abundant glycoproteins produced by osteoblasts, which compose the organic part of the bone and are essential for calcification. Hyperphosphatemia is involved in several phases of calcification: The final step in the mineralization process for bone formation is apoptosis. The presence of apoptosis is critical for bone mineralization. Apoptosis is the final common pathway necessary for the transition of the osteoblasts to mineralized bone. Phosphate induces osteoblast differentiation and apoptosis of vascular smooth muscle cells, resulting in calcification. Furthermore, the pro-apoptotic effect of phosphate is mediated through inhibition of survival pathways.

Conclusion

Most of the risk factors for AS are identical with the risk factors for atherosclerosis and may be targeted in patients with AS. However, it seems that the medical intervention in valve calcification must take place in very early stages of the disease and may be ineffective later. A possible explanation is that in early stages of the disease the inflammatory features are more prominent, while in later stages calcification and bone formation are dominant. The exact timing of medical therapy is highly important as different processes are involved in the course of the disease. Furthermore, defining the mechanistic domain in every phase and finding specific markers for disease progression are the foundation to possible therapeutic interventions to counter AS. The complexity of AS is illustrated in patients with RF.

Renal failure is a major risk factor for AS and patients with RF associated calcification have more severe and rapidly progressive disease than patients with "senile AS". Renal failure associated calcification is a complex process involving different pathways than "senile AS". Apart from the traditional risk factors and the importance of atherosclerosis, specific unique metabolic conditions as hyperphosphatemia, elevated PTH and decreased calcification inhibitors play an important role. Due to the difference in the pathogenesis of RF associated AS, RF population may react differently to medical intervention and therefore any intervention should be evaluated specifically in the renal failure milieu. Although patients with RF often have more advanced disease, targeting the metabolic abnormalities such is decreasing serum phosphate levels, or preventing hyperparathyroidism, in early stages may halt the rapid course of AS.

References

Aikawa E, Nahrendorf M, Sosnovik D, Lok VM, Jaffer FA, Aikawa M, Weissleder R. Multimodality molecular imaging identifies proteolytic and osteogenic activities in early aortic valve disease. Circulation. 2007;115(3):377–86.

Aronow WS, Ahn C, Kronzon I, Goldman ME. Association of coronary risk factors and use of statins with progression of mild valvular aortic stenosis in older persons. Am J Cardiol. 2001;88(6):693–5.

Bennett BJ, Scatena M, Kirk EA, Rattazzi M, Varon RM, Averill M, Schwartz SM, Giachelli CM, Rosenfeld ME. Osteoprotegerin inactivation accelerates advanced atherosclerotic lesion progression and calcification in older ApoE–/– mice. Arterioscler Thromb Vasc Biol. 2006;26(9):2117–24.

Bhakta M, Bruce C, Messika-Zeitoun D, Bielak L, Sheedy PF, Peyser P, Sarano M. Oral calcium supplements do not affect the progression of aortic valve calcification or coronary artery calcification. J Am Board Fam Med. 2009;22(6):610–6.

Boon A, Cheriex E, Lodder J, Kessels F. Cardiac valve calcification: characteristics of patients with calcification of the mitral annulus or aortic valve. Heart. 1997;78(5):472–4.

Briand M, Lemieux I, Dumesnil JG, Mathieu P, Cartier A, Despres JP, Arsenault M, Couet J, Pibarot P. Metabolic syndrome negatively influences disease progression and prognosis in aortic stenosis. J Am Coll Cardiol. 2006;47(11):2229–36.

Bucay N, Sarosi I, Dunstan CR, Morony S, Tarpley J, Capparelli C, Scully S, Tan HL, Xu W, Lacey DL, Boyle WJ, Simonet WS. Osteoprotegerin-deficient mice develop early onset osteoporosis and arterial calcification. Genes Dev. 1998;12(9):1260–8.

Caira FC, Stock SR, Gleason TG, McGee EC, Huang J, Bonow RO, Spelsberg TC, McCarthy PM, Rahimtoola SH, Rajamannan NM. Human degenerative valve disease is associated with up-regulation of low-density lipoprotein receptor-related protein 5 receptor-mediated bone formation. J Am Coll Cardiol. 2006;47(8):1707–12.

Chan KL, Ghani M, Woodend K, Burwash IG. Case-controlled study to assess risk factors for aortic stenosis in congenitally bicuspid aortic valve. Am J Cardiol. 2001;88(6):690–3.

Chui MC, Newby DE, Panarelli M, Bloomfield P, Boon NA. Association between calcific aortic stenosis and hypercholesterolemia: is there a need for a randomized controlled trial of cholesterol-lowering therapy? Clin Cardiol. 2001;24(1):52–5.

Cozzolino M, Dusso AS, Slatopolsky E. Role of calcium-phosphate product and bone-associated proteins on vascular calcification in renal failure. J Am Soc Nephrol. 2001;12(11):2511–6.

Deutscher S, Rockette HE, Krishnaswami V. Diabetes and hypercholesterolemia among patients with calcific aortic stenosis. J Chronic Dis. 1984;37(5):407–15.

Drolet MC, Arsenault M, Couet J. Experimental aortic valve stenosis in rabbits. J Am Coll Cardiol. 2003;41(7):1211–7.

Drolet MC, Roussel E, Deshaies Y, Couet J, Arsenault M. A high fat/high carbohydrate diet induces aortic valve disease in C57BL/6J mice. J Am Coll Cardiol. 2006;47(4):850–5.

Faggiano P, Antonini-Canterin F, Baldessin F, Lorusso R, D'Aloia A, Cas LD. Epidemiology and cardiovascular risk factors of aortic stenosis. Cardiovasc Ultrasound. 2006;4:27.

Giachelli CM. Vascular calcification: in vitro evidence for the role of inorganic phosphate. J Am Soc Nephrol. 2003;14(9 Suppl 4):S300–4.

Giachelli CM. Vascular calcification mechanisms. J Am Soc Nephrol. 2004;15(12):2959–64.

Goodman WG. Vascular calcification in chronic renal failure. Lancet. 2001;358(9288):1115–6.

Goodman WG. Calcium and phosphorus metabolism in patients who have chronic kidney disease. Med Clin North Am. 2005;89(3):631–47.

Gu X, Masters KS. Role of the MAPK/ERK pathway in valvular interstitial cell calcification. Am J Physiol. 2009;296(6):H1748–57.

Heiss A, DuChesne A, Denecke B, Grötzinger J, Yamamoto K, Renné T, Jahnen-Dechent W. Structural basis of calcification inhibition by alpha 2-HS glycoprotein/fetuin-A. J Biol Chem. 2003;278(15):13333–41.

Helske S, Syvaranta S, Lindstedt KA, Lappalainen J, Oorni K, Mayranpaa MI, Lommi J, Turto H, Werkkala K, Kupari M, Kovanen PT. Increased expression of elastolytic cathepsins S, K, and V and their inhibitor cystatin C in stenotic aortic valves. Arterioscler Thromb Vasc Biol. 2006;26(8):1791–8.

Hoagland PM, Cook EF, Flatley M, Walker C, Goldman L. Case–control analysis of risk factors for presence of aortic stenosis in adults (age 50 years or older). Am J Cardiol. 1985;55(6):744–7.

Jian B, Jones PL, Li Q, Mohler 3rd ER, Schoen FJ, Levy RJ. Matrix metalloproteinase-2 is associated with tenascin-C in calcific aortic stenosis. Am J Pathol. 2001;159(1):321–7.

Jian B, Narula N, Li QY, Mohler 3rd ER, Levy RJ. Progression of aortic valve stenosis: TGF-beta1 is present in calcified aortic valve cusps and promotes aortic valve interstitial cell calcification via apoptosis. Ann Thorac Surg. 2003;75(2):457–65; discussion 465–56.

Kaden JJ, Dempfle CE, Grobholz R, Tran HT, Kilic R, Sarikoc A, Brueckmann M, Vahl C, Hagl S, Haase KK, Borggrefe M. Interleukin-1 beta promotes matrix metalloproteinase expression and cell proliferation in calcific aortic valve stenosis. Atherosclerosis. 2003;170(2):205–11.

Kaden JJ, Vocke DC, Fischer CS, Grobholz R, Brueckmann M, Vahl CF, Hagl S, Haase KK, Dempfle CE, Borggrefe M. Expression and activity of matrix metalloproteinase-2 in calcific aortic stenosis. Z Kardiol. 2004a;93(2):124–30.

Kaden JJ, Bickelhaupt S, Grobholz R, Haase KK, Sarikoc A, Kilic R, Brueckmann M, Lang S, Zahn I, Vahl C, Hagl S, Dempfle CE, Borggrefe M. Receptor activator of nuclear factor kappaB ligand and osteoprotegerin regulate aortic valve calcification. J Mol Cell Cardiol. 2004b;36(1):57–66.

Kaden JJ, Kilic R, Sarikoc A, Hagl S, Lang S, Hoffmann U, Brueckmann M, Borggrefe M. Tumor necrosis factor alpha promotes an osteoblast-like phenotype in human aortic valve myofibroblasts: a potential regulatory mechanism of valvular calcification. Int J Mol Med. 2005;16(5):869–72.

Kalpakian MA, Mehrotra R. Vascular calcification and disordered mineral metabolism in dialysis patients. Semin Dial. 2007;20(2):139–43.

Kestenbaum B, Sampson JN, Rudser KD, Patterson DJ, Seliger SL, Young B, Sherrard DJ, Andress DL. Serum phosphate levels and mortality risk among people with chronic kidney disease. J Am Soc Nephrol. 2005;16(2):520–8.

Ketteler M, Bongartz P, Westenfeld R, Wildberger JE, Mahnken AH, Böhm R, Metzger T, Wanner C, Jahnen-Dechent W, Floege J. Association of low fetuin-A (AHSG) concentrations in serum with cardiovascular mortality in patients on dialysis: a cross-sectional study. Lancet. 2003;361(9360):827–33.

Koos R, Brandenburg V, Mahnken AH, Muhlenbruch G, Stanzel S, Gunther RW, Floege J, Jahnen-Dechent W, Kelm M, Kuhl HP. Association of fetuin-A levels with the progression of aortic valve calcification in non-dialyzed patients. Eur Heart J. 2009; 30(16):2054–61.

Lindroos M, Kupari M, Valvanne J, Strandberg T, Heikkila J, Tilvis R. Factors associated with calcific aortic valve degeneration in the elderly. Eur Heart J. 1994;15(7):865–70.

Menon V, Gul A, Sarnak MJ. Cardiovascular risk factors in chronic kidney disease. Kidney Int. 2005;68(4):1413–8.

Miller JD, Chu Y, Brooks RM, Richenbacher WE, Pena-Silva R, Heistad DD. Dysregulation of antioxidant mechanisms contributes to increased oxidative stress in calcific aortic valvular stenosis in humans. J Am Coll Cardiol. 2008;52(10):843–50.

Moe SM. Uremic vasculopathy. Semin Nephrol. 2004;24(5):413–6.

Mohler ER, Sheridan MJ, Nichols R, Harvey WP, Waller BF. Development and progression of aortic valve stenosis: atherosclerosis risk factors – a causal relationship? A clinical morphologic study. Clin Cardiol. 1991;14(12):995–9.

Morena M, Dupuy A-M, Jaussent I, Vernhet H, Gahide G, Klouche K, Bargnoux A-S, Delcourt C, Canaud B, Cristol J-P. A cut-off value of plasma osteoprotegerin level may predict the presence of coronary artery calcifications in chronic kidney disease patients. Nephrol Dial Transplant. 2009;24(11):3389–97.

Murray TM, Rao LG, Divieti P, Bringhurst FR. Parathyroid hormone secretion and action: evidence for discrete receptors for the carboxyl-terminal region and related biological actions of carboxyl-terminal ligands. Endocr Rev. 2005;26(1):78–113.

Nagata K, Ohashi K, Nakano T, Arita H, Zong C, Hanafusa H, Mizuno K. Identification of the product of growth arrest-specific gene 6 as a common ligand for Axl, Sky, and Mer receptor tyrosine kinases. J Biol Chem. 1996;271(47):30022–7.

Neves KR, Graciolli FG, dos Reis LM, Graciolli RG, Neves CL, Magalhaes AO, Custodio MR, Batista DG, Jorgetti V, Moyses RMA. Vascular calcification: contribution of parathyroid hormone in renal failure. Kidney Int. 2007;71(12):1262–70.

Ortlepp JR, Pillich M, Schmitz F, Mevissen V, Koos R, Weiss S, Stork L, Dronskowski R, Langebartels G, Autschbach R, Brandenburg V, Woodruff S, Kaden JJ, Hoffmann R. Lower serum calcium levels are associated with greater calcium hydroxyapatite deposition in native aortic valves of male patients with severe calcific aortic stenosis. J Heart Valve Dis. 2006;15(4):502–8.

Osman L, Chester AH, Amrani M, Yacoub MH, Smolenski RT. A novel role of extracellular nucleotides in valve calcification: a potential target for atorvastatin. Circulation. 2006a;114(1 Suppl):I566–72.

Osman L, Amrani M, Isley C, Yacoub MH, Smolenski RT. Stimulatory effects of atorvastatin on extracellular nucleotide degradation in human endothelial cells. Nucleosides Nucleotides Nucleic Acids. 2006b;25(9–11):1125–8.

Otto CM, Lind BK, Kitzman DW, Gersh BJ, Siscovick DS. Association of aortic-valve sclerosis with cardiovascular mortality and morbidity in the elderly [comment]. N Engl J Med. 1999;341(3):142–7.

Palta S, Pai AM, Gill KS, Pai RG. New insights into the progression of aortic stenosis: implications for secondary prevention. Circulation. 2000;101(21):2497–502.

Pecoits-Filho R, Lindholm B, Stenvinkel P. The malnutrition, inflammation, and atherosclerosis (MIA) syndrome – the heart of the matter. Nephrol Dial Transplant. 2002;17 Suppl 11:28–31.

Peltier M, Trojette F, Sarano ME, Grigioni F, Slama MA, Tribouilloy CM. Relation between cardiovascular risk factors and nonrheumatic severe calcific aortic stenosis among patients with a three-cuspid aortic valve. Am J Cardiol. 2003;91(1):97–9.

Pohle K, Maffert R, Ropers D, Moshage W, Stilianakis N, Daniel WG, Achenbach S. Progression of aortic valve calcification: association with coronary atherosclerosis and cardiovascular risk factors. Circulation. 2001;104(16):1927–32.

Price PA, Faus SA, Williamson MK. Warfarin causes rapid calcification of the elastic lamellae in rat arteries and heart valves. Arterioscler Thromb Vasc Biol. 1998;18(9):1400–7.

Rajamannan NM, Sangiorgi G, Springett M, Arnold K, Mohacsi T, Spagnoli LG, Edwards WD, Tajik AJ, Schwartz RS. Experimental hypercholesterolemia induces apoptosis in the aortic valve. J Heart Valve Dis. 2001;10(3):371–4.

Rajamannan NM, Subramaniam M, Springett M, Sebo TC, Niekrasz M, McConnell JP, Singh RJ, Stone NJ, Bonow RO, Spelsberg TC. Atorvastatin inhibits hypercholesterolemia-induced cellular proliferation and bone matrix production in the rabbit aortic valve. Circulation. 2002;105(22):2260–5.

Rajamannan NM, Subramaniam M, Stock SR, Stone NJ, Springett M, Ignatiev KI, McConnell JP, Singh RJ, Bonow RO, Spelsberg TC. Atorvastatin inhibits calcification and enhances nitric oxide synthase production in the hypercholesterolaemic aortic valve. Heart. 2005a;91(6):806–10.

Rajamannan NM, Subramaniam M, Caira F, Stock SR, Spelsberg TC. Atorvastatin inhibits hypercholesterolemia-induced calcification in the aortic valves via the Lrp5 receptor pathway. Circulation. 2005b;112(9 Suppl):I229–34.

Schoppet M, Preissner KT, Hofbauer LC. RANK ligand and osteoprotegerin: paracrine regulators of bone metabolism and vascular function. Arterioscler Thromb Vasc Biol. 2002;22(4):549–53.

Shao JS, Cheng SL, Pingsterhaus JM, Charlton-Kachigian N, Loewy AP, Towler DA. Msx2 promotes cardiovascular calcification by activating paracrine Wnt signals. J Clin Invest. 2005;115(5):1210–20.

Shuvy M, Abedat S, Beeri R, Danenberg HD, Planer D, Ben-Dov IZ, Meir K, Sosna J, Lotan C. Uraemic hyperparathyroidism causes a reversible inflammatory process of aortic valve calcification in rats. Cardiovasc Res. 2008;79(3):492–9.

Son BK, Kozaki K, Iijima K, Eto M, Kojima T, Ota H, Senda Y, Maemura K, Nakano T, Akishita M, Ouchi Y. Statins protect human aortic smooth muscle cells from inorganic phosphate-induced calcification by restoring gas6-Axl survival pathway. Circ Res. 2006;98(8):1024–31.

Stenvinkel P, Ketteler M, Johnson RJ, Lindholm B, Pecoits-Filho R, Riella M, Heimburger O, Cederholm T, Girndt M. IL 10, IL 6, and TNF-alpha: central factors in the altered cytokine network of uremia–the good, the bad, and the ugly. Kidney Int. 2005;67(4):1216–33.

Stewart BF, Siscovick D, Lind BK, Gardin JM, Gottdiener JS, Smith VE, Kitzman DW, Otto CM. Clinical factors associated with calcific aortic valve disease. Cardiovascular Health Study. J Am Coll Cardiol. 1997;29(3):630–4.

Tomson C. Vascular calcification in chronic renal failure. Nephron Clin Pract. 2003;93(4):c124–30.

Verberckmoes SC, Persy V, Behets GJ, Neven E, Hufkens A, Zebger-Gong H, Muller D, Haffner D, Querfeld U, Bohic S, De Broe ME, D'Haese PC. Uremia-related vascular calcification: more than apatite deposition. Kidney Int. 2007;71(4):298–303.

Wang AY-M, Woo J, Lam CW-K, Wang M, Chan IH-S, Gao P, Lui S-F, Li PK-T, Sanderson JE. Associations of serum fetuin-A with malnutrition, inflammation, atherosclerosis and valvular calcification syndrome and outcome in peritoneal dialysis patients. Nephrol Dial Transplant. 2005;20(8):1676–85.

Weiss RM, Ohashi M, Miller JD, Young SG, Heistad DD. Calcific aortic valve stenosis in old hypercholesterolemic mice. Circulation. 2006;114(19):2065–9.

Westenfeld R, Schafer C, Kruger T, Haarmann C, Schurgers LJ, Reutelingsperger C, Ivanovski O, Drueke T, Massy ZA, Ketteler M, Floege J, Jahnen-Dechent W. Fetuin-A protects against atherosclerotic calcification in CKD. J Am Soc Nephrol. 2009;20(6):1264–74.

Wilcox JN, Subramanian RR, Sundell CL, Tracey WR, Pollock JS, Harrison DG, Marsden PA. Expression of multiple isoforms of nitric oxide synthase in normal and atherosclerotic vessels. Arterioscler Thromb Vasc Biol. 1997;17(11):2479–88.

Wilmshurst PT, Stevenson RN, Griffiths H, Lord JR. A case–control investigation of the relation between hyperlipidaemia and calcific aortic valve stenosis. Heart. 1997;78(5):475–9.

Yang X, Fullerton DA, Su X, Ao L, Cleveland Jr JC, Meng X. Pro-osteogenic phenotype of human aortic valve interstitial cells is associated with higher levels of Toll-like receptors 2 and 4 and enhanced expression of bone morphogenetic protein 2. J Am Coll Cardiol. 2009;53(6):491–500.

Yao Q, Pecoits-Filho R, Lindholm B, Stenvinkel P. Traditional and non-traditional risk factors as contributors to atherosclerotic cardiovascular disease in end-stage renal disease. Scand J Urol Nephrol. 2004;38(5):405–16.

Zebboudj AF, Shin V, Boström K. Matrix GLA protein and BMP-2 regulate osteoinduction in calcifying vascular cells. J Cell Biochem. 2003;90(4):756–65.

Bicuspid Aortic Valve Disease: From Bench to Bedside

3

Philippe Sucosky and Nalini Marie Rajamannan

Introduction

The bicuspid aortic valve (BAV), which is an aortic valve with two functional leaflets instead of the normal three, is the most common congenital heart valve abnormality accounting for a large number of valve replacements in the United States. Although bicuspid aortic valve disease (BAVD) is more common with age, it is not an inevitable consequence of aging. Tricuspid aortic valve disease (TAVD) appears to be an actively regulated disease process that cannot be characterized simply as "senile" or "degenerative" (Rajamannan et al. 2003). BAVD covers a spectrum of disease from initial changes in the cell biology of the valve leaflets, through early calcification, tissue remodeling and aortic sclerosis, to outflow obstruction and aortic stenosis (Rajamannan 2011a). The later stages are characterized by fibrotic thickening of the valve leaflets and the formation of new blood vessels and calcium nodules – often including the formation of actual bone – throughout the valve leaflets but concentrated near the aortic surface. Epidemiological studies show that some of the risk factors for BAVD are similar to those for vascular atherosclerosis. Age, gender, and certain clinical factors are all associated with an increased risk of BAVD and TAVD. Clinical risk factors associated with the presence of BAVD include elevated low-density lipoprotein (LDL) cholesterol, but the association is relatively weak in those over 65 years old, the group at greatest risk of progressing to aortic stenosis. Other factors include smoking, hypertension, shorter height, lipoprotein (a) level, metabolic syndrome, type II diabetes, end-stage renal disease (but not mild to moderate renal disease), and imbalances in calcium or phosphate metabolism. However, the factors associated with disease initiation may differ from those that promote disease progression. Although aortic stenosis may occur in individuals with otherwise anatomically normal tricuspid aortic valves, congenital valve abnormalities markedly increase the risk as shown in Fig. 3.1. Nearly half of the individuals with aortic stenosis have a BAV.

Hemodynamic Mechanisms

Echocardiography initially revealed that the BAV orifice presents an elliptical shape, an intrinsic degree of stenosis, an eccentric systolic jet and abnormal downstream helical flow patterns. During the acceleration phase, the pressure

P. Sucosky, Ph.D. (✉)
Department of Aerospace and Mechanical Engineering,
University of Notre Dame,
Notre Dame, IN, USA
e-mail: philippe.sucosky@nd.edu

N.M. Rajamannan, M.D.
Department of Molecular Biology and Biochemistry,
Mayo Clinic, 200 First St SW,
Rochester 55905, MN, USA
e-mail: nrajamannan@gmail.com

N.M. Rajamannan (ed.), *Cardiac Valvular Medicine*,
DOI 10.1007/978-1-4471-4132-7_3,

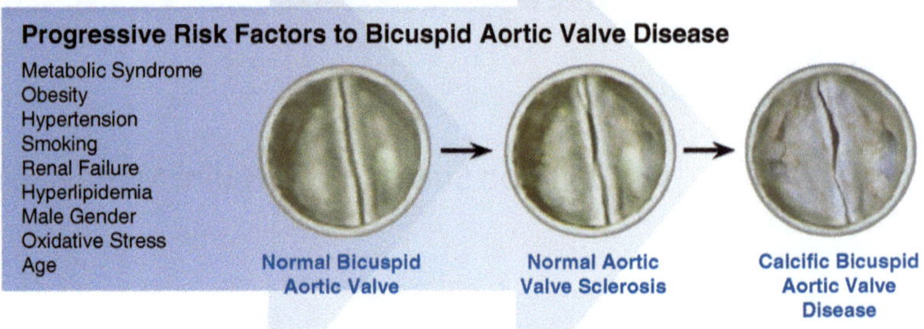

Fig. 3.1 Progression of bicuspid aortic valve disease secondary to clinical risk factors

gradient imposed across the valve produces a forward flow which contributes to the opening of the leaflets. Regardless of the anatomy, the flow downstream of the leaflets is divided into two regions: (1) a jet originating from the valvular orifice; and (2) a recirculation region marked by the presence of vortices located between the leaflet fibrosa and the wall of the aortic sinus. The emergence of a hemodynamic theory of BAV calcification has motivated the investigation of BAV hemodynamics at higher resolutions using computational approaches to understand the flow through the valve and its contribution to the mechanisms of valvular heart disease. A recent study implemented a fluid–structure interaction model to characterize the flow, leaflet dynamics and regional leaflet wall-shear stress in a normal TAV and in normal and calcified type-1 BAV anatomies (Chandra et al. 2011). The main findings from the study included: (1) the quantification of the local wall-shear stress experienced on both sides of normal and calcified TAV and BAV leaflets; and (2) the demonstration of the strong dependence of the leaflet hemodynamic stresses on valvular anatomy and leaflet calcification state. The comparison of the flow in TAV and BAV anatomies suggested the existence of a jet aligned along the centerline of the aorta in the TAV and a jet slightly skewed toward the non-coronary leaflet in the BAV (Fig. 3.2). Additionally, under a similar pressure gradient, the predicted TAV orifice was wider than the BAV orifice, regardless of the degree of BAV asymmetry. This computational model provided new evidence of the existence of abnormal hemodynamic stresses on BAV leaflets. The characterization of the regional leaflet wall-shear stress described in this paper is a critical and necessary step toward the validation/rejection of the hypothetical hemodynamic theory of CAVD in the BAV.

Molecular Mechanisms of BAVD

Although the causes for the development of BAV are unclear, genetic factors have been identified in some patients (Garg et al. 2005). Normally the aortic valve has a trileaflet structure. TAVD tends to develop at a later age than in individuals with BAV. BAVD tends to progress more rapidly for reasons that are just starting to emerge with the computational modeling approach described above. Human ex vivo BAV studies have demonstrated upregulation of Wnt3a/Lrp5 and osteogenic bone markers (Rajamannan 2011a; Caira et al. 2006). Several studies have confirmed the importance of Lrp5 regulation of bone formation in the aortic valve via the canonical Wnt pathway (Rajamannan et al. 2005; Rajamannan 2011b, c). The eNOS null mouse has a previously described bicuspid phenotype in approximately 25% of the population (Lee et al. 2000). When exposed to experimental hypercholesterolemia the bicuspid phenotype progressed more rapidly than the tricuspid eNOS null mouse phenotype (Rajamannan 2012). These

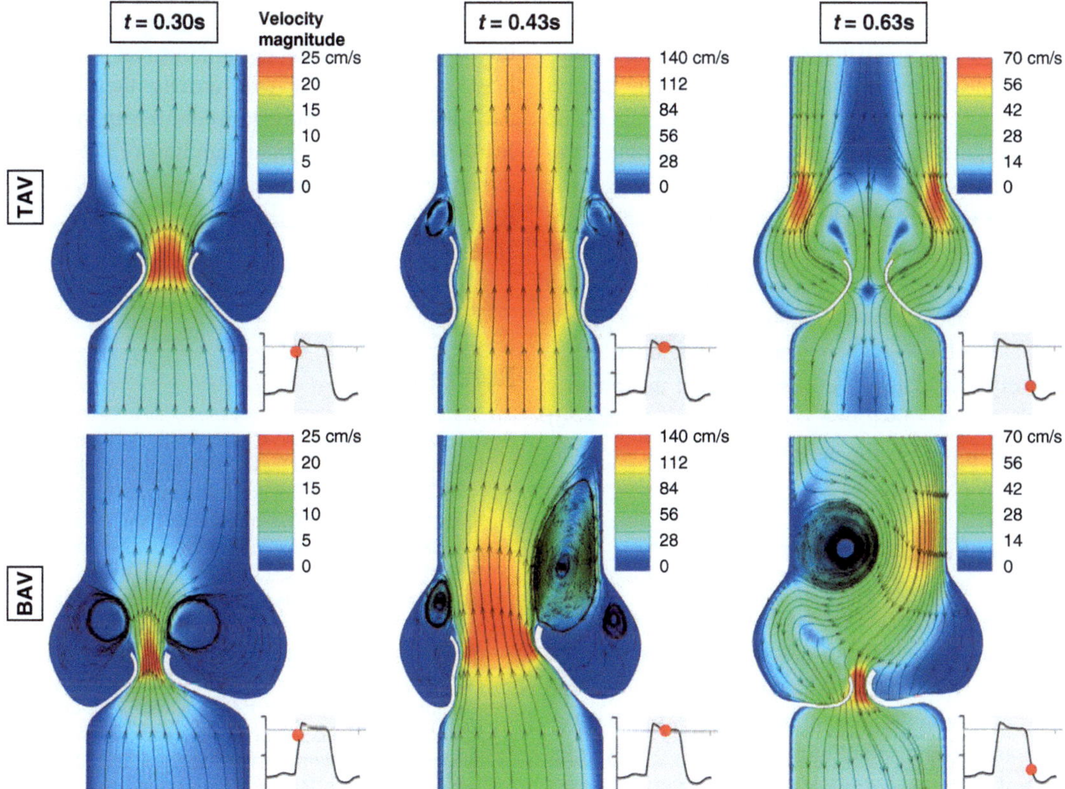

Fig. 3.2 Leaflet deformations, flow velocity and streamline fields predicted computationally in the TAV and type-1 BAV during the acceleration phase (t=0.30 s), at peak systole (t=0.43 s) and during the deceleration phase (t=0.63 s) (Reprinted with permission from Chandra et al. (2012))

experimental findings provide further evidence that not only an oxidative initiation event is critical but the flow through the abnormal valve accelerates this disease process.

Clinical Implications of BAVD and Aortic Root Abnormalities

Although still incompletely understood, the natural history of BAVD is severe aortic stenosis and associated ascending aortic dilatation. In addition to the increased risk for endocarditis, aortic dissection and severe aortic valve dysfunction are responsible for most fatal complications. Thus, early and precise recognition of this condition is mandatory. The American College of Cardiology/American Heart Association/ESC recommendations highlight the role of MRI and CT as complimentary tools to echocardiography for the diagnosis and surveillance of the morphology of the aortic valve and ascending aorta (Bonow et al. 2006; Vahanian et al. 2007).

Aortic dilatation is a common finding in patients with BAV. Up to 70% of these patients have echocardiographic evidence of aortic dilatation despite the absence of significant valve dysfunction (Nistri et al. 2008; Cecconi et al. 2006). If severe regurgitation is present, aortic dilatation is even more pronounced than in cases with stenotic or functionally normal BAV. The prognostic implications of aortic dilatation are that patients with a BAV are being increasingly recognized, as these patients are at ninefold higher risk of aortic dissection compared with patients who have normal valves. The fact that the aortic dilatation and dissection can occur out of proportion and even in the absence of hemodynamically significant stenosis or regurgitation has led many investigators to postulate the presence of a common underlying pathogenic mechanism involving the aortic wall and BAV. Several tissue abnormalities, including cystic medial degeneration, loss of elastic fibers, increased apoptosis, altered smooth muscle cell alignment, and more recently an increase in matrix metalloproteinases, have been described in the aortic wall of these patients (Boyum et al. 2004). Although the pathogenesis of aortic dilatation has not been completely elucidated, the possibility of an intrinsic aortic disease resulting in structural weakness of the aortic wall is the current hypothesis.

Clinical Presentation

The clinical suspicion of BAV is based on the physical finding of an ejection click or systolic murmur. It is also associated with other congenital cardiovascular anomalies such as patent ductus arteriosus, coarctation of aorta, ventricular septal defects, coronary anatomic variants, and other conditions such as Marfan's and Turner's syndromes. Quite often, the diagnosis of BAV is an incidental finding during an echocardiogram. A predictive accuracy of 93% has been reported for transthoracic two-dimensional echocardiography. Transesophageal echocardiography is an excellent tool for the evaluation of the valve and proximal thoracic aorta morphology, but it is not indicated for serial imaging. Cardiovascular MRI is emerging as a noninvasive modality that likely provides both high diagnostic sensitivity and specificity. The high spatial resolution and reproducibility of MRI angiography make this technique especially useful for the serial assessment and surveillance of the aorta (Ortiz et al. 2006).

In conclusion, a better understanding of the cellular mechanisms, including inflammation, bone formation, atherosclerotic-like processes, and aortic wall abnormalities, as well as the heritability and genetic predisposition for the disease will define the potential for targeted medical therapies in the future. Currently, the treatment of this condition is primarily surgical. Although combined valve and ascending aorta replacement has been the most common surgical approach in the past, the increased cumulative risk of thrombotic and embolic events among these young patients has led to more conservative approaches. In the future, better understanding of the hemodynamic and cellular mechanisms of BAVD will help to possibly slow the progression of this disease process.

References

Bonow RO, Carabello BA, Chatterjee K, de Leon Jr AC, Faxon DP, Freed MD, Gaasch WH, Lytle BW, Nishimura RA, O'Gara PT, O'Rourke RA, Otto CM, Shah PM, Shanewise JS, Smith Jr SC, Jacobs AK, Adams CD, Anderson JL, Antman EM, Fuster V, Halperin JL, Hiratzka LF, Hunt SA, Lytle BW, Nishimura R, Page RL, Riegel B. ACC/AHA 2006 guidelines for the management of patients with valvular heart disease: a report of the American College of Cardiology/American Heart Association Task Force on Practice Guidelines (writing Committee to Revise the 1998 guidelines for the management of patients with valvular heart disease) developed in collaboration with the Society of Cardiovascular Anesthesiologists endorsed by the Society for Cardiovascular Angiography and Interventions and the Society of Thoracic Surgeons. J Am Coll Cardiol. 2006;48(3):e1–148.

Boyum J, Fellinger EK, Schmoker JD, Trombley L, McPartland K, Ittleman FP, Howard AB. Matrix metalloproteinase activity in thoracic aortic aneurysms associated with bicuspid and tricuspid aortic valves. J Thorac Cardiovasc Surg. 2004;127(3):686–91.

Caira FC, Stock SR, Gleason TG, McGee EC, Huang J, Bonow RO, Spelsberg TC, McCarthy PM, Rahimtoola SH, Rajamannan NM. Human degenerative valve disease is associated with up-regulation of low-density lipoprotein receptor-related protein 5 receptor-mediated bone formation. J Am Coll Cardiol. 2006;47(8):1707–12.

Cecconi M, Nistri S, Quarti A, Manfrin M, Colonna PL, Molini E, Perna GP. Aortic dilatation in patients with bicuspid aortic valve. J Cardiovasc Med. 2006;7(1):11–20.

Chandra S, Rajamannan NM, Sucosky P. Computational assessment of bicuspid aortic valve wall-shear stress: implications for calcific aortic valve disease. Biomech Model Mechanobiol. 2011. doi:10.1007/s10237-012-0375-x

Chandra S, Rajamannan NM, Sucosky P. Computational assessment of bicuspid aortic valve wall-shear stress: implications for calcific aortic valve disease. Biomech Model Mechanobiol. 2012. doi:10.1007/s10237-012-0375-x.

Garg V, Muth AN, Ransom JF, Schluterman MK, Barnes R, King IN, Grossfeld PD, Srivastava D. Mutations in NOTCH1 cause aortic valve disease. Nature. 2005;437(7056):270–4.

Lee TC, Zhao YD, Courtman DW, Stewart DJ. Abnormal aortic valve development in mice lacking endothelial nitric oxide synthase. Circulation. 2000;101(20):2345–8.

Nistri S, Grande-Allen J, Noale M, Basso C, Siviero P, Maggi S, Crepaldi G, Thiene G. Aortic elasticity and size in bicuspid aortic valve syndrome. Eur Heart J. 2008;29(4):472–9.

Ortiz JT, Shin DD, Rajamannan NM. Approach to the patient with bicuspid aortic valve and ascending aorta aneurysm. Curr Treat Options Cardiovasc Med. 2006;8(6):461–7.

Rajamannan NM. Bicuspid aortic valve disease: the role of oxidative stress in Lrp5 bone formation. Cardiovasc Pathol. 2011a;20(3):168–76.

Rajamannan NM. The role of Lrp5/6 in cardiac valve disease: LDL-density-pressure theory. J Cell Biochem. 2011b;112:2222–9.

Rajamannan NM. The role of Lrp5/6 in cardiac valve disease: experimental hypercholesterolemia in the ApoE(–/–)/Lrp5(–/–) mice. J Cell Biochem. 2011c; 112(10):2987–91.

Rajamannan NM. Oxidative-mechanical stress signals stem cell niche mediated Lrp5 osteogenesis in eNOS(–/–) null mice. J Cell Biochem. 2012;113(5): 1623–34.

Rajamannan NM, Subramaniam M, Rickard D, Stock SR, Donovan J, Springett M, Orszulak T, Fullerton DA, Tajik AJ, Bonow RO, Spelsberg T. Human aortic valve calcification is associated with an osteoblast phenotype [see comment]. Circulation. 2003;107(17):2181–4.

Rajamannan NM, Subramaniam M, Caira F, Stock SR, Spelsberg TC. Atorvastatin inhibits hypercholesterolemia-induced calcification in the aortic valves via the Lrp5 receptor pathway. Circulation. 2005;112(9 Suppl):I229–34.

Vahanian A, Baumgartner H, Bax J, Butchart E, Dion R, Filippatos G, Flachskampf F, Hall R, Iung B, Kasprzak J, Nataf P, Tornos P, Torracca L, Wenink A. Guidelines on the management of valvular heart disease: the Task Force on the Management of Valvular Heart Disease of the European Society of Cardiology. Eur Heart J. 2007;28(2):230–68.

Experimental Evidence for the Role of Atherosclerosis in Calcific Aortic Valve Disease

4

Malayannan Subramaniam, Thomas C. Spelsberg, and Nalini Marie Rajamannan

Introduction

Calcific aortic stenosis is the most common indication for surgical valve replacement in the United States (www.sts.com). Currently, in 2012 surgical valve replacement is the number one indication for the treatment of this disease process (Bonow et al. 1998). For years, this disease has been described as a passive phenomena during which serum calcium attaches to the valve surface and binds to the leaflet to form nodules. Over decades, as aortic stenosis progresses, it will cause progressive left ventricular hypertrophy, left ventricular diastolic and systolic dysfunction, congestive heart failure, angina, arrhythmias, and syncope. Recent studies demonstrate an association between atherosclerotic risk factors and aortic valve disease. Although a unifying hypothesis for the role of atherosclerotic risk factors towards the mechanism of vascular and aortic valve disease is emerging, progress in studying the cell biology of this disease has been defining turning point in understanding the overall mechanisms.

In the past decade several epidemiologic data and experimental data has evolved to provide evidence that this disease process is not a passive phenomena but an active cellular biologic process that develops within the valve leaflet and causes a regulated bone formation to develop. Vascular atherosclerosis which was once thought to be a "degenerative process" is now an active biological process which can be targeted with medical therapy. Recently NHLBI, Working Group of Valvular Heart Disease, provided a consensus statement that the calcification in the aortic valve is not a degenerative process but an active biology (Rajamannan et al. 2011). A similar phenomena has occurred with our understanding of aortic valve disease with the growing number of clinical and experimental studies over the past decade. The growing evidence for the etiology of degenerative calcific aortic valve disease points towards a "response to injury" mechanism similar to what has been described for vascular atherosclerosis.

If the atherosclerotic hypothesis is present in the development of aortic stenosis then treatments used in slowing the progression of vascular atherosclerosis may be effective in patients with aortic valve disease. Current management of calcific aortic valve disease focuses on defining patients with valvular disease and the development of symptoms to determine the timing of surgical valve replacement. This chapter reviews the pathogenesis and the cellular targets for medical therapy in the management of patients with calcific aortic stenosis. It provides an overview of the emerging experimental and clinical studies important in the understanding of the cellular mechanisms of calcific aortic stenosis.

M. Subramaniam, Ph.D. (✉) • N.M. Rajamannan, M.D.
T.C. Spelsberg, Ph.D.
Department of Molecular Biology and Biochemistry,
Mayo Clinic, 200 First St SW,
Rochester 55905, MN, USA
e-mail: subramaniam.malayannan@mayo.edu

N.M. Rajamannan (ed.), *Cardiac Valvular Medicine*,
DOI 10.1007/978-1-4471-4132-7_4, © Springer-Verlag London 2013

The Role of Lipids and Atherosclerosis in Aortic Valve Disease

Vascular atherosclerosis has been described in the literature for hundreds of years (Stokes 1845). In 2010, the complexity of atherosclerosis and the different signaling pathways involved in the development of this pathology are under intense investigation including: (1) lipid signaling pathways in the vascular wall (Rye et al. 2003; Tabas 2002; Thukkani et al. 2003), (2) evaluation of an immune hypothesis for the mechanism of vascular inflammation (Koh et al. 2004; Cheitlin et al. 2003), (3) identifying cytokines, chemokines (Charo and Taubman 2004), (4) determining the effects of macrophages and T cell activation in the vessel wall (Tabas 2002; Adams et al. 2000) and (5) the effects of lipoprotein and insulin metabolism and their interactions with the vessel wall resulting in the multifactorial mechanisms of vascular atherosclerosis (Towler et al. 1998).

Emerging epidemiological studies are revealing convincing clinical evidence towards an atherosclerotic hypothesis for the cellular mechanism of this valvular lesion. Risk factors for calcific aortic valve disease have recently been described including male gender, hypertension, elevated levels of LDL, and smoking (Deutscher et al. 1984; Aronow et al. 1987; Mohler et al. 1991; Lindroos et al. 1994; Boon et al. 1997; Stewart et al. 1997; Wilmshurst et al. 1997; Chan et al. 2001; Aronow et al. 2001; Chui et al. 2001; Peltier et al. 2003). These risk factors are similar to those that promote the development of vascular atherosclerosis (Whyte 1976; Wilson et al. 1987; D'Agostino et al. 1989). Surgical pathological studies have identified or verified the presence of LDL (Olsson et al. 1999; O'Brien et al. 1996) and atherosclerosis in calcified human aortic valves, demonstrating similarities between the genesis of valvular and vascular disease and suggesting a common cellular mechanism of atherosclerosis in these tissues (O'Brien et al. 1996).

An important patient population to study the effects of accelerated atherosclerosis is the homozygous familial hypercholesterolemia (FH) population. Autopsy studies of these patients demonstrate a severe form of aortic stenosis associated with supravalvar narrowing in these patients (Sprecher et al. 1984). In this specific condition extremely high low density lipoprotein cholesterol (LDL-c) concentrations are seen without the other traditional risk factors for coronary artery disease. Recently, the proof of principle for the atherosclerotic process was demonstrated in a case report from 1949 (Rajamannan et al. 2003a). In this study, we described a patient with the diagnosis of familial hypercholesterolemia IIb and prominent skin xanthomas at the time of birth. The patient died of cardiac complications at age 7 and elevated cholesterol of over 900 mg/dl. We examined the cardiac pathology demonstrated coronary atherosclerosis and aortic valve atherosclerosis as shown in Fig. 4.1.

The histology in Fig. 4.1, demonstrates the development of atherosclerosis along the aortic surface of the aortic valve and in the lumen of the left circumflex (Used with permission) (Rajamannan et al. 2003a). This patient had total cholesterol over 900 mg/dl as measured in 1949 similar to lipid levels of patients with Familial Hypercholesterolemia. This study and previous studies of this patient population have provided the descriptive proof of atherosclerosis involving the vascular and valvular structures. The data from this index case has been shown in other autopsy and clinical studies from patients with Familial Hypercholesterolemia providing further proof that this disease involves a similar pathophysiology of vascular atherosclerosis (Sprecher et al. 1984; Rajamannan et al. 2003a; Buja et al. 1979; Kawaguchi et al. 1999, 2003).

Experimental Models of Valvular Atherosclerosis

There are emerging experimental studies evaluating the effects of experimental hypercholesterolemia on atherosclerosis in the aortic valves (Drolet et al. 2003; Rajamannan et al. 2001, 2002; Sarphie 1986; Sarphie 1985a, b). The rabbit model of treatment with a high cholesterol diet has been used for many years in the field of vascular atherosclerosis. Our laboratory has developed the rabbit model of experimental

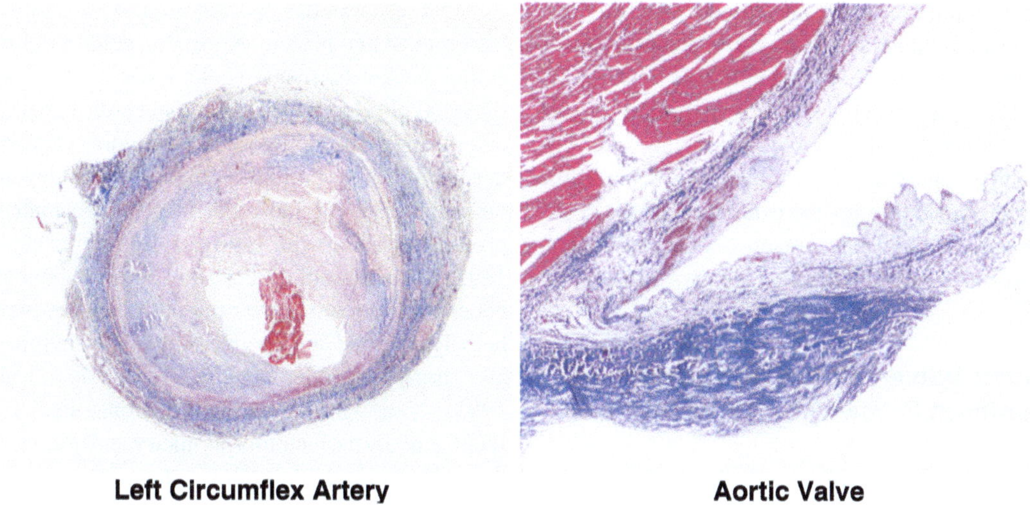

Fig. 4.1 Atherosclerosis in the circumflex artery and the aortic valve in a patient with familial hypercholesterolemia (Reprinted with permission from Rajamannan et al. (2003a))

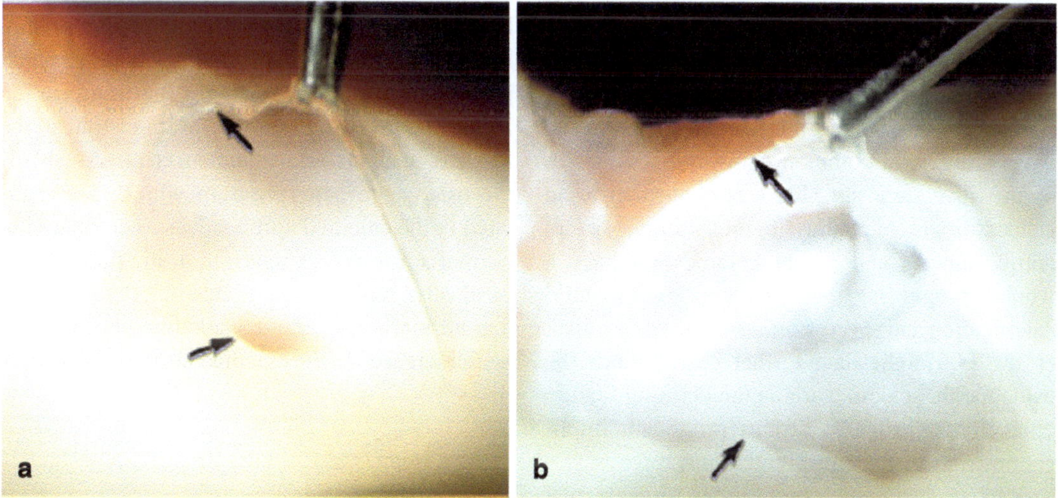

Fig. 4.2 Experimental hypercholesterolemia in the aortic valve (Reprinted with permission from Rajamannan et al. (2001))

hypercholesterolemia inducing valvular heart disease. Early studies demonstrate that the vascular lesion in the rabbit aorta from experimental hypercholesterolemia has a similar atherosclerotic lesion of that of the aortic valve. Figure 4.2, demonstrates the aorta versus the aortic valve from an experimental hypercholesterolemia rabbit model of atherosclerosis (Rajamannan et al. 2001). The valve and aorta were surgically removed from a rabbit which was fed a 1% cholesterol diet for 8 weeks. Figure 4.2, Panel A, is the normal aorta and the aortic valve demonstrating a clear aortic valve leaflet and normal appearing aorta. Figure 4.2, Panel b, is the hypercholesterolemic aorta and aortic valve marked exudative lesions along the aortic surface of the valve and extending along the aorta. Further analysis of this early aortic valve lesion identified apoptosis and cellular proliferation present in the atherosclerotic valve lesion (Rajamannan et al. 2001). Drolet et al., have also tested an experimental diet including Vitamin D and hypercholesterolemia in mice and found that the diet induces a hemodynamic early stenotic lesion within the aortic valve leaflets (Drolet et al. 2003). Atherosclerosis and lipid infiltration are the hallmarks of vascular atherosclerosis. The rabbit and genetic mouse models will serve as the future foundation for the evaluation of the cellular pathways and mechanisms of the development of valvular heart disease.

Aortic Valve Calcification as the Final Common Pathway to Aortic Stenosis

Understanding calcification is the key to the success of understanding aortic valve stenosis. Calcification is a common feature of vascular atherosclerotic plaques and stenotic aortic valves. The presence of calcification may lead to clinical vascular complications, including myocardial infarction, impaired vascular tone, and coronary insufficiency caused by loss of aortic recoil (Becker et al. 2005). Calcification in the aortic valve is the final common pathway that leads to aortic valve stenosis. This was confirmed in an echocardiographic study demonstrating severe aortic stenosis and severe calcification have a worse prognosis than patients with mild calcification and severe aortic stenosis (Rosenhek et al. 2000). The data further corroborates the evidence that calcification is the defining feature clinically for prognostic future prognostic implications for this patients population.

Recent intriguing observations suggest that rapid advancement in our understanding of the basic mechanisms involved in the initiation and progression of vascular and valvular calcification is now possible. Historically, cardiovascular calcification was considered a degenerative process leading to passive accumulation of calcium phosphate. New findings strongly suggest that ectopic mineralization is part of an active ongoing process, rather than the result of passive degeneration. The concept of regulated vascular calcification suggests the presence of cellular and molecular determinants of ectopic calcification, natural inhibitors of ectopic calcification, and regulators of bone resorption.

Most research has evolved around descriptive histological and protein expression studies delineating the development of calcification in the aortic valve. Studies have shown that cardiovascular calcification is composed of hydroxyapatite deposited on a bone-like matrix of collagen, osteopontin (OP), and other minor bone matrix proteins (Mohler et al. 1997, 2001; O'Brien et al. 1995). In addition, osteopontin expression has been demonstrated in the mineralization zones of heavily calcified aortic valves obtained at autopsy and surgery (Mohler et al. 2001; O'Brien et al. 1995). Our laboratory has demonstrated by RTPCR analysis, histomorphometry and microCT that an osteoblast-like cellular phenotype is present in calcified aortic valves removed at the time of surgical valve replacement (Rajamannan et al. 2003b). We tested mRNA from calcified vs. normal aortic valves to determine osteoblast markers in calcified aortic valves including: osteopontin, bone sialoprotein, osteocalcin, alkaline phosphatase and the osteoblast specific transcription factor Cbfa1. Figure 4.3, demonstrates the RTPCR analysis (Rajamannan et al. 2003b) of the osteogenic gene program which is upregulated in the calcified aortic valves as compared to normal aortic valves removed at the time of surgical valve replacement. Figure 4.3, demonstrates that all markers except for alkaline phosphatase, were increased in the calcified aortic valves when

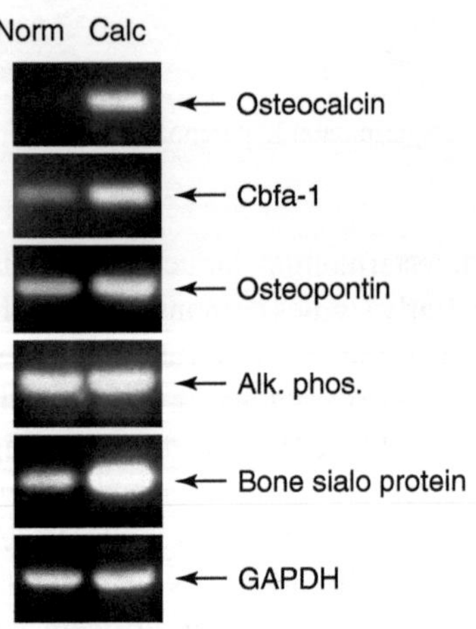

Fig. 4.3 Osteogenic gene markers in the calcified aortic valve tissues (Rajamannan et al. 2003b)

compared to the non-calcified controls indicating that a regulated bone formation process is occurring at the level of RNA expression.

These *ex vivo* and *in vivo* models have provided a basic novel understanding of the development of calcification in the aortic valve and may represent parallel signaling pathways that are present in aortic valve myofibroblast cells and osteoblast cells. Furthermore, these studies demonstrate that the aortic valve has an actual bone biology instead of a passive degenerative process.

Lrp5 Signaling Pathway in the Development of Valvular Heart Disease

Studies have recently shown that different mutations in Lrp5 develop a high bone mass phenotype and an osteoporosis phenotype implicating this coreceptor and the canonical Wnt signaling pathway in bone formation and bone mass regulation (Gong et al. 2001; Little et al. 2002). Our laboratory and others have demonstrated in experimental animal models that atherosclerotic bone matrix protein expression in the aortic valve and vasculature are regulated by the Lrp5 pathway in the presence of elevated hypercholesterolemia (Rajamannan et al. 2005a; Shao et al. 2005). The LDL receptor-related protein 5 (Lrp5), a co-receptor of LDL receptor family, has been discovered as an important receptor in the activation of skeletal bone formation via binding to the secreted glycoprotein Wnt and activating beta catenin to induce bone formation. Therefore, we hypothesized that the underlying mechanism of degenerative valve disease may be related to the activation of the Lrp5 receptor in the spectrum of osteoblast differentiation within human diseased valve leaflets. The most common location of degenerative valves is the left side of the heart. Myxomatous mitral valve lesions causing mitral regurgitation are believed to be caused by progressive thickening due to activated myofibroblasts (Rabkin et al. 2001). Recent evidence suggests that aortic valve develops calcification secondary to an osteoblast differentiation pathway (Rajamannan et al. 2003b). Finally, bicuspid aortic valve valves develop calcification similar to that of tricuspid aortic stenosis but at an earlier age (Roberts and Ko 2005). Figure 4.4, demonstrates the immunohistochemistry stains for the osteoblast signaling markers: Lrp5, Wnt3 and PCNA. Figure 4.4, Panels A1, A2, B1 and B2, demonstrates a mild amount of Lrp5 and Wnt3 staining in the control valves and in the areas of hypertrophic chondrocytes in the mitral valves. Lrp5 and Wnt3 staining was increased in the calcified aortic valves (Fig. 4.4, Panels A3, A4, B3, and B4). Figure 4.4, Panels C3 and C4, demonstrates the presence of an increase in PCNA protein expression in the calcified valve as compared to Fig. 4.4, Panels C1 and C2 (Control valves) which demonstrate a decrease in PCNA protein staining.

This study (Caira et al. 2006) demonstrates that the Lrp5/Wnt3 signaling markers are present in the calcified aortic valve greater than the degenerative mitral valve. These data provide the first evidence of a mechanistic pathway for the initiation of bone differentiation in degenerative valve lesions which is expressed in the mitral valve as a cartilage phenotype, and in the calcified aortic valve as a bone phenotype. These results indicate that there is a continuum of an earlier stage of osteoblast bone differentiation in the mitral valves as compared to the calcified aortic valves. In normal adult skeleton bone the initiation of bone formation occurs with the development of a cartilaginous template which eventually mineralizes and forms calcified bone. In this process the mitral valve expresses an early cartilage formation and the aortic valve demonstrates the mineralized osteoblast phenotype. The process follows the spectrum of normal skeletal bone formation. This is the first study to demonstrate the presence of chondrocytes in mitral valves, and osteoblasts in aortic valves implicating this pathologic mechanism in the development of mitral regurgitation in degenerative myxomatous mitral valves and stenosis in calcific aortic valves. These findings may be secondary to an osteoblast differentiation process that is mediated by the Lrp5/Wnt3 pathway followed by an active endochondral bone formation mechanism in the development of heart valve disease. These data provide the first evidence of a mechanistic pathway for the initiation of bone differentiation in degenerative valve

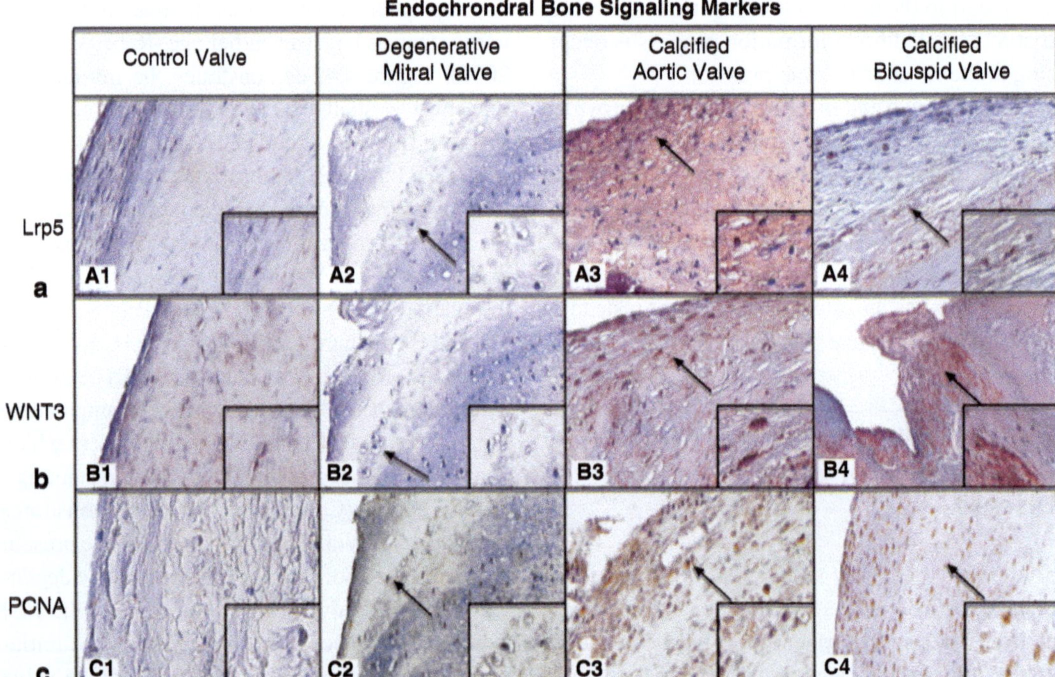

Fig. 4.4 Endochondral bone signaling markers in valvular heart disease: mitral and aortic (Reprinted with permission from Caira et al. (2006))

lesions which is expressed in the mitral valve as a cartilage phenotype and in the calcified aortic valve as a bone phenotype (Caira et al. 2006).

Statins as a Potential Therapy for Atherosclerotic Aortic Valve Disease

Although valve replacement and catheter based therapies are the current treatment of choice for severe critical aortic stenosis, future insights into the mechanisms of calcification and its progression may indicate a role for lipid lowering therapy in modifying the rate of progression of stenosis. Several members of the HMG CoA reductase agents, long recognized as effective in lowering cholesterol levels and reducing cardiovascular risk, recently have been shown to have significant effects on cardiovascular mortality and atherosclerosis. There are a growing number of studies from retrospective echo databases which have demonstrated that statin therapy may slow the progression of this disease process (Aronow et al. 2001; Bellamy et al. 2002; Pohle et al. 2001; Shavelle et al. 2002; Novaro et al. 2001). Figure 4.5, demonstrates the potential mechanism by which lipids regulate the differentiation of the valve myofibroblast cell to a bone like phenotype and the use of statins in the slowing of progression of this atherosclerotic disease. HMG CoA reductase inhibitors may provide an innovative therapeutic approach by employing both lipid lowering and possible non-lipid lowering effects to forestall critical stenosis in the aortic valve (Rajamannan 2010). Despite the increasing prevalence of this condition and the growing epidemiological evidence demonstrating the clinical risk factors, very little is known regarding the cellular mechanisms of calcific aortic stenosis. Furthermore, there are no established medial treatments indicated for calcific aortic stenosis. If cholesterol is a causative risk factor, then medications may have a pivotal role in the management of aortic valve disease. The understanding of medical therapy in aortic valve disease may slow the progression of stenosis and will decrease the number of aortic valve replacements in the future.

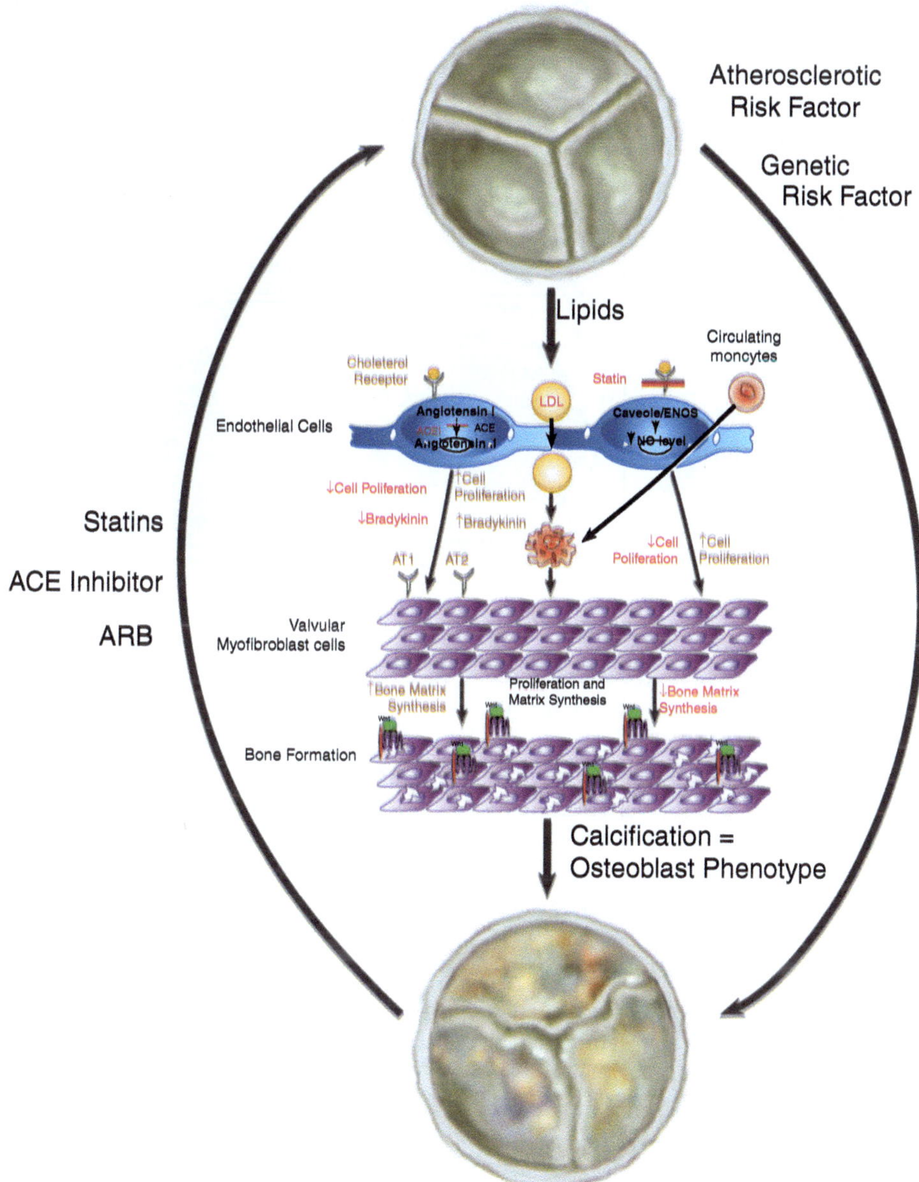

Fig. 4.5 Cellular targets for medical therapy in calcific aortic valve disease (Reprinted with permission from Rajamannan (2010))

Experimental Hypercholesterolemic Rabbit Model Testing Statins in Atherosclerotic Aortic Valves

Our laboratory has developed models of experimental hypercholesterolemia and aortic valve atherosclerosis and valve calcification. We tested if calcification was developing in the aortic valve. To test this hypothesis we tested the rabbit model for 6 months with and without statins to allow the valves to mineralize (Rajamannan et al. 2005b). Furthermore, identification of the intermediate signaling steps between lipid accumulation, cellular proliferation, and calcification have not been

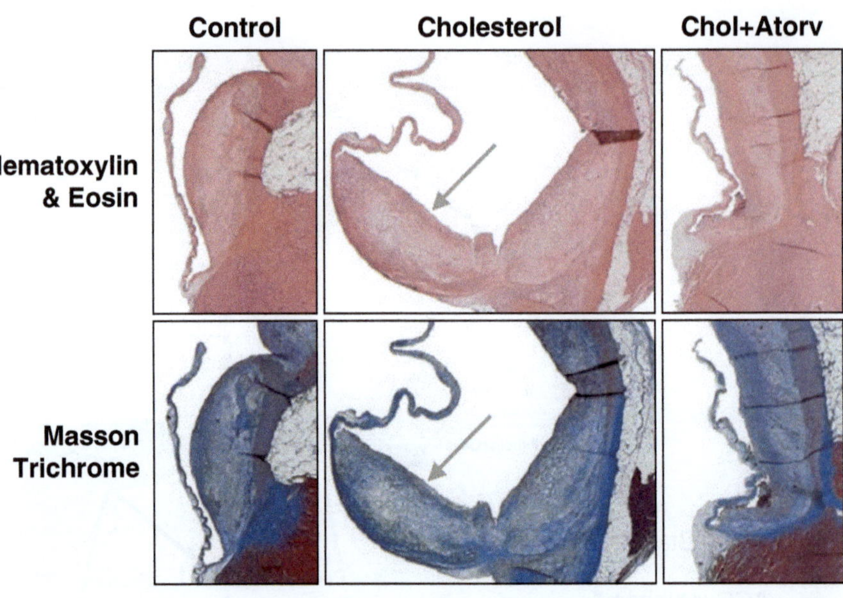

Fig. 4.6 Chronic experimental hypercholesterolemia induces mineralization in the aortic valve and statins slow progression (Rajamannan et al. 2005a)

clearly established. Studying the signaling pathways in disease processes help to develop future targeted therapies for aortic stenosis. Figure 4.6, demonstrates the normal aortic valve surface from control animals appeared thin and intact, with a smooth endothelial cell layer covering the entire surface and a thin collagen layer in the spongiosa layer of the valve, as demonstrated by Hematoxylin and Eosin stain and Masson Trichrome stain (Rajamannan et al. 2005a). There was also an increase in the blue collagen trichrome stain, mineralization, Lrp5 expression and cellular proliferation in the hypercholesterolemic aortic valves. The atorvastatin treated rabbits demonstrated a marked decrease in the amount of atherosclerotic plaque burden, and these changes were most pronounced at the base of the leaflets. This study extends our original study demonstrating atherosclerosis and cell proliferation in a short term cholesterol feeding in the rabbit model to demonstrate the findings in a long term lower concentration of cholesterol feeding.

Summary

Calcific Aortic Stenosis is an active biologic process with the initial atherosclerotic lesion progressing via different stages to severe stenosis associated with calcification to translate the treatment strategies for treatment disease.

References

Adams LD, Geary RL, McManus B, Schwartz SM. A comparison of aorta and vena cava medial message expression by cDNA array analysis identifies a set of 68 consistently differentially expressed genes, all in aortic media. Circ Res. 2000;87(7):623–31.

Aronow WS, Schwartz KS, Koenigsberg M. Correlation of serum lipids, calcium, and phosphorus, diabetes mellitus and history of systemic hypertension with presence or absence of calcified or thickened aortic cusps or root in elderly patients. Am J Cardiol. 1987;59(9):998–9.

Aronow WS, Ahn C, Kronzon I, Goldman ME. Association of coronary risk factors and use of statins with progression of mild valvular aortic stenosis in older persons. Am J Cardiol. 2001;88(6):693–5.

Becker CR, Majeed A, Crispin A, Knez A, Schoepf UJ, Boekstegers P, Steinbeck G, Reiser MF. CT measurement of coronary calcium mass: impact on global cardiac risk assessment. Eur Radiol. 2005;15(1):96–101.

Bellamy MF, Pellikka PA, Klarich KW, Tajik AJ, Enriquez-Sarano M. Association of cholesterol levels, hydroxymethylglutaryl coenzyme-A reductase inhibitor treatment, and progression of aortic stenosis in the community. [Comment]. J Am Coll Cardiol. 2002;40(10):1723–30.

Bonow RO, Carabello B, de Leon Jr AC, Edmunds Jr LH, Fedderly BJ, Freed MD, Gaasch WH, McKay CR, Nishimura RA, O'Gara PT, O'Rourke RA, Rahimtoola SH, Ritchie JL, Cheitlin MD, Eagle KA, Gardner TJ,

Garson Jr A, Gibbons RJ, Russell RO, Ryan TJ, Smith Jr SC. Guidelines for the management of patients with valvular heart disease: executive summary. A report of the American College of Cardiology/American Heart Association Task Force on practice guidelines (Committee on management of patients with valvular heart disease). Circulation. 1998;98(18):1949–84.

Boon A, Cheriex E, Lodder J, Kessels F. Cardiac valve calcification: characteristics of patients with calcification of the mitral annulus or aortic valve. Heart. 1997;78(5):472–4.

Buja LM, Kovanen PT, Bilheimer DW. Cellular pathology of homozygous familial hypercholesterolemia. Am J Pathol. 1979;97:327–57.

Caira FC, Stock SR, Gleason TG, McGee EC, Huang J, Bonow RO, Spelsberg TC, McCarthy PM, Rahimtoola SH, Rajamannan NM. Human degenerative valve disease is associated with up-regulation of low-density lipoprotein receptor-related protein 5 receptor-mediated bone formation. J Am Coll Cardiol. 2006;47(8):1707–12.

Chan KL, Ghani M, Woodend K, Burwash IG. Case-controlled study to assess risk factors for aortic stenosis in congenitally bicuspid aortic valve. Am J Cardiol. 2001;88(6):690–3.

Charo IF, Taubman MB. Chemokines in the pathogenesis of vascular disease. Circ Res. 2004;95(9):858–66.

Cheitlin M, Armstrong W, Aurigemma G, Beller G, Bierman F, Davis J, Douglas P, Faxon D, Gillam L, Kimball T, Kussmaul W, Pearlman A, Philbrick J, Rakowski H, Thys D, Antman E, Smith S, Alpert J, Gregoratos G, Anderson J, Hiratzka L, Faxon D, Hunt S, Fuster V, Jacobs A, Gibbons R, Russell R. ACC/AHA/ASE 2003 guideline update for the clinical application of echocardiography: summary article: a report of the American College of Cardiology/American Heart Association Task Force on Practice Guidelines (ACC/AHA/ASE Committee to Update the 1997 Guidelines for the Clinical Application of Echocardiography). J Am Soc Echocardiogr. 2003;16(10):1091–110.

Chui MC, Newby DE, Panarelli M, Bloomfield P, Boon NA. Association between calcific aortic stenosis and hypercholesterolemia: is there a need for a randomized controlled trial of cholesterol-lowering therapy? Clin Cardiol. 2001;24(1):52–5.

D'Agostino RB, Kannel WB, Belanger AJ, Sytkowski PA. Trends in CHD and risk factors at age 55–64 in the Framingham Study. Int J Epidemiol. 1989;18(3 Suppl 1):S67–72.

Deutscher S, Rockette HE, Krishnaswami V. Diabetes and hypercholesterolemia among patients with calcific aortic stenosis. J Chronic Dis. 1984;37(5):407–15.

Drolet MC, Arsenault M, Couet J. Experimental aortic valve stenosis in rabbits. J Am Coll Cardiol. 2003;41(7):1211–7.

Gong Y, Slee RB, Fukai N, Rawadi G, Roman-Roman S, Reginato AM, Wang H, Cundy T, Glorieux FH, Lev D, Zacharin M, Oexle K, Marcelino J, Suwairi W, Heeger S, Sabatakos G, Apte S, Adkins WN, Allgrove J, Arslan-Kirchner M, Batch JA, Beighton P, Black GC, Boles RG, Boon LM, Borrone C, Brunner HG, Carle GF, Dallapiccola B, De Paepe A, Floege B, Halfhide ML, Hall B, Hennekam RC, Hirose T, Jans A, Juppner H, Kim CA, Keppler-Noreuil K, Kohlschuetter A, LaCombe D, Lambert M, Lemyre E, Letteboer T, Peltonen L, Ramesar RS, Romanengo M, Somer H, Steichen-Gersdorf E, Steinmann B, Sullivan B, Superti-Furga A, Swoboda W, van den Boogaard MJ, Van Hul W, Vikkula M, Votruba M, Zabel B, Garcia T, Baron R, Olsen BR, Warman ML, Osteoporosis-Pseudoglioma Syndrome Collaborative Group. LDL receptor-related protein 5 (LRP5) affects bone accrual and eye development. Cell. 2001;107(4):513–23.

Kawaguchi A, Miyatake K, Yutani C, Beppu S, Tsushima M, Yamamura T, Yamamoto A. Characteristic cardiovascular manifestation in homozygous and heterozygous familial hypercholesterolemia. Am Heart J. 1999;137:410–8.

Kawaguchi A, Yutani C, Yamamoto A. Hypercholesterolemic valvulopathy: an aspect of malignant atherosclerosis. Ther Apher Dial. 2003;7(4):439–43.

Koh KP, Wang Y, Yi T, Shiao SL, Lorber MI, Sessa WC, Tellides G, Pober JS. T cell-mediated vascular dysfunction of human allografts results from IFN-{gamma} dysregulation of NO synthase. J Clin Invest. 2004;114(6):846–56.

Lindroos M, Kupari M, Valvanne J, Strandberg T, Heikkila J, Tilvis R. Factors associated with calcific aortic valve degeneration in the elderly. Eur Heart J. 1994; 15(7):865–70.

Little RD, Carulli JP, Del Mastro RG, Dupuis J, Osborne M, Folz C, Manning SP, Swain PM, Zhao SC, Eustace B, Lappe MM, Spitzer L, Zweier S, Braunschweiger K, Benchekroun Y, Hu X, Adair R, Chee L, FitzGerald MG, Tulig C, Caruso A, Tzellas N, Bawa A, Franklin B, McGuire S, Nogues X, Gong G, Allen KM, Anisowicz A, Morales AJ, Lomedico PT, Recker SM, Van Eerdewegh P, Recker RR, Johnson ML. A mutation in the LDL receptor-related protein 5 gene results in the autosomal dominant high-bone-mass trait. Am J Hum Genet. 2002;70(1):11–9.

Mohler ER, Sheridan MJ, Nichols R, Harvey WP, Waller BF. Development and progression of aortic valve stenosis: atherosclerosis risk factors–a causal relationship? A clinical morphologic study. Clin Cardiol. 1991;14(12):995–9.

Mohler 3rd ER, Adam LP, McClelland P, Graham L, Hathaway DR. Detection of osteopontin in calcified human aortic valves. Arterioscler Thromb Vasc Biol. 1997;17(3):547–52.

Mohler 3rd ER, Gannon F, Reynolds C, Zimmerman R, Keane MG, Kaplan FS. Bone formation and inflammation in cardiac valves. Circulation. 2001;103(11):1522–8.

Novaro GM, Tiong IY, Pearce GL, Lauer MS, Sprecher DL, Griffin BP. Effect of hydroxymethylglutaryl coenzyme a reductase inhibitors on the progression of calcific aortic stenosis. Circulation. 2001;104(18):2205–9.

O'Brien KD, Kuusisto J, Reichenbach DD, Ferguson M, Giachelli C, Alpers CE, Otto CM. Osteopontin is expressed in human aortic valvular lesions [comment]. Circulation. 1995;92(8):2163–8.

O'Brien KD, Reichenbach DD, Marcovina SM, Kuusisto J, Alpers CE, Otto CM. Apolipoproteins B, (a), and E accumulate in the morphologically early lesion of 'degenerative' valvular aortic stenosis. Arterioscler Thromb Vasc Biol. 1996;16(4):523–32.

Olsson M, Thyberg J, Nilsson J. Presence of oxidized low density lipoprotein in nonrheumatic stenotic aortic valves. Arterioscler Thromb Vasc Biol. 1999;19(5):1218–22.

Peltier M, Trojette F, Sarano ME, Grigioni F, Slama MA, Tribouilloy CM. Relation between cardiovascular risk factors and nonrheumatic severe calcific aortic stenosis among patients with a three-cuspid aortic valve. Am J Cardiol. 2003;91(1):97–9.

Pohle K, Maffert R, Ropers D, Moshage W, Stilianakis N, Daniel WG, Achenbach S. Progression of aortic valve calcification: association with coronary atherosclerosis and cardiovascular risk factors. [See comment]. Circulation. 2001;104(16):1927–32.

Rabkin E, Aikawa M, Stone JR, Fukumoto Y, Libby P, Schoen FJ. Activated interstitial myofibroblasts express catabolic enzymes and mediate matrix remodeling in myxomatous heart valves. Circulation. 2001;104(21):2525–32.

Rajamannan NM. Mechanisms of aortic valve calcification: the LDL-density-radius theory: a translation from cell signaling to physiology. Am J Physiol Heart Circ Physiol. 2010;298(1):H5–15.

Rajamannan NM, Sangiorgi G, Springett M, Arnold K, Mohacsi T, Spagnoli LG, Edwards WD, Tajik AJ, Schwartz RS. Experimental hypercholesterolemia induces apoptosis in the aortic valve. J Heart Valve Dis. 2001;10(3):371–4.

Rajamannan NM, Subramaniam M, Springett M, Sebo TC, Niekrasz M, McConnell JP, Singh RJ, Stone NJ, Bonow RO, Spelsberg TC. Atorvastatin inhibits hypercholesterolemia-induced cellular proliferation and bone matrix production in the rabbit aortic valve. Circulation. 2002;105(22):2260–5.

Rajamannan NM, Edwards WD, Spelsberg TC. Hypercholesterolemic aortic-valve disease. N Engl J Med. 2003a;349(7):717–8.

Rajamannan NM, Subramaniam M, Rickard D, Stock SR, Donovan J, Springett M, Orszulak T, Fullerton DA, Tajik AJ, Bonow RO, Spelsberg T. Human aortic valve calcification is associated with an osteoblast phenotype. Circulation. 2003b;107(17):2181–4.

Rajamannan NM, Subramaniam M, Caira FC, Stock SR, Spelsberg TC. Atorvastatin inhibits hypercholesterolemia-induced calcification in the aortic valves via the Lrp5 receptor pathway. Circulation. 2005a;112(9 Suppl):I229–34.

Rajamannan NM, Subramaniam M, Stock SR, Stone NJ, Springett M, Ignatiev KI, McConnell JP, Singh RJ, Bonow RO, Spelsberg TC. Atorvastatin inhibits calcification and enhances nitric oxide synthase production in the hypercholesterolaemic aortic valve. Heart. 2005b;91(6):806–10.

Rajamannan NM, Evans FJ, Aikawa E, Grande-Allen KJ, Demer LL, Heistad DD, Simmons CA, Masters KS, Mathieu P, O'Brien KD, Schoen FJ, Towler DA, Yoganathan AP, Otto CM. Calcific aortic valve disease: not simply a degenerative process: a review and agenda for research from the National Heart and Lung and Blood Institute Aortic Stenosis Working Group. Executive summary: calcific aortic valve disease-2011 update. Circulation. 2011;124(16):1783–91.

Roberts WC, Ko JM. Frequency by decades of unicuspid, bicuspid, and tricuspid aortic valves in adults having isolated aortic valve replacement for aortic stenosis, with or without associated aortic regurgitation. Circulation. 2005;111(7):920–5.

Rosenhek R, Binder T, Porenta G, Lang I, Christ G, Schemper M, Maurer G, Baumgartner H. Predictors of outcome in severe, asymptomatic aortic stenosis. N Engl J Med. 2000;343(9):611–7.

Rye KA, Wee K, Curtiss LK, Bonnet DJ, Barter PJ. Apolipoprotein A-II Inhibits high density lipoprotein remodeling and lipid-poor apolipoprotein A-I formation. J Biol Chem. 2003;278(25):22530–6.

Sarphie TG. Anionic surface properties of aortic and mitral valve endothelium from New Zealand white rabbits. Am J Anat. 1985a;174:145–60.

Sarphie TG. Surface responses of aortic valve endothelia from diet-induced, hypercholesterolemic rabbits. Atherosclerosis. 1985b;54(3):283–99.

Sarphie TG. A cytochemical study of the surface properties of aortic and mitral valve endothelium from hypercholesterolemic rabbits. Exp Mol Pathol. 1986;44:281–96.

Shao JS, Cheng SL, Pingsterhaus JM, Charlton-Kachigian N, Loewy AP, Towler DA. Msx2 promotes cardiovascular calcification by activating paracrine Wnt signals. J Clin Invest. 2005;115(5):1210–20.

Shavelle DM, Takasu J, Budoff MJ, Mao S, Zhao XQ, O'Brien KD. HMG CoA reductase inhibitor (statin) and aortic valve calcium. [Comment]. Lancet. 2002;359(9312):1125–6.

Sprecher DL, Schaefer EJ, Kent KM, Gregg RE, Zech LA, Hoeg JM, McManus B, Roberts WC, Brewer Jr HB. Cardiovascular features of homozygous familial hypercholesterolemia: analysis of 16 patients. Am J Cardiol. 1984;54(1):20–30.

Stewart BF, Siscovick D, Lind BK, Gardin JM, Gottdiener JS, Smith VE, Kitzman DW, Otto CM. Clinical factors associated with calcific aortic valve disease. Cardiovascular Health Study. J Am Coll Cardiol. 1997;29(3):630–4.

Stokes W. The diseases of the heart and aorta. Dublin: Hodges & Smith; 1845. p. 211–2.

Tabas I. Consequences of cellular cholesterol accumulation: basic concepts and physiological implications. J Clin Invest. 2002;110(7):905–11.

Thukkani AK, McHowat J, Hsu FF, Brennan ML, Hazen SL, Ford DA. Identification of alpha-chloro fatty aldehydes and unsaturated lysophosphatidylcholine molecular species in human atherosclerotic lesions. Circulation. 2003;108(25):3128–33.

Towler DA, Bidder M, Latifi T, Coleman T, Semenkovich CF. Diet-induced diabetes activates an osteogenic gene regulatory program in the aortas of low density lipoprotein receptor-deficient mice. J Biol Chem. 1998;273(46):30427–34.

Whyte HM. The relative importance of the major risk factors in atherosclerotic and other diseases. Aust N Z J Med. 1976;6(5):387–93.

Wilmshurst PT, Stevenson RN, Griffiths H, Lord JR. A case–control investigation of the relation between hyperlipidaemia and calcific aortic valve stenosis. Heart. 1997;78(5):475–9.

Wilson PW, Castelli WP, Kannel WB. Coronary risk prediction in adults (the Framingham Heart Study). Am J Cardiol. 1987;59(14):91G–4.

The Electrocardiogram as a Risk Predictor in Asymptomatic Aortic Stenosis

5

Anders M. Greve and Kristian Wachtell

Calcific aortic stenosis (AS) shares several etiological factors and histopathological changes with vascular atherosclerosis and the two diseases often coincide (Otto et al. 1994). Observed cardiovascular event rates might therefore differ substantially despite equal AS severity in the presence of additional vascular disease, such as atherosclerosis or hypertension (Otto et al. 1999; Briand et al. 2005). Moreover, cardiac response to the same pressure load may not be uniform in otherwise comparable patients (Awtry and Davidoff 2011). As such, is the development of left ventricular (LV) hypertrophy in response to increased afterload, the result of a complex dynamic process which involves mechanical, genes, molecular and biochemical factors (Devereux and Roman 1999). Thus, sole reliance on echocardiographic AS severity and symptoms might prove insufficient to identify all AS patients whose prognosis could be improved by earlier aortic valve replacement or other available therapy. A simple and reproducible score, which encapsulates the sum of AS and coexisting risk factors is therefore needed for reliable prognostication in these patients. In turn, this may allow for improved prediction of the safety of continued watchful waiting prior to the occurrence of potentially irreversible or fatal cardiac damage. The electrocardiogram, a low-cost and easily repeatable examination, is appealing in this context, as it is feasible for mass examination and sensitive to changes in cardiac structure and function induced by valvular- as well as vascular disease (Greve et al. 2011a; Wachtell et al. 2000; Nesto and Kowalchuk 1987). The purpose of this chapter is therefore to review the potential role of classic electrocardiography as a widely available tool for risk stratification in the growing population of patients with calcific aortic valve disease.

A.M. Greve, M.D. (✉)
K. Wachtell, M.D., Ph.D., DrMedSci
Department of Cardiology,
The Heart Center, Rigshospitalet,
Copenhagen, Denmark

Department of Cardiology, Gentofte Hospital,
Hellerup, Denmark

University of Copenhagen,
Copenhagen, Denmark
e-mail: greve_anders@hotmail.com

Changes in the Electrocardiogram Reflecting Cardiac Pressure Load

The Development of Electrocardiographic Abnormalities

LV outflow resistance depends on the global hemodynamic load ([Z_{va} = systolic arterial pressure + mean net transaortic gradient]/[stroke volume index]) (Otto 2006). The relations between LV afterload, wall-stress, and cardiac burden are schematized in Fig. 5.1 (Heart-Valve-Arterial interaction model). The changes in the hearts structure and function following chronic pressure load and calcific aortic valve disease per se are, as reflected in the electrocardiogram, given in Fig. 5.2. The order by which these maladaptations

N.M. Rajamannan (ed.), *Cardiac Valvular Medicine*,
DOI 10.1007/978-1-4471-4132-7_5,

Fig. 5.1 Global left ventricular load in aortic stenosis

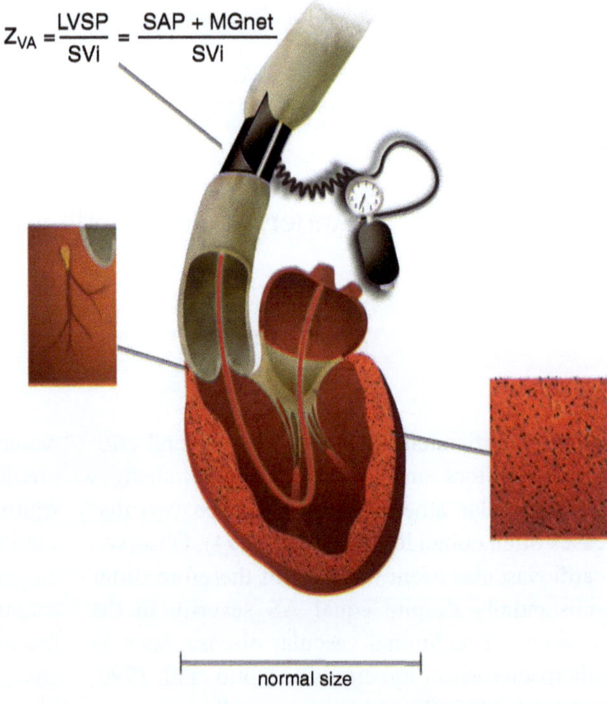

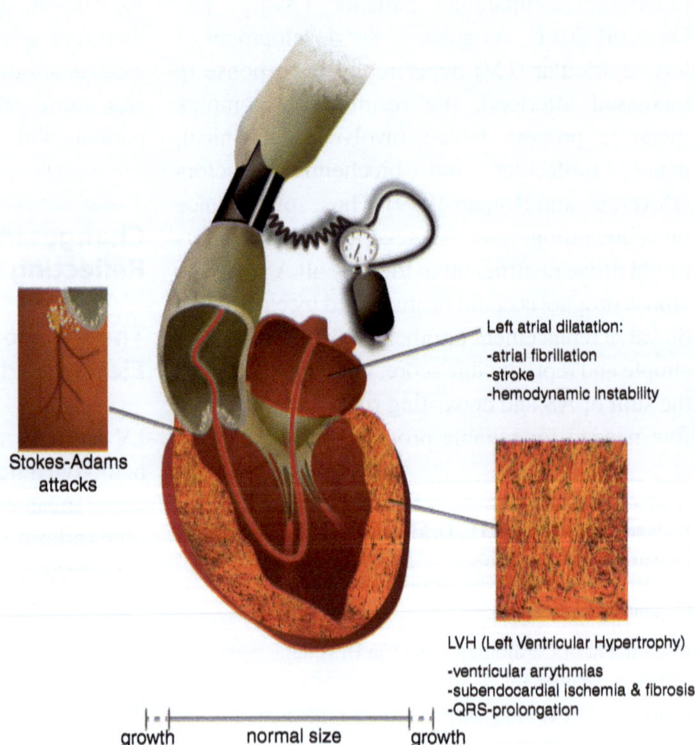

Fig. 5.2 Electrocardiographic abnormalities reflecting cardiac response to pressure load

occur is not known to follow any specific pattern, i.e. atrial fibrillation might occur prior to the development of LV hypertrophy and vice versa. Furthermore, relations between valvular pathology and cardiac abnormalities are non-linear, as they depend on age, body stature and comorbid status (Cramariuc et al. 2008). Some patients with preserved LV systolic function might have aortic valve areas in the severe ranges but no other signs (mean gradient <30 mmHg) indicating critical AS (Jander et al. 2011). Whether or not additional electrocardiographic signs of myocardial damage for the same AS severity relate to the presence of true rather than low gradient "severe" AS is unknown. However, in some, particularly the obese or very old, a lack of electrocardiographic signals indicating advanced AS should alert the clinician of possible confounding factors such as a relative voltage deficiency or shifted anatomy. Similarly, the electrocardiogram is not a reliable test for AS severity in itself, as it can show severe LV hypertrophy in mild AS due to concomitant hypertension. For simplicity, the electrocardiographic changes associated with increased blood pressure and AS per se, will first be presented in the order they appear as the electrical impulse travels from the sinus node to the distal Purkinje fibers and then as the potential prognostic implications of the respective electrocardiographic findings.

Atrial Fibrillation and Atrial Abnormalities

Left atrial size is in patients with normal systolic function a barometer of LV filling pressure (Simek et al. 1995). Accordingly, left atrial volume and function are independently associated with AS severity and LV dimensions (Dalsgaard et al. 2008). Given its thin walled structure, left atrial size is, however, expected to increase already in earlier stages of AS and be influenced by arterial stiffness, relating to older age and/or concomitant vascular disease such as hypertension. This might suggest that left atrial abnormalities are not good markers of AS severity per se. Notwithstanding, the additional presence of left atrial abnormalities in later AS seems associated with LV and atrial pressure overload (Dalsgaard et al. 2010; Bang et al. 2012). Moreover, the morphology and function of the left atrium is at all times heavily dependent upon appropriate opening and closure of the mitral valve during cardiac cycle. Backwards pressure- and/or volume induced stretch of atrial myocytes may lead to atrial fibrosis and disturbances in neuro-hormonal control systems. This can be seen as increased supraventricular ectopic activity and eventually the development of sustained atrial fibrillation. Intra-atrial blocks, noticed as changes in p-wave duration and orientation, may arise if the fibrotic patches are located within Bachmann's bundle. Similarly, atrial dilatation and increased anatomical distance from sinus to atrioventricular node might also lead to alterations in atrial depolarization patterns and predisposition to atrial arrhythmia (Roberts-Thomson et al. 2008). Increased load on atrial myocytes during the active contractile phase may lead to abnormal p-wave repolarization, which is probably suggestive of more advanced backwards failure.

Cardiac Conduction Delay

As the electrical impulse arrives at the atrioventricular node it comes into close anatomical proximity with the aortic valve. Particularly in later stages of calcific AS, pathology may therefore extend into the conductive system resulting in hindered atrioventricular conduction and potentially complete heart block. However, although histopathological studies are supportive of such a link between AS and atrioventricular conduction delay (Nair et al. 1984), it seems likely that the individual anatomy and specific localization of calcific nodules have a large influence on this relation. Moving through the interventricular septum and into the intraventricular conduction system, electrical conduction properties now become increasingly dependent upon myocardial structure and function. In the natural history of AS, LV wall stress increases with progressive valvular disease initiating numerous adaptive processes, which will eventually result in cardiac pump failure. This process can take decades and the path leading to, if ever, terminal AS is individual depending on a vast spectrum of mechanisms, risk factors and their combinations (Rajamannan et al. 2011). Nevertheless, there seems to be a common pathway through which initial LV hypertrophy via subendocardial ischemia and fibrosis leads to LV dilatation and eventually impaired LV systolic function and heart failure (Herrmann et al. 2011). The electrocardiogram is not a specific test for visualizing these changes, but longer QRS-duration may reflect the early extent of intra-myocardial fibrosis, and later mainly changes in LV diameter and wall thickness (Dhingra et al. 2005). On the molecular level, cardiac conduction velocity is influenced by connexins and ion-channels, which in turn are governed by activity in regulatory systems such as the renin-angiotensin system (Kasi et al. 2007). Thus, in AS patients without other reasons for intraventricular conduction delay, longer QRS-duration could be an early sign of subclinical cardiac damage due to AS and increased afterload as a whole (Cameron et al. 1983). Although, intraventricular blocks may occur with normal LV pressures as a physiologic phenomenon, a degenerative process within the conductive system itself or result from Q-waves and lesions to the conductive fibers following a coronary occlusion.

Left Ventricular Hypertrophy and Strain Patterns

Now within the LV structure, the electrocardiographic patterns are normally dominated by the LV de- and repolarization. As indicated above, LV response to increased pressure load is, however, very complex, involving regional changes in LV mass, myocardial energy consumption and delivery of oxygenated blood to cardiac myocytes. Concentric LV hypertrophy due to elevated afterload is often viewed as a compensatory mechanism in order to apply the increased wall stress over a larger wall area to overcome the increased afterload (Grossman et al. 1975). Indeed, it is likely that small adaptations in LV structure are needed to preserve systemic blood pressure and flow to vital organs. However, the balance between a favorable increase in LV work capacity and the vicious spiral of LV hypertrophy is delicate. As such are the correlates of LV hypertrophy in AS probably dependent upon the duration of increased LV afterload, additional hypertension and whether or not this can be timely reduced, such as with the treatment of hypertension or aortic valve replacement (Borer et al. 1983; Garcia et al. 2007). LV hypertrophy and ensuing changes in cardiac homeostasis can be measured by several electrocardiographic criteria (Prineas et al. 1982). The biology underlying electrocardiographic LV hypertrophy is not completely understood, but most likely involves maladaptive changes in LV geometry as well as increases in myocardial volume (Bacharova et al. 2010; Wiegerinck et al. 2006; Thiry et al. 1975). LV hypertrophy raises myocardial oxygen consumption, which at rest is compensated by a proportional increase in coronary blood flow (Rowe et al. 1961). This can be achieved by a dilatation of existing coronary vasculature and/or neovascular growth. However, although these measures do elevate total absolute flow, compensatory dilatation of coronary artery lumen may be insufficient to match regional increases in LV mass (Villari et al. 1992). Similarly, myocardial volume might increase to a greater extent than arterioles and capillaries, and increases in LV wall stress can further increase myocardial oxygen demand (Tomanek et al. 1986; van den Heuvel et al. 2000). This concurs with evidence of reduced coronary flow reserve in AS patients with LV hypertrophy, which particularly under dynamic activity may result in regional mismatches between myocardial oxygen consumption and demand (Nadell et al. 1983). These relative flow insufficiencies will due to cardiac anatomy be most marked in the subendocardium. ST-segment depression and T-wave inversion in leads V_{4-6} is believed to reflect the acute and chronic effects of LV hypertrophy induced subendocardial ischemia (Pichard et al. 1981).

Prognostic Implications of Electrocardiographic Abnormalities

Predicting future risks of cardiovascular events is notoriously difficult. This is particularly true among asymptomatic patients in earlier disease stages, as the final cause of morbidity and mortality might be completely different from that initially studied. Similarly, in asymptomatic AS, there is a prolonged period in which risk of adverse events due to AS is very low and endpoints will therefore often be driven by more rapidly accelerating sicknesses. However, a seemingly non-valvular event can have a decisive impact on future risks of valve related outcomes, i.e. reduced LV systolic function following a myocardial infarction might lead to secondary decompensated AS despite unchanged valvular pathology *per se*. For the clinician facing an asymptomatic patient with AS and no perceived need for aortic valve replacement, guidelines support continued watchful waiting in the majority but at the same time a search for high-risk patients who may warrant closer follow-up and/or referral for more advanced diagnostic techniques (Bonow et al. 2006). Ideal risk stratification should therefore identify; (1) the risk of AS being a sole or the primary cause of poor prognosis and; (2) the risk of secondary decompensation due to AS in combination with one or more comorbidities. The electrocardiogram can be useful for predicting some of these risks, as it may detect cardiac pathology with various etiologies in initially asymptomatic AS with or without critical outflow obstruction at that given time.

Atrial Fibrillation

Pre- or perioperative atrial fibrillation is an independent predictor of late mortality after aortic valve replacement (Greve et al. 2011b; Tjang et al. 2007; Levy et al. 2006; Filardo et al. 2010). However, few studies have dealt with the prognostic implications of atrial fibrillation in asymptomatic AS not scheduled for surgery (Fuster et al. 2011). Epidemiological data indicate a relation between atrial fibrillation and AS severity, but its prevalence in milder AS seems only moderately higher than in comparable background population (Otto 2006). Atrial fibrillation is therefore, particularly in early AS, most likely a marker of older and generally sicker patients rather than more severe AS per se. This is further supported by rates of stroke and heart failure in asymptomatic mild to moderate AS with additional atrial fibrillation (Fig, 5.3), which seem comparable to that expected in non-valvular atrial fibrillation (Greve et al. 2011b). In patients with established AS, rate of new-onset atrial fibrillation is ~1.2%/year prior to aortic valve replacement, most frequent in those with reduced LV systolic function and/or increased LV mass (Greve et al. 2011b). The development of atrial fibrillation in more advanced AS could therefore be a sign of cardiac decompensation and thus the need for aortic valve replacement. Moreover, atrial filling is likely to be of incremental importance for maintaining a normal cardiac output as LV diastolic filling is hindered with increasing wall stiffness in progressed aortic valve disease.

Cardiac Conduction Delay

Substantial evidence links QRS abnormalities to risk of cardiovascular morbidity and mortality in the general population and in various cardiovascular diseases (Dhingra et al. 2006; Brembilla-Perrot et al. 1999; Wang et al. 2008). Notably, longer QRS duration has been shown to be predictive of sudden cardiac death in the general population as well as in subjects with structural heart disease (Aro et al. 2011; Dhar et al. 2008). A pathophysiological mechanism may involve that longer QRS duration reflects abnormal myocardial depolarization and/or a higher threshold for termination of spontaneously occurring ventricular arrhythmia (Nagai et al. 2009). The predictive value of longer QRS duration of risk of sudden cardiac death is interesting in AS, since observational studies have indicated a real risk of sudden cardiac death in these patients (Pellikka et al. 2005; Carabello 2002). However, there is

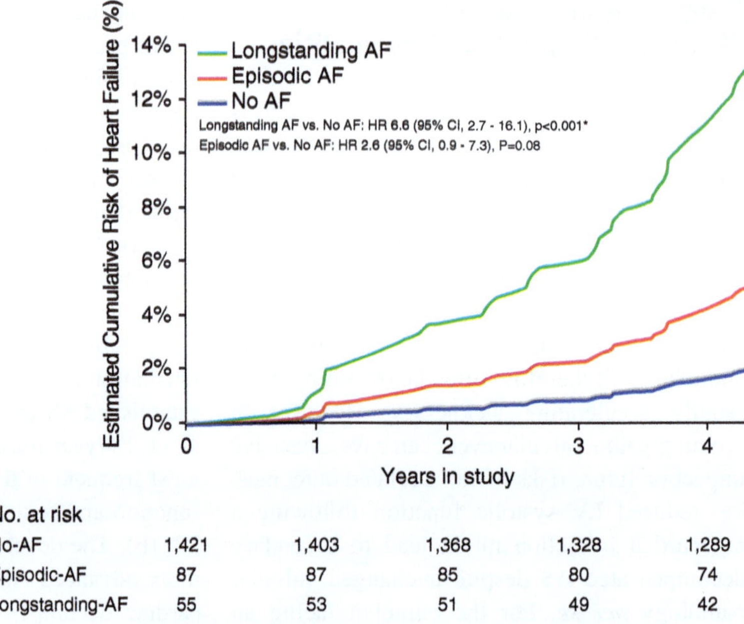

	0	1	2	3	4
No-AF	1,421	1,403	1,368	1,328	1,289
Episodic-AF	87	87	85	80	74
Longstanding-AF	55	53	51	49	42

* Abbreviations: AF: Atrial fibrillation, HR: Hazard ratio, CI: Confidence interval

Fig. 5.3 Estimated cumulative risk of heart failure (vertical axis) in patients with no-, episodic- and longstanding atrial fibrillation at baseline: during 4.3 years of follow-up (horizontal axis) (Reprinted with permission from Greve et al. (2011b))

limited mechanistic data on sudden cardiac death in AS. Literature describes at least two pathways relating to whether or not cardiac arrhythmia is a primary or secondary phenomenon, i.e. subsequent to an abnormal Bezold-Jarisch reflex with hypotension and bradyarrhythmia (Sorgato et al. 1998). In theory, secondary arrhythmias might be expected to have a relatively larger impact in later AS, where aortic pressures are more dependent upon LV outflow obstruction. Delayed cardiac activation, as a measure of pressure induced myocardial damage, is therefore probably related to the risk of primary arrhythmic death likely to have a relatively larger role in earlier asymptomatic AS (Sorgato et al. 1996). In the clinical setting, there are, however, often comorbidities, such as ischemic heart disease, which could be an important etiology of sudden cardiac death potentially unrelated to AS severity (Otto et al. 1999). Furthermore, longer QRS duration might not only reflect AS induced myocardial damage, as similar correlates with sudden cardiac death can be found in patients with increased afterload due to hypertension (Morin et al. 2009). Finally, QRS durations of ≥120 ms may, especially in healthier subjects, overlap with isolated degenerative changes in conductive fibers (Cheng et al. 2010). The clinical message might therefore be that patients with short QRS durations have a lower risk of arrhythmic death during watchful waiting in asymptomatic AS (Fig. 5.4) (Greve et al. 2012a).

Left Ventricular Hypertrophy and Strain Patterns

The classic electrocardiographic patterns of LV strain and LV hypertrophy are independent predictors of poor prognosis and death in AS patients on the waiting list for aortic valve replacement (Lund et al. 1996). Moreover, electrocardiographic signs of LV strain and LV hypertrophy have been shown to be associated with a shorter asymptomatic period before onset of symptoms requiring aortic valve replacement (Pellikka et al. 2005; Hering et al. 2004). In long term follow-up of initially asymptomatic patients with mild to moderate AS, cardiovascular event rates were considerably higher in those with additional electrocardiographic LV strain and LV hypertrophy (Greve et al. 2012b). In the latter study, observed incidences of myocardial

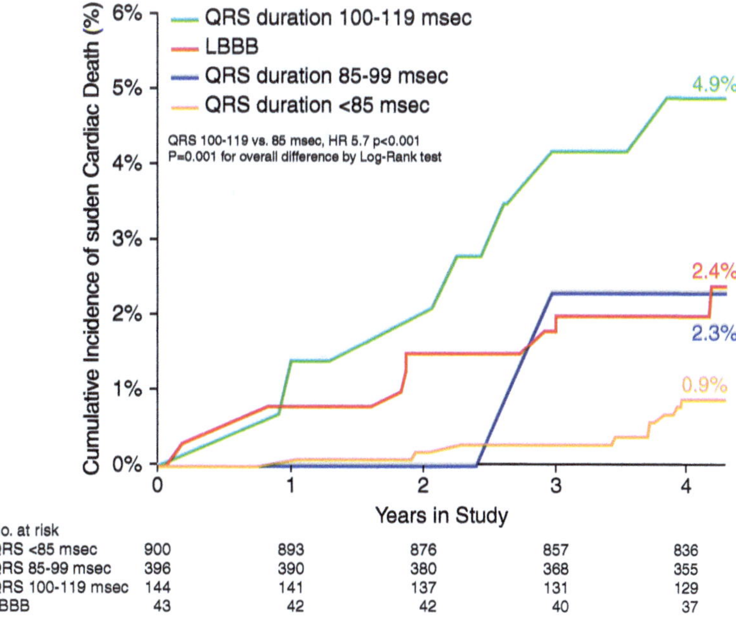

Fig. 5.4 Rate of sudden cardiac death by QRS group (Reprinted with permission from Greve et al. (2012a))

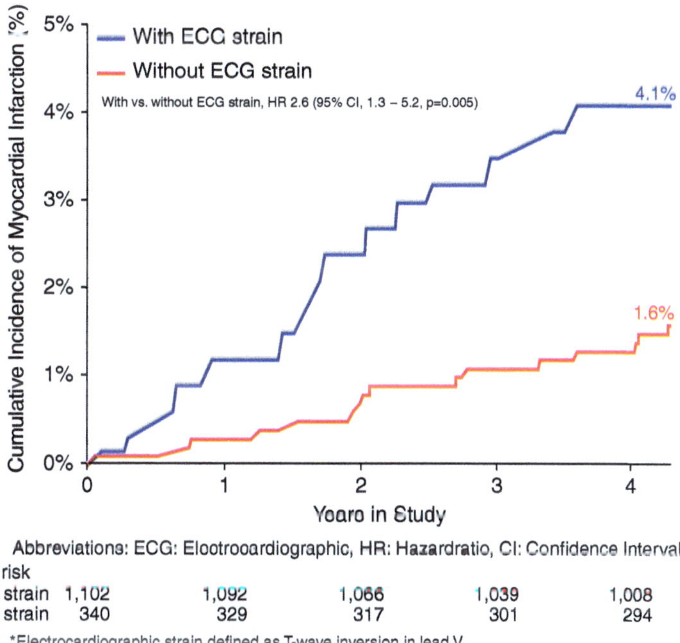

Fig. 5.5 Incidence of myocardial infarction (vertical axis) in patients with and without baseline ECG left ventricular strain during 4.3 years of follow-up (horizontal axis) (Reprinted with permission from Greve et al. (2012b))

infarction and relations to increased myocardial oxygen consumption, were consistent with electrocardiographic LV strain indicating subendocardial ischemia and reduced coronary flow reserve (Fig. 5.5). Similarly, electrocardiographic LV hypertrophy as a marker of the individual response to increased afterload, identified patients with a more than tenfold increase in the risk of heart failure (Fig. 5.6). Thus, low-cost and easily accessible electrocardiographic LV strain and LV hypertrophy data provide valuable tools for risk stratification in AS. Whether or not

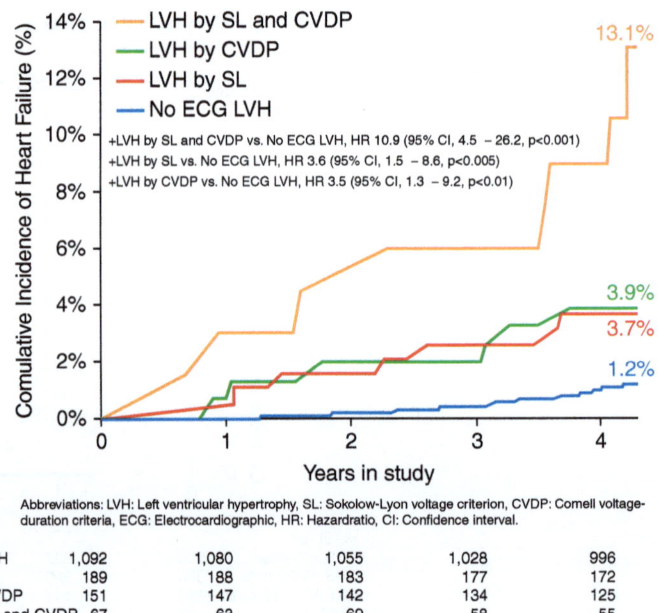

Fig. 5.6 Incidence of heart failure (vertical axis) in patients with and without baseline ECG left ventricular hypertrophy during 4.3 years of follow-up (horizontal axis) (Reprinted with permission from Greve et al. (2012b))

these electrocardiographic abnormalities results from AS and thus correlates with the need for aortic valve replacement is more uncertain, but merits further study.

A Normal Electrocardiogram

The above subchapters underscore that prognostication in AS involves a complex interplay between known and lesser studied factors. Indeed, there is probably no single variable that can be used to define the clinical fate of individual AS patients as competing risk factors might relate to entirely different mechanisms. In long term follow-up of initially asymptomatic mild to moderate AS, the number of abnormalities on a resting 12-lead electrocardiograms, as detected by annual reexamination, related to a stepwise worsening of prognosis (Greve et al. 2012b). This might suggest that assessment of electrocardiographic signs of myocardial damage contains a sum of biologic information, which could be helpful for the development of pertinent risk stratification scores in asymptomatic AS.

Interplay Between Electrocardiography and Other Modalities

It is evident that aortic valve disease involves a complex interplay between the valvular apparatus, the vasculature and the heart itself. Ideally this would suggest that each patient should undergo a complete examination of the entire cardiovascular system combined with genetic profiling and multiple tests for comorbidities. However, in the clinical setting it is not possible or cost-effective to submit all patients with aortic valve disease, ranging from early lesions to very severe AS, to advanced and often expensive imaging and invasive hemodynamic testing. Echocardiographic examination supplemented with exercise testing and/or biomarkers, is currently the clinical standard for measuring AS severity (Otto 2006). However, each modality has its own strengths and weaknesses, indicating that they are likely to be separately helpful, rather than competitors, in building on the basic information obtained by the electrocardiogram (Table 5.1).

Table 5.1 Translating electrocardiographic abnormalities into biology

Modality	Comments
Echocardiography	Limited by flow dependent nature of valve opening, very dependent upon user angling the probe correctly at the jet stream
Magnetic resonance imaging	Expensive, special training, but reference for detecting cardiac response to AS, i.e. myocardial fibrosis, systolic/diastolic measures, perfusion etc
Computer tomography	Radiation, interesting for possible measure of calcific infiltration into conduction system, particularly in transcatheter aortic-valve implantation (TAVI) where anatomic displacement of calcium might cause heart blocks
Invasive measures	Fractional flow reserve in AS with LV hypertrophy, LV pressures
Biomarkers	Natriuretic peptides vary widely between reexaminations, markers of calcification
Genes	Interesting in special families, role in general population uncertain, interesting if genes can suggest that some patients react to LV pressure load differently from others and or that aortic valve pathology will progress at a faster rate

Conclusion

Despite the fact that AS is a valvular disease it cannot be considered independently. Comorbidities, genes and therapeutic interventions are crucial factors for determining the prognostic impact of AS in individual patients. The electrocardiogram can be useful in trying to determine how the individual heart copes with the same AS severity. In the future, as more advanced techniques become available for clinical research, this might help us to a better understanding of the pathobiology underlying diverging prognoses in seemingly similar patients with asymptomatic AS.

References

Aro AL, Anttonen O, Tikkanen JT, Junttila MM, Kerola T, Rissanen HA, Reunanen A, Huikuri HV. Intraventricular conduction delay in a standard 12-lead electrocardiogram as a predictor of mortality in general population. Circ Arrhythm Electrophysiol. 2011;4(5):704–10.

Awtry E, Davidoff R. Low-flow/low-gradient aortic stenosis. Circulation. 2011;124:e739–41.

Bacharova L, Szathmary V, Kovalcik M, Mateasik A. Effect of changes in left ventricular anatomy and conduction velocity on the QRS voltage and morphology in left ventricular hypertrophy: a model study. J Electrocardiol. 2010;43:200–8.

Bang CN, Dalsgaard M, Greve AM, Køber L., Egstrup K, Gohlke-Baerwolf C, Ray S, Wachtell K. Left atrial size and function as predictors of new-onset atrial fibrillation in patients with asymptomatic aortic stenosis. J Am Coll Cardiol. 2012;59:E2026.

Bonow RO, Carabello BA, Chatterjee K, de Leon ACJ, Faxon DP, Freed MD, Gaasch WH, Lytle BW, Nishimura RA, O'Gara PT, O'Rourke RA, Otto CM, Shah PM, Shanewise JS, Smith Jr SC, Jacobs AK, Adams CD, Anderson JL, Antman EM, Fuster V, Halperin JL, Hiratzka LF, Hunt SA, Lytle BW, Nishimura R, Page RL, Riegel B. ACC/AHA 2006 guidelines for the management of patients with valvular heart disease: a report of the American College of Cardiology/American Heart Association Task Force on Practice Guidelines (writing Committee to Revise the 1998 guidelines for the management of patients with valvular heart disease) developed in collaboration with the Society of Cardiovascular Anesthesiologists endorsed by the Society for Cardiovascular Angiography and Interventions and the Society of Thoracic Surgeons. J Am Coll Cardiol. 2006;48:e1–148.

Borer JS, Jason M, Devereux RB, Fisher J, Green MV, Bacharach SL, Pickering T, Laragh JH. Function of the hypertrophied left ventricle at rest and during exercise. Hypertension and aortic stenosis. Am J Med. 1983;75:34–9.

Brembilla-Perrot B, Houriez P, Claudon O, Preiss JP, De La Chaise AT. Evolution of QRS duration after myocardial infarction: clinical consequences. Pacing Clin Electrophysiol. 1999;22:1466–75.

Biland M, Dumesnil JG, Kadem L, Tonguc AG, Rieu R, Garcia D, Pibarot P. Reduced systemic arterial compliance impacts significantly on left ventricular afterload and function in aortic stenosis: implications for diagnosis and treatment. J Am Coll Cardiol. 2005;46: 291–8.

Cameron JS, Myerburg RJ, Wong SS, Gaide MS, Epstein K, Alvarez TR, Gelband H, Guse PA, Bassett AL. Electrophysiologic consequences of chronic experimentally induced left ventricular pressure overload. J Am Coll Cardiol. 1983;2:481–7.

Carabello BA. Evaluation and management of patients with aortic stenosis. Circulation. 2002;105:1746–50.

Cheng S, Larson MG, Keyes MJ, McCabe EL, Newton-Cheh C, Levy D, Benjamin EJ, Vasan RS, Wang TJ.

Relation of QRS width in healthy persons to risk of future permanent pacemaker implantation. Am J Cardiol. 2010;106:668–72.

Cramariuc D, Rieck AE, Staal EM, Wachtell K, Eriksen E, Rossebo AB, Gerdts E. Factors influencing left ventricular structure and stress-corrected systolic function in men and women with asymptomatic aortic valve stenosis (a SEAS Substudy). Am J Cardiol. 2008;101:510–5.

Dalsgaard M, Egstrup K, Wachtell K, Gerdts E, Cramariuc D, Kjaergaard J, Hassager C. Left atrial volume in patients with asymptomatic aortic valve stenosis (the Simvastatin and Ezetimibe in Aortic Stenosis study). Am J Cardiol. 2008;101:1030–4.

Dalsgaard M, Kjaergaard J, Pecini R, Iversen KK, Kober L, Moller JE, Grande P, Clemmensen P, Hassager C. Predictors of exercise capacity and symptoms in severe aortic stenosis. Eur J Echocardiogr. 2010;11:482–7.

Devereux RB, Roman MJ. Left ventricular hypertrophy in hypertension: stimuli, patterns, and consequences. Hypertens Res. 1999;22:1–9.

Dhar R, Alsheikh-Ali AA, Estes III NA, Moss AJ, Zareba W, Daubert JP, Greenberg H, Case RB, Kent DM. Association of prolonged QRS duration with ventricular tachyarrhythmias and sudden cardiac death in the Multicenter Automatic Defibrillator Implantation Trial II (MADIT-II). Heart Rhythm. 2008;5:807–13.

Dhingra R, Ho NB, Benjamin EJ, Wang TJ, Larson MG, D'Agostino Sr RB, Levy D, Vasan RS. Cross-sectional relations of electrocardiographic QRS duration to left ventricular dimensions: the Framingham Heart Study. J Am Coll Cardiol. 2005;45:685–9.

Dhingra R, Pencina MJ, Wang TJ, Nam BH, Benjamin EJ, Levy D, Larson MG, Kannel WB, D'Agostino Sr RB, Vasan RS. Electrocardiographic QRS duration and the risk of congestive heart failure: the Framingham Heart Study. Hypertension. 2006;47:861–7.

Filardo G, Hamilton C, Hamman B, Hebeler Jr RF, Adams J, Grayburn P. New-onset postoperative atrial fibrillation and long-term survival after aortic valve replacement surgery. Ann Thorac Surg. 2010;90:474–9.

Fuster V, Ryden LE, Cannom DS, Crijns HJ, Curtis AB, Ellenbogen KA, Halperin JL, Kay GN, Le Huezey JY, Lowe JE, Olsson SB, Prystowsky EN, Tamargo JL, Wann LS. 2011 ACCF/AHA/HRS focused updates incorporated into the ACC/AHA/ESC 2006 Guidelines for the management of patients with atrial fibrillation: a report of the American College of Cardiology Foundation/ American Heart Association Task Force on Practice Guidelines developed in partnership with the European Society of Cardiology and in collaboration with the European Heart Rhythm Association and the Heart Rhythm Society. J Am Coll Cardiol. 2011;57:e101–98.

Garcia D, Pibarot P, Kadem L, Durand LG. Respective impacts of aortic stenosis and systemic hypertension on left ventricular hypertrophy. J Biomech. 2007;40:972–80.

Greve AM, Gerdts E, Boman K, Gohlke-Baerwolf C, Rossebo AB, Hammer-Hansen S, Kober L, Willenheimer R, Wachtell K. Differences in cardiovascular risk profile between electrocardiographic hypertrophy versus strain in asymptomatic patients with aortic stenosis (from SEAS Data). Am J Cardiol. 2011a;108:541–7.

Greve AM, Gerdts E, Boman K, Gohlke-Baerwolf C, Rossebo AB, Nienaber CA, Ray S, Egstrup K, Pedersen TR, Kober L, Willenheimer R, Wachtell K. Prognostic importance of atrial fibrillation in asymptomatic aortic stenosis: the Simvastatin and Ezetimibe in aortic stenosis study. Int J Cardiol. 2011.

Greve AM, Gerdts E, Boman K, Gohlke-Baerwolf C, Rossebo AB, Devereux RB, Køber L, Ray S, Willenheimer R, Wachtell K. Impact of QRS duration and morphology on the risk of sudden cardiac death in asymptomatic patients with aortic stenosis: the simvastatin and ezetimibe in aortic stenosis study. J Am Coll Cardiol. 2012a;59(13):1142–9.

Greve AM, Boman K, Gohlke-Baerwolf C, Kesaniemi YA, Nienaber C, Ray S, Egstrup K, Rossebo AB, Devereux RB, Kober L, Willenheimer R, Wachtell K. Clinical implications of electrocardiographic left ventricular strain and hypertrophy in asymptomatic patients with aortic stenosis: the Simvastatin and Ezetimibe in aortic stenosis study. Circulation. 2012b;125:346–53.

Grossman W, Jones D, McLaurin LP. Wall stress and patterns of hypertrophy in the human left ventricle. J Clin Invest. 1975;56:56–64.

Hering D, Piper C, Horstkotte D. Influence of atypical symptoms and electrocardiographic signs of left ventricular hypertrophy or ST-segment/T-wave abnormalities on the natural history of otherwise asymptomatic adults with moderate to severe aortic stenosis: preliminary communication. J Heart Valve Dis. 2004;13:182–7.

Herrmann S, Stork S, Niemann M, Lange V, Strotmann JM, Frantz S, Beer M, Gattenlohner S, Voelker W, Ertl G, Weidemann F. Low-gradient aortic valve stenosis myocardial fibrosis and its influence on function and outcome. J Am Coll Cardiol. 2011;58:402–12.

Jander N, Minners J, Holme I, Gerdts E, Boman K, Brudi P, Chambers JB, Egstrup K, Kesaniemi YA, Malbecq W, Nienaber CA, Ray S, Rossebo A, Pedersen TR, Skjaerpe T, Willenheimer R, Wachtell K, Neumann FJ, Gohlke-Barwolf C. Outcome of patients with low-gradient "severe" aortic stenosis and preserved ejection fraction. Circulation. 2011;123:887–95.

Kasi VS, Xiao HD, Shang LL, Iravanian S, Langberg J, Witham EA, Jiao Z, Gallego CJ, Bernstein KE, Dudley Jr SC. Cardiac-restricted angiotensin-converting enzyme overexpression causes conduction defects and connexin dysregulation. Am J Physiol Heart Circ Physiol. 2007;293:H182–92.

Levy F, Garayalde E, Quere JP, Ianetta-Peltier M, Peltier M, Tribouilloy C. Prognostic value of preoperative atrial fibrillation in patients with aortic stenosis and low ejection fraction having aortic valve replacement. Am J Cardiol. 2006;98:809–11.

Lund O, Nielsen TT, Emmertsen K, Flo C, Rasmussen B, Jensen FT, Pilegaard HK, Kristensen LH, Hansen OK. Mortality and worsening of prognostic profile during waiting time for valve replacement in aortic stenosis. Thorac Cardiovasc Surg. 1996;44:289–95.

Morin DP, Oikarinen L, Viitasalo M, Toivonen L, Nieminen MS, Kjeldsen SE, Dahlof B, John M, Devereux RB, Okin PM. QRS duration predicts sudden cardiac death in hypertensive patients undergoing intensive medical therapy: the LIFE study. Eur Heart J. 2009;30:2908–14.

Nadell R, DePace NL, Ren JF, Hakki AH, Iskandrian AS, Morganroth J. Myocardial oxygen supply/demand ratio in aortic stenosis: hemodynamic and echocardiographic evaluation of patients with and without angina pectoris. J Am Coll Cardiol. 1983;2:258–62.

Nagai T, Kurita T, Satomi K, Noda T, Okamura H, Shimizu W, Suyama K, Aihara N, Kobayashi J, Kamakura S. QRS prolongation is associated with high defibrillation thresholds during cardioverter-defibrillator implantations in patients with hypertrophic cardiomyopathy. Circ J. 2009;73:1028–32.

Nair CK, Aronow WS, Stokke K, Mohiuddin SM, Thomson W, Sketch MH. Cardiac conduction defects in patients older than 60 years with aortic stenosis with and without mitral anular calcium. Am J Cardiol. 1984;53:169–72.

Nesto RW, Kowalchuk GJ. The ischemic cascade: temporal sequence of hemodynamic, electrocardiographic and symptomatic expressions of ischemia. Am J Cardiol. 1987;59:23C–30.

Otto CM. Valvular aortic stenosis: disease severity and timing of intervention. J Am Coll Cardiol. 2006;47:2141–51.

Otto CM, Kuusisto J, Reichenbach DD, Gown AM, O'Brien KD. Characterization of the early lesion of 'degenerative' valvular aortic stenosis. Histological and immunohistochemical studies. Circulation. 1994;90:844–53.

Otto CM, Lind BK, Kitzman DW, Gersh BJ, Siscovick DS. Association of aortic-valve sclerosis with cardiovascular mortality and morbidity in the elderly. N Engl J Med. 1999;341:142–7.

Pellikka PA, Sarano ME, Nishimura RA, Malouf JF, Bailey KR, Scott CG, Barnes ME, Tajik AJ. Outcome of 622 adults with asymptomatic, hemodynamically significant aortic stenosis during prolonged follow-up. Circulation. 2005;111:3290–5.

Pichard AD, Gorlin R, Smith H, Ambrose J, Meller J. Coronary flow studies in patients with left ventricular hypertrophy of the hypertensive type. Evidence for an impaired coronary vascular reserve. Am J Cardiol. 1981;47:547–54.

Prineas RJ, Crowe RS, Blackburn H. The Minnesota code manual of electrocardiographic findings. Bristol: John Wright; 1982. p. 298.

Rajamannan NM, Evans FJ, Aikawa E, Grande-Allen KJ, Demer LL, Heistad DD, Simmons CA, Masters KS, Mathieu P, O'Brien KD, Schoen FJ, Towler DA, Yoganathan AP, Otto CM. Calcific aortic valve disease: not simply a degenerative process: a review and agenda for research from the National Heart and Lung and Blood Institute Aortic Stenosis Working Group. Executive summary: calcific aortic valve disease-2011 update. Circulation. 2011;124:1783–91.

Roberts-Thomson KC, Stevenson IH, Kistler PM, Haqqani HM, Goldblatt JC, Sanders P, Kalman JM. Anatomically determined functional conduction delay in the posterior left atrium relationship to structural heart disease. J Am Coll Cardiol. 2008;51:856–62.

Rowe GG, Castillo CA, Maxwell GM, Crumpton CW. A hemodynamic study of hypertension including observations on coronary blood flow. Ann Intern Med. 1961;54:405–12.

Simek CL, Feldman MD, Haber HL, Wu CC, Jayaweera AR, Kaul S. Relationship between left ventricular wall thickness and left atrial size: comparison with other measures of diastolic function. J Am Soc Echocardiogr. 1995;8:37–47.

Sorgato A, Faggiano P, Simoncelli U, Rusconi C. Prevalence of late potentials in adult aortic stenosis. Int J Cardiol. 1996;53:55–9.

Sorgato A, Faggiano P, Aurigemma GP, Rusconi C, Gaasch WH. Ventricular arrhythmias in adult aortic stenosis: prevalence, mechanisms, and clinical relevance. Chest. 1998;113:482–91.

Thiry PS, Rosenberg RM, Abbott JA. A mechanism for the electrocardiogram response to left ventricular hypertrophy and acute ischemia. Circ Res. 1975;36:92–104.

Tjang YS, van HY, Korfer R, Grobbee DE, van der Heijden GJ. Predictors of mortality after aortic valve replacement. Eur J Cardiothorac Surg. 2007;32:469–74.

Tomanek RJ, Palmer PJ, Peiffer GL, Schreiber KL, Eastham CL, Marcus ML. Morphometry of canine coronary arteries, arterioles, and capillaries during hypertension and left ventricular hypertrophy. Circ Res. 1986;58:38–46.

van den Heuvel AF, van Veldhuisen DJ, van der Wall EE, Blanksma PK, Siebelink HM, Vaalburg WM, van Gilst WH, Crijns HJ. Regional myocardial blood flow reserve impairment and metabolic changes suggesting myocardial ischemia in patients with idiopathic dilated cardiomyopathy. J Am Coll Cardiol. 2000;35:19–28.

Villari B, Hess OM, Moccetti D, Vassalli G, Krayenbuehl HP. Effect of progression of left ventricular hypertrophy on coronary artery dimensions in aortic valve disease. J Am Coll Cardiol. 1992;20:1073–9.

Wachtell K, Bella JN, Liebson PR, Gerdts E, Dahlof B, Aalto T, Roman MJ, Papademetriou V, Ibsen H, Rokkedal J, Devereux RB. Impact of different partition values on prevalences of left ventricular hypertrophy and concentric geometry in a large hypertensive population: the LIFE study. Hypertension. 2000; 35:6–12.

Wang NC, Maggioni AP, Konstam MA, Zannad F, Krasa HB, Burnett Jr JC, Grinfeld L, Swedberg K, Udelson JE, Cook T, Traver B, Zimmer C, Orlandi C, Gheorghiade M. Clinical implications of QRS duration in patients hospitalized with worsening heart failure and reduced left ventricular ejection fraction. JAMA. 2008;299:2656–66.

Wiegerinck RF, Verkerk AO, Belterman CN, van Veen TA, Baartscheer A, Opthof T, Wilders R, de Bakker JM, Coronel R. Larger cell size in rabbits with heart failure increases myocardial conduction velocity and QRS duration. Circulation. 2006;113:806–13.

6 Exercise Testing in Aortic Stenosis and in Mitral Regurgitation

Patrizio Lancellotti and Julien Magne

Introduction

The European Society of Cardiology (ESC) and the American College of Cardiology/American Heart Association (ACC/AHA) have placed renewed emphasis on the role of exercise testing to provide objective evidence of exercise capacity and symptom status in patients with valvular heart disease (Vahanian et al. 2007; Bonow et al. 2006). Exercise testing represents the first choice over pharmacological stress for risk stratification in asymptomatic patients with aortic stenosis (AS) or degenerative mitral regurgitation (MR) (Pierard and Lancellotti 2007; Picano et al. 2009). It has been shown to provide insights regarding exertional symptoms disproportionate to resting hemodynamics in patients with functional ischemic MR. When combined with echocardiography, although treadmill or bicycle may be used, supine bicycle exercise is the recommended technique in valvular heart diseases. Semi-supine exercise echocardiography offers the advantage that Doppler information, in addition to assessment of regional wall motion, can be evaluated during the different steps of the test (Rosca et al. 2011).

P. Lancellotti, M.D., Ph.D. (✉) • J. Magne, Ph.D.
Department of Cardiology, Heart Valve Clinic,
University Hospital Sart Tilman, University of Liège,
Liège, Belgium
e-mail: plancellotti@chu.ulg.ac.be

Exercise Testing: Protocols

A symptom-limited graded exercise test is recommended. At least 80% of the age-predicted heart rate should be reached in the absence of symptoms. The test is adapted to the clinical condition and should be performed under supervision. Treadmill exercise is the most commonly used test in UK and in US, while upright bicycle test is the preferred approach in the rest of Europe. It is performed according the ACC/AHA practice guidelines using a Bruce modified protocol (Gibbons et al. 1997). When combined with per-exercise imaging, the test is performed on a dedicated tilting exercise table. Classically, the initial workload of 25 W is maintained for 2 min and the workload is increased every 2 min by 25 W. An increase by 10 W seems to be more appropriate in old patients with AS or in subjects with secondary MR and heart failure symptoms. Blood pressure and a 12-lead electrocardiogram are recorded at rest and at each step of the test. The patient should be frequently questioned for symptoms. Exercise test is interrupted promptly when the target heart rate is reached or in case of typical chest pain, limiting breathlessness, dizziness, muscular exhaustion, hypotension (drop in systolic blood pressure ≥20 mmHg), or significant ventricular arrhythmia. To note, isolated abnormalities in the ST (>2 mm ST depression, horizontal or downsloping) segment is rarely a reason to stop the stress exam, especially in patients with AS or primary MR. The test is considered abnormal if the patient presented ≥1 of the following

N.M. Rajamannan (ed.), *Cardiac Valvular Medicine*,
DOI 10.1007/978-1-4471-4132-7_6, © Springer-Verlag London 2013

Table 6.1 Contra-indications to perform an exercise stress test in patients in valvular heart diseases

Truly symptomatic aortic stenosis
Physical or mental disability to adequately perform an exercise stress test
Clear indications for surgery, except in secondary mitral regurgitation
High blood pressure (systolic > 200 mmHg or diastolic > 110 mmHg)
Uncontrolled or symptomatic arrhythmias
Systemic illness

criteria: angina, evidence of dyspnea, dizziness, syncope or near-syncope, ≥2 mm ST segment depression in comparison to baseline levels, fall in blood pressure below baseline value and complex ventricular arrhythmias (ventricular tachycardia, more than four premature ventricular complexes in a row) (Lancellotti et al. 2008a). Contra-indications to exercise testing are listed in Table 6.1.

Exercise Echocardiography: Data Acquisition

Exercise echocardiography enables the assessment of various echocardiographic parameters related to the valve, the hemodynamic, and the left ventricle (LV) (Fig. 6.1). As some valve-related exercise changes are evanescent, peak exercise imaging is mandatory. Unless change in E/e'- an estimate of LV filling pressure- that is obtained at low level exercise (around 100 bpm), all others parameters should be obtained throughout the test. The kinetic of changes in aortic pressure gradients in AS and in transtricuspid pressure gradient in MR need to be assessed (Magne et al. 2011a; Lancellotti et al. 2009). A rapid increase in pressure gradients can indicate a more severe disease process. Worsening in wall motion from baseline classically indicates an ischemic insult. The absence of LV contractile reserve is characterized by a small change in LV ejection fraction or in long-axis function (derived from tissue Doppler imaging or 2D speckle tracking) (Lancellotti et al. 2008a, b, 2009; Magne et al. 2011a; Donal et al. 2011).

Asymptomatic Severe Aortic Stenosis

Indications

AS is a prevalent condition and a progressive disease (Lancellotti et al. 2010). When symptoms appear, usually after a long asymptomatic period, prompt surgical replacement of the aortic valve is warranted (Vahanian et al. 2007; Bonow et al. 2006). The risk of sudden death is very low in asymptomatic patients, even with severe AS (Monin et al. 2009). It may nevertheless occur soon after the onset of symptoms or if the waiting period for surgery is too long. Moreover, symptomatic status can be difficult to establish especially in elderly patients, who may ignore their symptoms or may reduce their level of physical activity to avoid or minimize symptoms. Thus, exercise testing could be useful to unmask symptoms in patients with severe AS who claim to be asymptomatic or who have equivocal symptoms. A recent meta-analysis confirmed that symptom-limited stress testing is safe and has an important prognostic value (Rafique et al. 2009). Exercise testing is strongly advocated in the ESC guidelines (Vahanian et al. 2007), whereas it is a class IIb recommendation in the ACC/AHA guidelines (Bonow et al. 2006). In AS, the clinical value of exercise echocardiography is still limited. It may however refine the risk stratification of asymptomatic AS patients. To note, exercise testing is contraindicated in truly symptomatic AS patients (Vahanian et al. 2007; Bonow et al. 2006).

Prognostic Value of Exercise Test

Changes in clinical and electrocardiographic parameters during treadmill exercise test have recently proved to influence the prognosis and subsequent clinical decision making in asymptomatic AS patients (Table 6.2). Approximately one third of patients who claim to be asymptomatic develop symptoms on exercise (Amato et al. 2001; Alborino et al. 2002; Das et al. 2005; Lancellotti et al. 2005a; Marechaux et al. 2007, 2010). The occurrence of exercise-limiting

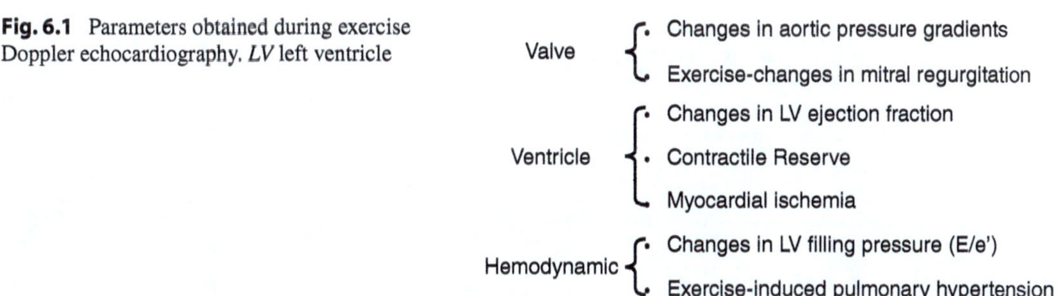

Fig. 6.1 Parameters obtained during exercise Doppler echocardiography. *LV* left ventricle

Table 6.2 Impact on outcomes and clinical decision making of exercise testing in patients with asymptomatic AS

			Impact on clinical decision (AVR)	
Stress data	Parameters	Impact on outcome	ESC guidelines	ACC/AHA guidelines
Clinical	Symptoms (dizziness, dyspnea at low workload, angina, syncope)	Onset of symptoms (Das et al. 2005), cardiac-related death, aortic valve replacement dictated by symptoms (Amato et al. 2001; Lancellotti et al. 2005a)	Class I (C)	Class IIb (C)
	Abnormal blood pressure response (fall in blood pressure)		Class IIa (C)	Class IIb (C)
Electrocardiographic	Ventricular arrhythmias	Onset of symptoms, cardiac-related death, aortic valve replacement dictated by symptoms (Amato et al. 2001; Alborino et al. 2002; Lancellotti et al. 2005a)	Class IIa	Class IIb
	ST depression (≥2 mm)		–	–
Echocardiographic	Increase in mean aortic pressure gradient: >18 mmHg (18) or 20 mmHg (19)	Spontaneous symptoms, cardiac-related death, aortic valve replacement dictated by symptoms (Lancellotti et al. 2005a; Marechaux et al. 2010), hospitalization for heart failure (Lancellotti et al. 2005a)	–	–
	Decrease (19)/smaller (20) increase in LV ejection fraction	Spontaneous symptoms, cardiac-related death (Marechaux et al. 2010), abnormal exercise test (Marechaux et al. 2007)	–	–

LV left ventricle

symptoms (dizziness, dyspnea at low workload, angina or syncope) predicts the rapid development of symptoms in daily life, cardiac death (including sudden death) and need for aortic valve replacement (Amato et al. 2001; Alborino et al. 2002; Das et al. 2005; Lancellotti et al. 2005a), particularly in patients <70 years and physically active (Das et al. 2005). Dizziness during a treadmill test has a higher positive predictive value for development of symptoms during the next year (Das et al. 2005). The occurrence of rapidly reversible dyspnea at high workloads (close to the age-gender predicted maximum workloads) is usually considered to be normal. Abnormal blood pressure response (<20 mmHg increase in systolic blood pressure) and ST-depression (>2 mm, horizontal or downsloping) during exercise do not seem to improve the accuracy of the test (Das et al. 2005).

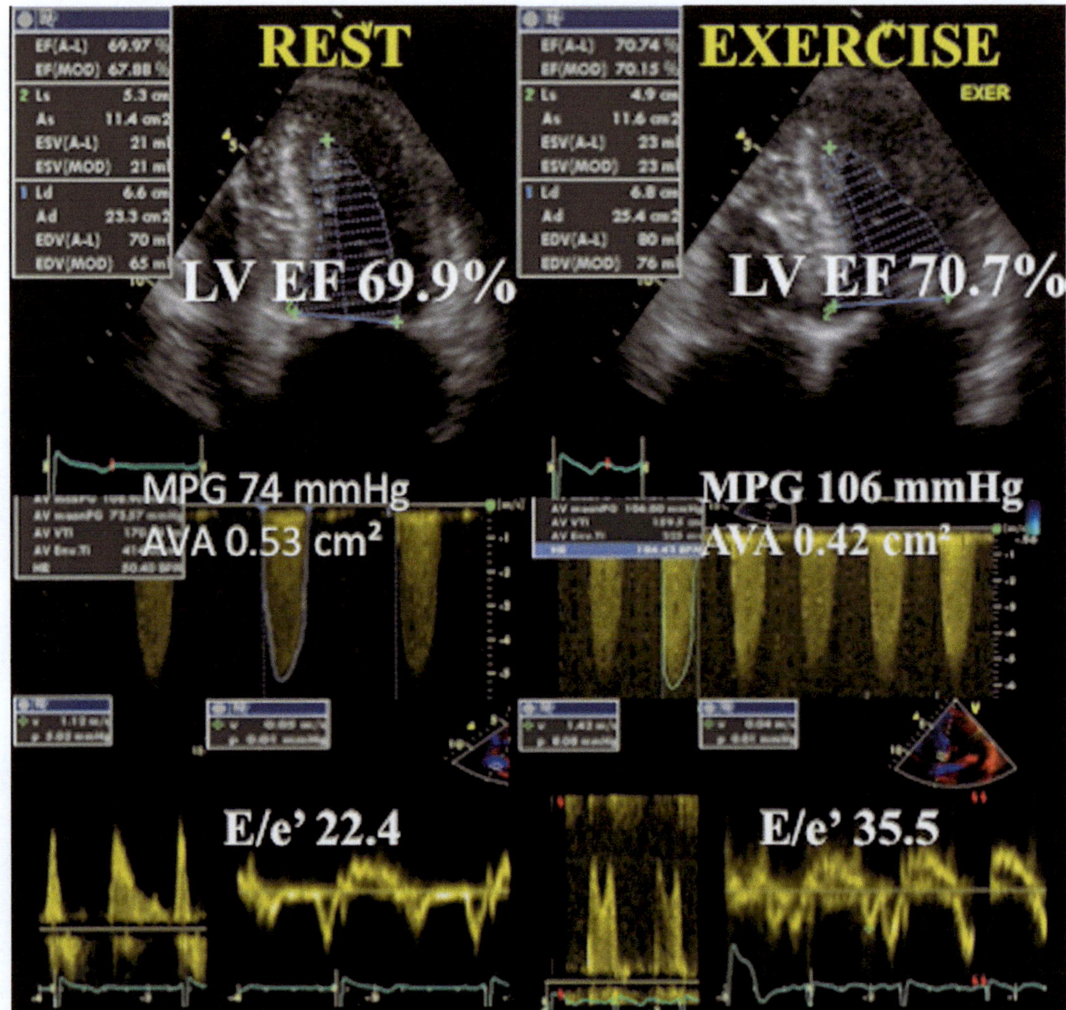

Fig. 6.2 Two dimensional echocardiography and Doppler findings in a patient with asymptomatic severe aortic stenosis, absence of contractile reserve and increase of trans-aortic pressure gradient with exercise. This patient has a fixed severe AS, with no increase in aortic valve area at exercise. *AVA* aortic valve area, *LVEF* left ventricular ejection fraction, *MPG* mean aortic pressure gradient

Clinical Value of Exercise Echocardiography

In asymptomatic moderate-severe AS (valve area <1.2 cm^2), exercise-induced changes in LV function or in AS indices are predictive of the outcome. Whatever the results of exercise test, an increase in mean aortic pressure gradient by ≥18–20 mmHg during exercise is associated with an increased risk of cardiac-related events (Lancellotti et al. 2005a; Marechaux et al. 2010). To note, the increase in pressure gradient reflects the presence of either a more severe AS (the more severe is the stenosis at rest, the higher is the increase in gradients for a given flow rate during exercise) or a non-compliant and rigid aortic valve (no or minimal enlargement of aortic valve orifice area during test) (Leurent et al. 2009) (Fig. 6.2). Patients with a decrease or a smaller increase in LV ejection fraction or in long-axis function (2D strain) during exercise are more likely to exhibit an abnormal response to exercise and cardiac-related events during follow-up (Lancellotti et al. 2005a, 2008a, b, 2009, 2010;

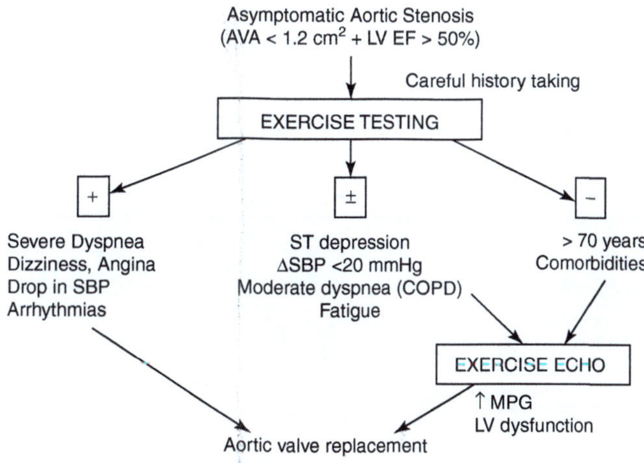

Fig. 6.3 Usefulness of exercise test in asymptomatic aortic stenosis. *AVA* aortic valve area, *COPD* chronic obstructive pulmonary disease, *LV* left ventricle, *MPG* mean aortic pressure gradient, *SBP* systolic blood pressure

Magne et al. 2011a; Donal et al. 2011; Monin et al. 2009; Rafique et al. 2009; Amato et al. 2001; Alborino et al. 2002; Das et al. 2005; Marechaux et al. 2007, 2010). Limiting symptoms on exercise testing relate in part to blunted changes in systolic blood pressure, which is the witness that peripheral demands (abnormal vascular adaptation) exceed the rise in cardiac output (substantial pump failure) (Lancellotti et al. 2008a, 2009; Laskey et al. 2009; Weisenberg et al. 2008). Increase in LV filling pressure –E/e′- also contributes to limited exercise capacity and symptoms in patients with severe AS (Dalsgaard et al. 2009).

Impact on Clinical Decision-Making

In asymptomatic severe AS, if the exercise test is abnormal, particularly if it shows symptom development or asymptomatic hypotension, aortic valve replacement represents a class IIbC indication in the ACC/AHA guidelines (Bonow et al. 2006). Conversely, in the ESC guidelines, surgery is highly recommended in physically active patients younger than 70 years old with exercise-induced symptoms (IC), is reasonable in patients with fall in systolic blood pressure below baseline value during test (IIaC), and may be considered in case of significant ventricular arrhythmia (Table 6.2) (Vahanian et al. 2007). Abnormal exercise Doppler echocardiography can also possibly favour early valve replacement. It might be useful in asymptomatic patients with moderate-severe AS and preserved LV ejection fraction to improve risk stratification. Both patients with inconclusive or negative exercise test but with comorbidities and over 70 years old might benefit from a comprehensive exercise echocardiographic evaluation (Fig. 6.3). More confirmatory data are needed to support incorporating this technique in the daily management of asymptomatic patients with AS.

Mitral Regurgitation

MR is the second most frequent valve disease in Europe after AS. Since the decline in the incidence of rheumatic valve disease over the past decades, its origin is nowadays predominantly degenerative (61%), followed by rheumatic (14%) and ischemic functional disease (7%) (Iung et al. 2003). However, the incidence of functional MR is expected to increase, due to the concomitant growing prevalence of obesity, metabolic disorders and coronary artery disease, and improvement in the treatment of acute myocardial infarction. According to its etiology and mechanism, MR can be classified as primary MR, resulting from valvular lesions (e.g. prolapse, flail or rheumatic disease), and secondary MR (i.e. ischemic and functional non-ischemic MR). The management and the prognosis of these two MR entities are considerably diverse. In this regard, the usefulness and the indications of exercise echocardiography should be exclusively studied.

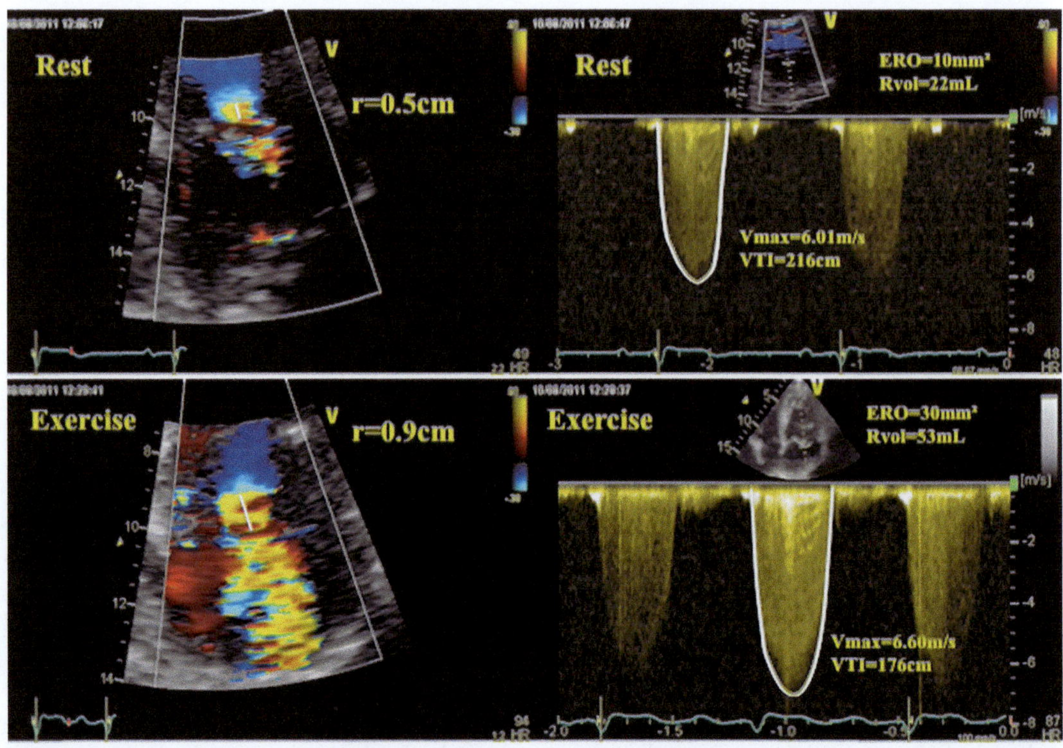

Fig. 6.4 Two dimensional echocardiography and Doppler findings in a patient with mild primary mitral regurgitation and developing moderate mitral regurgitation at peak exercise. *ERO* effective regurgitant orifice area, *Rvol* regurgitant volume, *Vmax* maximal velocity of regurgitant jet, *VTI* velocity-time integral

Asymptomatic Primary MR

Indications

The management of primary MR is currently one of the most controversial topic in the field of valvular heart diseases (Enriquez-Sarano and Sundt 2010; Gillam and Schwartz 2010). Both ACC/AHA and ESC class I indications for surgery in patients with primary MR are based on the presence of symptoms, the degree of LV dysfunction (LVEF < 60%) and/or the degree of LV dilatation (LV diameter ≥40 mm or >45 mm) (Vahanian et al. 2007; Bonow et al. 2006). The presences of atrial fibrillation (AF) and/or pulmonary hypertension (PHT) are considered as class IIa indications, with a level of evidence C. These recommendations result in two schools of thoughts opposing "early elective surgery", where the patients is referred to surgery regardless the presence of symptoms, LV dysfunction or dilation, AF or PHT, *vs.* "watchful waiting", suggesting to operate patients only when the criteria of the current guidelines are reached. The use of exercise echocardiography can potentially reconcile these approaches. Recent studies emphasized that primary MR can be dynamic and significantly increase during exercise (Fig. 6.4). More than 50% of patients with moderate MR can develop severe MR during exercise (Magne et al. 2011b) (Table 6.3). In addition, the exercise-induced increase in MR is well associated with the development of exercise PHT (Magne et al. 2010b). Performing an exercise Doppler echocardiography is a class IIa (ACC/AHA guidelines) recommendation in patients with asymptomatic severe MR to assess exercise capacity and the effect of exercise on pulmonary artery pressure (Bonow et al. 2006). Nevertheless, the ESC guidelines only recommend exercise echocardiography to evaluate LV contractile reserve. According to the guidelines and our own experience, exercise echocardiography in primary MR could be

Table 6.3 Impact on outcomes and clinical decision making of exercise testing in patients with asymptomatic primary MR

			Management	
Stress data	Parameters	Impact on outcome	ESC guidelines	ACC/AHA guidelines
Clinical	Exercise tolerance	Reduced cardiac event-free survival in patients with impaired functional capacity (Messika-Zeitoun et al. 2006)	–	Class IIa (C)
Echocardiographic	Increase in MR severity	Reduced symptom-free survival (Magne et al. 2010a, b) in primary MR	–	–
	Increase in systolic PAP	Reduced survival, survival-free of cardiac HF (Lancellotti et al. 2005a, b) in secondary MR	–	Class IIa (C)
	Absence of contractile reserve	Reduced cardiac-event-free survival (Magne et al. 2011b)	Recommended without specific level	–

MR mitral regurgitation, *HF* heart failure, *PAP* pulmonary arterial pressure

recommended (1) in asymptomatic patients with moderate or severe MR and no LV dysfunction or dilatation, (2) in patients with moderate or severe MR with no or mild symptoms and/or early signs of LV dysfunction (LVEF: 65–60%) or LV dilatation (LV end-systolic diameter: 40–45 mm), and (3) in patients with asymptomatic moderate or severe MR at high risk of developing exercise PHT (Magne et al. 2011a).

Prognostic Value of Exercise Test

The decision to submit an asymptomatic patient to an early mitral valve surgery should be adequately assessed prior to surgery and should be made in dedicated experienced centers. Exercise echocardiography may help to better stratify the global risk of patients with asymptomatic severe MR. Exercise tolerance itself is a marker of occurrence of symptoms and LV dysfunction in these patients (Supino et al. 2007). Surgery may also be considered in patients with exercise-induced systolic pulmonary arterial pressure >60 mmHg (Table 6.3) and a high likelihood of valve repair (ACC/AHA: class IIa). In asymptomatic MR, the development of exercise PHT is associated with threefold decrease in symptom-free survival. Exercise PHT was found to be more accurate than resting PHT to identify patients at high risk to more frequently and more rapidly develop symptoms during follow-up. Consistently, exercise-induced marked increase in MR (effective regurgitant orifice area >10 mm^2 or regurgitant volume >15 ml) is also a powerful marker of reduced symptom-free survival. At 2-year, only 30% of patients developing higher degree of MR during exercise remained asymptomatic (Magne et al. 2010a).

Clinical Value of Exercise Echocardiography

Although exercise test alone (i.e. without echocardiography) may help to identify a subset of patients with reduced functional capacity (<84% of maximal predicted VO_2) and thus with higher rate of cardiovascular events (Messika-Zeitoun et al. 2006), the use of exercise echocardiography may have several clinical implications. The evaluation of LV contractile reserve is recommended by the ESC guidelines (Table 6.2). Previous reports have demonstrated that patients with an exercise-induced increase in LVEF < 4% (Leung et al. 1996; Lee et al. 2005) can be considered as having no LV contractile reserve. These patients had high risk of postoperative LV dysfunction and poor outcome. More recently, limited exercise LV longitudinal contractile recruitment assessed by 2D speckle-tracking analysis and global longitudinal strain (GLS) has been shown to predict postoperative LV dysfunction in patients with primary MR (Lancellotti et al. 2008b). Assessed either with changes in LVEF or with changes in GLS, LV contractile reserve appears to be clinically useful (Table 6.2). Nevertheless, recent data showed around one third of discrepancies between the two methods (LVEF or GLS) in evaluating the presence of LV contractile reserve in asymptomatic patients (Magne et al. 2011b). Indeed, LV contractile reserve by GLS is correlated with BNP level and cardiovascular events, whereas changes in LVEF was neither associated with BNP nor with outcome. Consequently, the clinical value of LV contractile reserve is probably better when assessed using 2D speckle tracking and GLS.

Impact on Clinical Decision-Making

In the debate opposing "early surgery" *vs.* "watchful waiting", the use of exercise echocardiography may be very relevant in asymptomatic patients in order to identify those at higher risk of developing symptoms and cardiovascular events. Patients who exhibit exercise-induced marked increase in MR or exercise-induced PHT, and those without LV contractile reserve represent a subset of high-risk patients in whom prompt surgery, to prevent adverse LA remodeling, irreversible LV damage, and morbid events could potentially be indicated. Conversely, asymptomatic severe MR without any signs of LV dilation or dysfunction, showing LV longitudinal recruitment during exercise and no PHT could be safely follow-up.

Secondary MR

Indications

Secondary MR (i.e. functional ischemic or non-ischemic) resulting from a complex LV remodelling process is associated with a poor prognosis. Rarely, exercise-induced increase in MR occurs as a consequence of acute transient ischemia. This type of MR may be easily identified by exercise stress echocardiography and should indicate coronary angiography to demonstrate or exclude a significant coronary stenosis, on the right coronary or circumflex coronary artery. In chronic secondary MR, the mitral valve itself is usually normal and the imbalance between the LV closing and tethering forces, related to LV dysfunction, produces MR. Exercise echocardiography may reveal the dynamic component of secondary MR. In this regard, exercise echocardiography might be considered in four clinical settings (Pierard and Lancellotti 2007): (1) patients with LV dysfunction who present exertional dyspnoea out of the proportion of resting LV dysfunction and/or the degree of mitral regurgitation, (2) patients in whom acute pulmonary oedema occurs without an obvious causes (Pierard and Lancellotti 2004), (3) for stratifying the risk of mortality and heart failure in the individual patients, (4) before surgical revascularisation in patients with moderate MR (Pierard and Lancellotti 2007) and (5) after surgery, to explain abnormally elevated systolic pulmonary arterial pressure and sustained PHT (Magne et al. 2008; Kubota et al. 2006).

Prognostic Value of Exercise Test

In secondary MR, an effective regurgitant orifice area ≥20 mm^2 at rest should be considered as severe due to its impact on cardiac mortality (Grigioni et al. 2001). Similarly, an increase in effective regurgitant orifice area by ≥13 mm^2 (Table 6.2 and Fig. 6.5) during exercise is associated with poor outcome (Lancellotti et al. 2003a). Importantly, the extent of exercise-induced changes in MR is unrelated to resting MR severity (Lancellotti et al. 2003b). It has also been demonstrated that patients who develop acute pulmonary edema have a parallel increase in MR severity and in pulmonary arterial pressure at exercise compared to patients with similar LV dysfunction and no acute episode of pulmonary oedema (Magne et al. 2011b). In addition, some patients may have a decrease in MR during exercise, reflecting the presence of contractile recruitment of viable myocardium. This infrequent phenomenon is associated with a good prognosis (Lancellotti et al. 2003b).

Clinical Value of Exercise Echocardiography

Following myocardial infarction, patients with secondary MR have more severe LV dysfunction compared to those without associated MR, which may lead to greater mortality risk and greater risk of developing heart failure (Grigioni et al. 1999, 2001, 2005). The role of exercise echocardiography in secondary MR is to determine the extent of dysfunctional but viable hibernating myocardium. Dobutamine stress echocardiography is

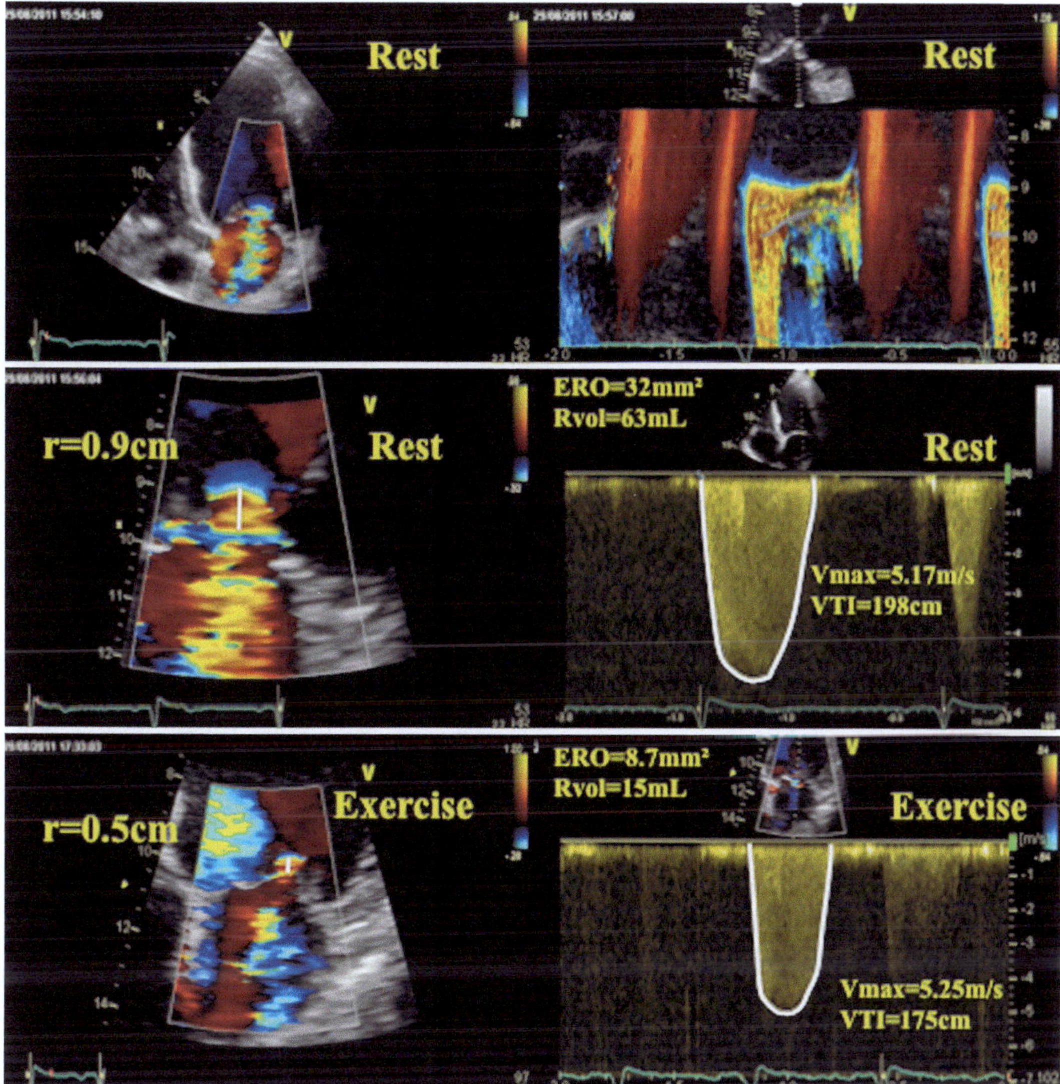

Fig. 6.5 Two dimensional echocardiography and Doppler findings in a patient with severe secondary mitral regurgitation following anterior myocardial infarction and developing mild-moderate mitral regurgitation at peak exercise. *ERO* effective regurgitant orifice area, *Rvol* regurgitant volume, *Vmax* maximal velocity of regurgitant jet, *VTI* velocity-time integral

very accurate to predict the likelihood of recovery of LV function and the extent of LV reverse remodeling following revascularization. Although changes in MR severity can be evaluated under dobutamine, its pharmacological effect on loading conditions is a major confounding variable. Importantly, due to the decrease in LV volume and in tethering forces, and also due to the increase in inotropy (resulting in improvement in closing forces), MR usually decreases during dobutamine test. Consequently, the dynamic component of secondary MR and its consequences are better evaluated with exercise echocardiography. The extent of the severity of secondary MR varies dynamically in accordance with changes LV regional wall motion, and annular size and the balance of tethering versus closing forces applied on the mitral leaflets. Hence, the severity of MR assessed by Doppler echocardiography at rest does not necessarily reflect the severity of MR that develops during exercise. Exercise stress echocardiography has been shown to unmask hemodynamically significant MR in patients with ischemic LV systolic dysfunction and only mild to moderate MR at rest, and in doing so to identify patients at higher risk for heart failure and death (Pierard and Lancellotti 2004; Lancellotti et al. 2003a).

Impact on Clinical Decision-Making

The management of patients with secondary MR is challenging (Levine and Schwammenthal 2005). Medical treatment of heart failure is mandatory. Cardiac resynchronization therapy has been shown to reduce ischemic MR both at rest and at exercise (Lancellotti et al. 2008c). The indications of combined surgery-coronary arterial bypass graft, combined with undersized mitral annuloplasty remain controversial. Ongoing trials on surgical treatment of moderate and severe ischemic MR will probably give a partial answer. Meanwhile, patients with significant increase in secondary MR during exercise (effective regurgitant orifice area ≥13 mm^2) should be considered as a subset at higher risk of poor outcome. In these patients, any effort targeting to improve the myocardial function, to reduce the LV remodelling and, in turn, to decrease the MR severity and its dynamic component should be performed. Furthermore, additional mitral valve repair or replacement (with chordal sparing) is probably beneficial. Conversely, patients with moderate MR at rest and only mild increase or with decrease in MR severity during exercise may be left without valve surgery. These recommendations need be validated in a large prospective trial.

References

Alborino D, Hoffmann JL, Fournet PC, Bloch A. Value of exercise testing to evaluate the indication for surgery in asymptomatic patients with valvular aortic stenosis. J Heart Valve Dis. 2002;11:204–9.

Amato MC, Moffa PJ, Werner KE, Ramires JA. Treatment decision in asymptomatic aortic valve stenosis: role of exercise testing. Heart. 2001;86:381–6.

Bonow RO, Carabello BA, Chatterjee K, et al. ACC/AHA 2006 guidelines for the management of patients with valvular heart disease: a report of the American College of Cardiology/American Heart Association Task Force on Practice Guidelines (writing Committee to Revise the 1998 guidelines for the management of patients with valvular heart disease) developed in collaboration with the Society of Cardiovascular Anesthesiologists endorsed by the Society for Cardiovascular Angiography and Interventions and the Society of Thoracic Surgeons. J Am Coll Cardiol. 2006;48:e1–148.

Dalsgaard M, Kjaergaard J, Pecini R, et al. Left ventricular filling pressure estimation at rest and during exercise in patients with severe aortic valve stenosis: comparison of echocardiographic and invasive measurements. J Am Soc Echocardiogr. 2009;22:343–9.

Das P, Rimington H, Chambers J. Exercise testing to stratify risk in aortic stenosis. Eur Heart J. 2005;26:1309–13.

Donal E, Thebault C, O'Connor K, et al. Impact of aortic stenosis on longitudinal myocardial deformation during exercise. Eur J Echocardiogr. 2011;12:235–41.

Enriquez-Sarano M, Sundt III TM. Early surgery is recommended for mitral regurgitation. Circulation. 2010;121:804–12.

Gibbons RJ, Balady GJ, Beasley JW. ACC/AHA Guidelines for Exercise Testing. A report of the American College of Cardiology/American Heart Association Task Force on Practice Guidelines (Committee on Exercise Testing). J Am Coll Cardiol. 1997;30:260–311.

Gillam LD, Schwartz A. Primum non nocere: the case for watchful waiting in asymptomatic "severe" degenerative mitral regurgitation. Circulation. 2010;121:813–21.

Grigioni F, Basmadjian A, Enriquez-Sarano M. Ischemic mitral regurgitation: impact on outcome and implications of quantitative measurements. Circulation. 1999;100:1–378.

Grigioni F, Enriquez-Sarano M, Zehr KJ, Bailey KR, Tajik AJ. Ischemic mitral regurgitation. Long-term outcome and prognostic implications with quantitative Doppler assessment. Circulation. 2001;103:1759–64.

Grigioni F, Detaint D, Avierinos JF, Scott C, Tajik J, Enriquez-Sarano M. Contribution of ischemic mitral regurgitation to congestive heart failure after myocardial infarction. J Am Coll Cardiol. 2005;45:260–7.

Iung B, Baron G, Butchart EG, et al. A prospective survey of patients with valvular heart disease in Europe: the Euro Heart Survey on Valvular Heart Disease. Eur Heart J. 2003;24(13):1231–43.

Kubota K, Otsuji Y, Ueno T. Functional mitral stenosis following surgical annuloplasty for ischemic mitral regurgitation [abstr]. J Am Coll Cardiol. 2006;47:279A–279-A.

Lancellotti P, Troisfontaines P, Toussaint AC, Pierard LA. Prognostic importance of exercise-induced changes in mitral regurgitation in patients with chronic ischemic left ventricular dysfunction. Circulation. 2003a;108:1713–7.

Lancellotti P, Lebrun F, Pierard LA. Determinants of exercise-induced changes in mitral regurgitation in patients with coronary artery disease and left ventricular dysfunction. J Am Coll Cardiol. 2003b;42:1921–8.

Lancellotti P, Lebois F, Simon M, Tombeux C, Chauvel C, Pierard LA. Prognostic importance of quantitative exercise Doppler echocardiography in asymptomatic valvular aortic stenosis. Circulation. 2005a;112:I377–82.

Lancellotti P, Gerard PL, Pierard LA. Long-term outcome of patients with heart failure and dynamic functional mitral regurgitation. Eur Heart J. 2005b;26:1528–32.

Lancellotti P, Karsera D, Tumminello G, Lebois F, Pierard LA. Determinants of an abnormal response to exercise in patients with asymptomatic valvular aortic stenosis. Eur J Echocardiogr. 2008a;9(3):338–43.

Lancellotti P, Cosyns B, Zacharakis D, et al. Importance of left ventricular longitudinal function and functional reserve in patients with degenerative mitral regurgitation: assessment by two-dimensional speckle tracking. J Am Soc Echocardiogr. 2008b;21:1331–6.

Lancellotti P, Marwick T, Pierard LA. How to manage ischaemic mitral regurgitation. Heart. 2008c;94:1497–502.

Lancellotti P, Moonen M, Garweg C, Pierard LA. Image. Afterload mismatch revealed by an exercise biphasic response in aortic stenosis. Arch Cardiovasc Dis. 2009;102:593–4.

Lancellotti P, Donal E, Magne J, et al. Risk stratification in asymptomatic moderate to severe aortic stenosis: the importance of the valvular, arterial and ventricular interplay. Heart. 2010;96:1364–71.

Laskey WK, Kussmaul III WG, Noordergraaf A. Systemic arterial response to exercise in patients with aortic valve stenosis. Circulation. 2009;119:996–1004.

Lee R, Haluska B, Leung DY, Case C, Mundy J, Marwick TH. Functional and prognostic implications of left ventricular contractile reserve in patients with asymptomatic severe mitral regurgitation. Heart. 2005;91:1407–12.

Leung D, Griffin B, Stewart W, Cosgrove D, Thomas J, Marwick T. Left Ventricular function after valve repair for chronic mitral regurgitation: predictive Value of preoperative assessment of contractile reserve by exercise echocardiography. J Am Coll Cardiol. 1996;28:1198–205.

Leurent G, Donal E, de Place C, et al. Argument for a Doppler echocardiography during exercise in assessing asymptomatic patients with severe aortic stenosis. Eur J Echocardiogr. 2009;10:69–73.

Levine RA, Schwammenthal E. Ischemic mitral regurgitation on the threshold of a solution: from paradoxes to unifying concepts. Circulation. 2005;112:745–58.

Magne J, Sénéchal M, Mathieu P, Dumesnil JG, Dagenais F, Pibarot P. Restrictive annuloplasty for ischemic mitral regurgitation may induce functional mitral stenosis. J Am Coll Cardiol. 2008;51:1692–701.

Magne J, Lancellotti P, Pierard LA. Exercise-induced changes in degenerative mitral regurgitation. J Am Coll Cardiol. 2010a;56:300–9.

Magne J, Lancellotti P, Pierard LA. Exercise pulmonary hypertension in asymptomatic degenerative mitral regurgitation. Circulation. 2010b;122:33–41.

Magne J, Lancellotti P, O'Connor K, Van de Heyning CM, Szymanski C, Pierard LA. Prediction of exercise pulmonary hypertension in asymptomatic degenerative mitral regurgitation. J Am Soc Echocardiogr. 2011a;24:1004–12.

Magne J, O'Connor K, Mahjoub H, et al. Evaluation and impact on outcome of left ventricular contractile reserve in asymptomatic degenerative mitral regurgitation. Eur Heart J. 2011b;32((Suppl)):170.

Marechaux S, Ennezat PV, LeJemtel TH, et al. Left ventricular response to exercise in aortic stenosis: an exercise echocardiographic study. Echocardiography. 2007;24:955–9.

Marechaux S, Hachicha Z, Bellouin A, et al. Usefulness of exercise-stress echocardiography for risk stratification of true asymptomatic patients with aortic valve stenosis. Eur Heart J. 2010;31:1390–7.

Messika-Zeitoun D, Johnson BD, Nkomo V, et al. Cardiopulmonary exercise testing determination of functional capacity in mitral regurgitation: physiologic and outcome implications. J Am Coll Cardiol. 2006;47:2521–7.

Monin JL, Lancellotti P, Monchi M, et al. Risk score for predicting outcome in patients with asymptomatic aortic stenosis. Circulation. 2009;120:69–75.

Picano E, Pibarot P, Lancellotti P, Monin JL, Bonow RO. The emerging role of exercise testing and stress echocardiography in valvular heart disease. J Am Coll Cardiol. 2009;54:2251–60.

Pierard LA, Lancellotti P. The role of ischemic mitral regurgitation in the pathogenesis of acute pulmonary edema. N Engl J Med. 2004;351:1627–34.

Pierard LA, Lancellotti P. Stress testing in valve disease. Heart. 2007;93:766–72.

Rafique AM, Biner S, Ray I, Forrester JS, Tolstrup K, Siegel RJ. Meta-analysis of prognostic value of stress testing in patients with asymptomatic severe aortic stenosis. Am J Cardiol. 2009;104:972–7.

Rosca M, Lancellotti P, Magne J, Pierard LA. Stress testing in valvular heart disease: clinical benefit of echocardiographic imaging. Expert Rev Cardiovasc Ther. 2011;9:81–92.

Supino PG, Borer JS, Schuleri K, et al. Prognostic value of exercise tolerance testing in asymptomatic chronic nonischemic mitral regurgitation. Am J Cardiol. 2007;100:1274–81.

Vahanian A, Baumgartner H, Bax J, et al. Guidelines on the management of valvular heart disease: The Task Force on the Management of Valvular Heart Disease of the European Society of Cardiology. Eur Heart J. 2007;28:230–68.

Weisenberg D, Shapira Y, Vaturi M, et al. Does exercise echocardiography have an added value over exercise testing alone in asymptomatic patients with severe aortic stenosis? J Heart Valve Dis. 2008;17:376–80.

Detection of Calcium in the Aortic Valve by Non-invasive Imaging

7

Antonia Delgado Montero, Alexandra Gonçalves, Nalini M. Rajamannan, and José Luis Zamorano

Introduction

The development and adaptation of previous and novel non-invasive image techniques are making possible a complete evaluation of the aortic valve (AV) as well as the study of the origin and progression of its disease from different points of view: molecular, anatomical, functional (Aikawa and Otto 2012). Calcium early detection and quantification plays a significant role in the study of calcified aortic valve disease (CAVD), as it has shown relation with the aortic valve disease development, grade of severity and progression. In patients with mild to moderate aortic stenosis (AS), moderate to severe aortic valve calcification has a significantly faster hemodynamic AS progression rate compared to patients with only mild or no aortic valve calcification (Rosenhek et al. 2000). Its presence is a predictor of worse clinical outcome, it is related to the severity of possible concomitant coronary atherosclerosis disease (CAD) (Otto et al. 1999); and finally it is a potential target to evaluate medical treatment efficacy (Rajamannan et al. 2011). These facts have been measured in a few studies in which different methods were employed to assess aortic calcification, often without a reference test to quantify the extent of aortic valve calcification (Rosenhek et al. 2000).

Echocardiography

Echocardiography is the actual clinical standard for CAVD study, giving us a reliable anatomical and functional description. By means of 2-Dimension imaging and Doppler, it allows us to estimate the valve fibrosis and calcium, the leaflet anatomy and mobility and the severity of the disease, as well as associated alterations in left ventricle and aorta. We can detect different stages from the calcific valve disease process, from AV sclerosis to the different grades of AV stenosis. AV sclerosis is defined by focal areas of valve thickening, typically located in the leaflet center with commissural sparing and normal leaflet mobility, without significant obstruction to left ventricular outflow, with an aortic velocity <2.5 m/s (Freeman and Otto 2005). AV stenosis implies obstruction to outflow, and its grades (mild, moderate and severe) are based on the

A. Delgado Montero, M.D. (✉)
J.L. Zamorano, M.D., Ph.D., FESC
Cardiology Department,
University Hospital Ramón y Cajal, Madrid, Spain
e-mail: antudm458@yahoo.es

A. Gonçalves, M.D.
Cardiology Department,
University Hospital Ramón y Cajal, Madrid, Spain

Hospital S. João/University of Porto Medical School,
Porto, Portugal

N.M. Rajamannan, M.D.
Department of Molecular Biology and Biochemistry,
Mayo Clinic, 200 First St SW, Rochester,
55905 MN, USA

Department of Aerospace Engineering,
University of Notre Dame, South Bend, IN, USA

N.M. Rajamannan (ed.), *Cardiac Valvular Medicine*,
DOI 10.1007/978-1-4471-4132-7_7, © Springer-Verlag London 2013

echocardiographic estimation of aortic valve area by continuity equation, mean pressure gradient, and aortic jet velocity (Baumgartner et al. 2009).

The severity of valve calcification can be graded semi-quantitatively, as mild (few areas of dense echogenicity with little acoustic shadowing), moderate, or severe (extensive thickening and increased echogenicity with a prominent acoustic shadow). The degree and extent of valve calcification by echo is an independent predictor of clinical outcome. Patients with no or mild valvular calcification have higher rates of event-free survival compared to those with moderate or severe calcification (Rosenhek et al. 2000).

Echocardiography is the most widely used image method, easily available, highly reproducible, cost effective, and safe for the patient. However, it has some important disadvantages as its high interobserver variability, bad image quality when poor acoustic window, and poor sensibility and resolution in detecting early stages in the CAVD. It is limited with regard of quantification of valve calcification, since it uses indirect signs, such as increased echogenicity and thickening of the aortic leaflets; with a modest correlation with calcium detection by CT (Otto et al. 1999).

CT

Aortic valve disease can be assessed with current Multislice (or Multirow Detector) or Electron Beam (also known as ultrafast) Computer Tomography (MDCT or EBCT) technology. Initially evaluated for noninvasive coronary angiography, as well as for detection and quantification of calcified and noncalcified coronary plaques; this technique has been adapted for aortic valve characterization.

CT is a rapid, noninvasive, sensitive, reproducible and accurate method with which anatomy study of the aortic valve can be assessed: number of leaflets, pattern and quantity of calcification, presence of vegetations or abcesses, relation with the coronary arteries. This information will be useful for determining the etiology of the AS, for planning a surgical replacement and for assessment of a validated valve orifice area in AS by planimetry (Willmann et al. 2002).

The quantification of aortic valve calcium (AVC) score is made with a simple protocol, there is no need of medication or contrast, and the level of radiation is relatively low (about 2 mSv). It can be performed in the absence of ECG gating. To analize the images, there are different protocolized quantifying systems, either the Agatston or volumetric scoring methods, used in a similar manner to that used for coronary artery calcium scoring (Agatston et al. 1990; Callister et al. 1998). Further evaluation of aortic valve and coronary arteries will involve the use of iodinated contrast agent and a retrospective or prospective enhanced ECG-gated protocol, with image reconstruction to obtain multidetector CT images of the aortic valve during systole or the coronary arteries lumen in diastole. The level of radiation in this case will vary depending on the technique between 6 and 13 mSv (Feuchtner et al. 2006).

Different clinical studies have shown the reproducibility and accuracy of AVC score by CT (Kizer et al. 2001; Budoff et al. 2002, 2006). The MESA study (Multi-Ethnic Study of Atherosclerosis), conducted since year 2000, has assessed the interreader, intrareader and interscan variability of CT measurements of AVC in 99 patients randomly selected from the total cohort (4–5%, 13.8% and 8% respectively). This study is investigating the prevalence, prognostic value, and progression of subclinical cardiovascular disease in a population-based sample of 6,814 men and women aged 45–84 years. AVC is one of the measurements evaluated, using the same method as for coronary calcification. A total calcium score was assessed in every patient, determined by summing the Agatston and volume scores of all individual lesions.

The high reproducibility in AVC measurement by cardiac CT will allow serial measurements for detecting changes over time. The importance of this study lies in the valuable information that we will adquire regarding the relationship between AVC with known and suspected risk factors, and the prognostic potential of AVC in predicting subsequent cardiovascular events, independently of other cardiovascular risk factors and calcified coronary plaque (Katz et al. 2006).

CT can directly and quantificably measure the AVC load or weight, which can be used as a derivate of AS presence, severity and progression of AS (Kizer et al. 2001). A calcium score >1,650 Agatson Units (AU) is indicative of severe AS with a sensitivity and specificity ≥80% (Cueff et al. 2011). AVC score measured by CT has also shown AVC relationship with bicuspid aortic valve (BAV); these patients are more likely to have severe calcification, which develops at an earlier age than tricuspid AV and is linked to aortic stenosis (Hope et al. 2011).

These findings have significant clinical implications: patients who incidentally are found to have calcified AV in a chest CT done for any reason, specially if they are young, should undergo further image tests to assess the aortic valve. CT has already been used to evaluate the effect of medical treatment on AS hemodynamic progression and outcome.

Multi-detector CT has also gained prominence during the last years as an important imaging method in Transcatheter Aortic Valvular Replacement procedure, complementary to echo. CT allows correct patient screening with 3-Dimensional measurements from the aortic root and valve annulus anatomy, root orientation and iliofemoral access. Additionally, it provides a useful tool for follow-up. AV calcification is being evaluated as a possible predictor for procedural complications and bad outcome in TAVR (Leipsic et al. 2011).

The main advantage of AVC measurement by CT is that it is not influenced by the hemodynamic conditions and it is thus particularly useful in presence of low LV outflow status. It provides useful information in cases of bad echocardiographic acoustic window. The disadvantage of CT calcium scoring is exposure to ionizing radiation (1–3 mSv per exam), which limits serial short-time interval follow-up. This radiation risk is however a less important issue in the elderly patients who represent an important proportion of the AS population (Cueff et al. 2011). Furthermore, the use of contrast agent must be taken into account in case of using enhanced techniques, especially in old people with a high prevalence of poor renal function. CT accuracy lies in high sensibility of detecting established calcium in the valve, but it still lacks for detecting very early deposit.

Cardiac MR

Cardiac magnetic resonance imaging is an accurate radiation free diagnostic method with a high sensitivity in measurement of AV area, although its ability to detect calcium (specially in small quantity) on the aortic valves is limited. Its high resolution allows visualization of detailed cardiac anatomy as well as functional studies such as flow measurement, ejection fraction, volume quantification and viability (late enhancement) (John et al. 2003). Recent techniques like Steady-State Free Precession (SSFP) make possible excellent direct measurement of AV area by planimetry. Despite its accuracy, MR is still an expensive technique with low availability, and is limited in patients with metallic devices, arrhythmia or claustrophobia.

PET

There is a more novel technic recently incorporated in AV disease assessment: positron emission tomography (PET), which has allowed to a better understanding of CAVD pathophisiology. This technic is based in the detection of gamma rays emitted by a positron-emitting isotope of natural elements (radiotracer). These tracers reach the body on biologically active molecules like glucose-analogues, which are used as metabolic substrates. The concentration of tracer imaged gives tissue metabolic activity, in terms of regional glucose uptake.

Currently, PET together with CT has been used to image the AV using two specific radiotracers, 18F-FDG (18F-fluorodeoxyglucose, a glucose analogue) and 18F-NaF (18F-sodium fluoride, a marker of active tissue calcification), which target inflammation and calcification respectively.

FDG uptake is increased in patients with mild or moderate AS, but not in severe cases of AS; in these first stages its signal level is associated with the degree of calcification. It has also been observed an increased tracer signal in patients with faster progression of AV disease. These findings support the concept of AS as an active inflammatory condition (Marincheva-Savcheva

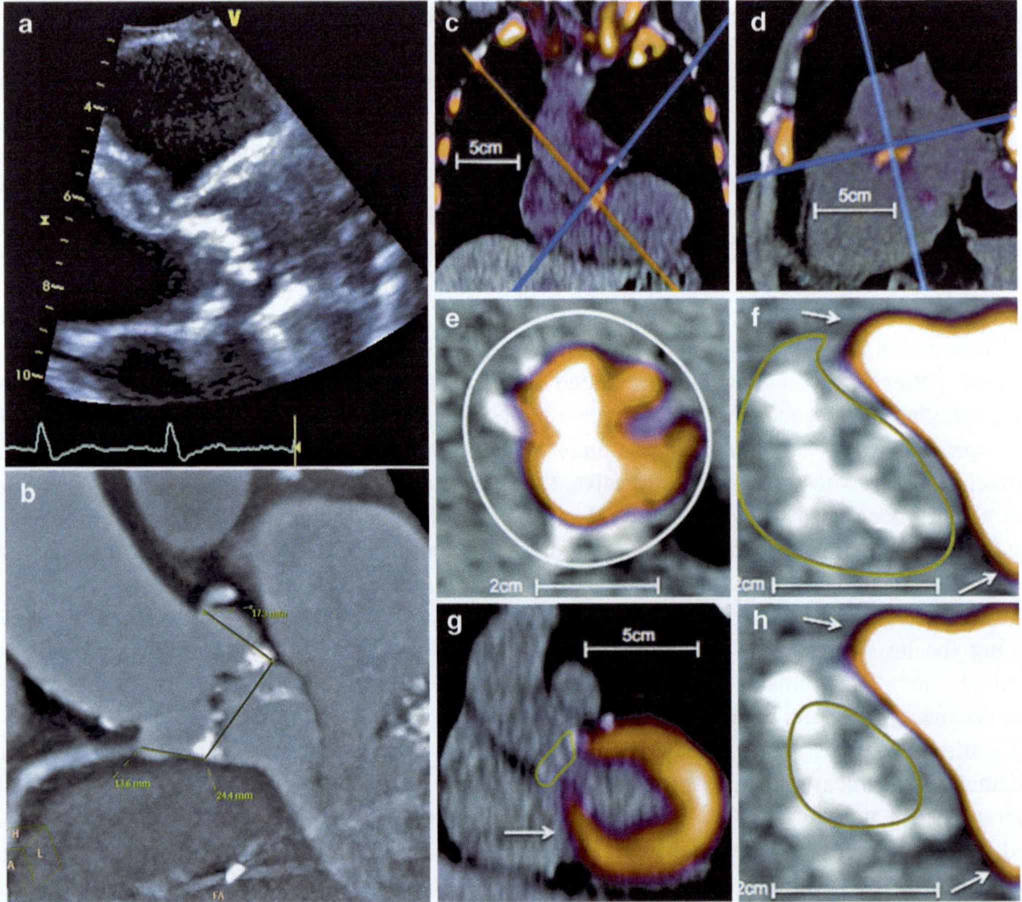

Fig. 7.1 (**a**) 2D Echo demonstrating calcification in the aortic valve, long axis parasternal view, (**b**) CT demonstrating calcification in the aortic valve, long axis view, (**c–h**) PET imaging, modified with permission demonstrating calcification by PET imaging (Budoff et al. 2006)

et al. 2011). Subsequent research studies have used both tracers related to inflammation and calcification, showing calcification as the predominant process affecting the valve in the later stages of the disease (Dweck et al. 2012). Figure 7.1 demonstrates and example of echo, CT and PET scanning to image calcification in the aortic valve.

These first studies have shown an excellent inter and intraobserver agreement, although more studies are needed to confirm and validate these results. The potential benefits of these radiotracers are its function as local biomarkers of disease activity, as well as predictors of disease progression. So far, PET is the highest sensible method for AVC measurement, as it detects the early molecular activity. This novel technique is being developed as a research tool, with no current use in clinical practice.

Summary

There is a high variation in the AVC detection sensitivity and current availability of the different non-invasive image techniques, with continuous improvements and developments. Recent studies have used molecular imaging techniques to evaluate the mecanism of calcification (New and Aikawa 2011). There will be future exciting studies in this field, with the aim of developing high-resolution and high-sensitivity imaging modalities that will allow us to understand and monitor the process of AVD from its origin. This way we will be able of confronting the disease with appropriate treatment.

References

Agatston AS, Janowitz WR, Hildner FJ, Zusmer NR, Viamonte Jr M, Detrano R. Quantification of coronary artery calcium using ultrafast computed tomography. J Am Coll Cardiol. 1990;15(4):827–32.

Aikawa E, Otto CM. Look more closely at the valve: imaging calcific aortic valve disease. Circulation. 2012;125(1):76–86.

Baumgartner H, Hung J, Bermejo J, Chambers JB, Evangelista A, Griffin BP, Iung B, Otto CM, Pellikka PA, Quiñones M. Echocardiographic assessment of valve stenosis: EAE/ASE recommendations for clinical practice. J Am Soc Echocardiogr. 2009;22(1):1–23.

Budoff MJ, Mao S, Takasu J, Shavelle DM, Zhao XQ, O'Brien KD. Reproducibility of electron-beam CT measures of aortic valve calcification. Acad Radiol. 2002;9(10):1122–7.

Budoff MJ, Takasu J, Katz R, Mao S, Shavelle DM, O'Brien KD, Blumenthal RS, Carr JJ, Kronmal R. Reproducibility of CT measurements of aortic valve calcification, mitral annulus calcification, and aortic wall calcification in the multi-ethnic study of atherosclerosis. Acad Radiol. 2006;13(2):166–72.

Callister TQ, Cooil B, Raya SP, Lippolis NJ, Russo DJ, Raggi P. Coronary artery disease: improved reproducibility of calcium scoring with an electron-beam CT volumetric method. Radiology. 1998;208:807–14.

Cueff C, Serfaty JM, Cimadevilla C, Laissy JP, Himbert D, Tubach F, Duval X, Iung B, Enriquez-Sarano M, Vahanian A, Messika-Zeitoun D. Measurement of aortic valve calcification using multislice computed tomography: correlation with haemodynamic severity of aortic stenosis and clinical implication for patients with low ejection fraction. Heart. 2011;97(9):721–6.

Dweck MR, Jones C, Joshi NV, Fletcher AM, Richardson H, White A, Marsden M, Pessotto R, Clark JC, Wallace WA, Salter DM, McKillop G, van Beek EJ, Boon NA, Rudd JH, Newby DE. Assessment of valvular calcification and inflammation by positron emission tomography in patients with aortic stenosis. Circulation. 2012;125(1):76–86.

Feuchtner GM, Dichtl W, Friedrich GJ, Frick M, Alber H, Schachner T, Bonatti J, Mallouhi A, Frede T, Pachinger O, Neddenzur D, Müller S. Multislice computed tomography for detection of patients with aortic valve stenosis and cuantification of severity. J Am Coll Cardiol. 2006;47(7):1410–7.

Freeman RV, Otto CM. Spectrum of calcific aortic valve disease: pathogenesis, disease progression, and treatment strategies. Circulation. 2005;111:3316–26.

Hope MD, Urbania TH, Yu JP, Chitsaz S, Tseng E. Incidental aortic valve calcification on CT scans significance for bicuspid and tricuspid valve disease. Acad Radiol. 2011;19(5):542–7.

John AS, Dill T, Brandt RR, Rau M, Ricken W, Bachmann G, Hamm CW. Magnetic resonance to assess the aortic valve area in aortic stenosis: how does it compare to current diagnostic standards? J Am Coll Cardiol. 2003;42:519–26.

Katz R, Wong ND, Kronmal R, Takasu J, Shavelle DM, Probstfield JL, Bertoni AG, Budoff MJ, O'Brien KD. Features of the metabolic syndrome and diabetes mellitus as predictors of aortic valve calcification in the multi-ethnic study of atherosclerosis. Circulation. 2006;113(17):2113–9.

Kizer JR, Gefter WB, de Lemos AS, Scoll BJ, Wolfe ML, Mohler ER. Electron beam computed tomography for the quantification of aortic valvular calcification. J Heart Valve Dis. 2001;10(3):361–6.

Leipsic J, Gurvitch R, Labounty TM, Min JK, Wood D, Johnson M, Ajlan AM, Wijesinghe N, Webb JG. Multidetector computed tomography in transcatheter aortic valve implantation. JACC Cardiovasc Imaging. 2011;4(4):416–29.

Marincheva Savcheva G, Subramanian S, Qadir S, Figueroa A, Truong Q, Vijayakumar J, Brady TJ, Hoffmann U, Tawakol A. Imaging of the aortic valve using fluorodeoxyglucose positron emission tomography increased valvular fluorodeoxyglucose uptake in aortic stenosis. J Am Coll Cardiol. 2011;57(25):2507–15.

New SE, Aikawa E. Molecular imaging insights into early inflammatory stages of arterial and aortic valve calcification. Circ Res. 2011;108:1381–91.

Otto CM, Lind BK, Kitzman DW, Gersh BJ, Siscovick DS. Association of aortic-valve sclerosis with cardiovascular mortality and morbidity in the elderly. N Engl J Med. 1999;341(3):142–7.

Rajamannan NM, Evans FJ, Aikawa E, Grande-Allen KJ, Demer LL, Heistad DD, Simmons CA, Masters KS, Mathieu P, O'Brien KD, Schoen FJ, Towler DA, Yoganathan AP, Otto CM. Calcific aortic valve disease: not simply a degenerative process. Circulation. 2011,124:1783–91.

Rosenhek R, Binder T, Porenta G, Lang I, Christ G, Schemper M, Maurer G, Baumgartner H. Predictors of outcome in severe, asymptomatic aortic stenosis. N Engl J Med. 2000;343(9):611–7.

Willmann JK, Weishaupt D, Lachat M, Kobza R, Roos JE, Seifert B, Lüscher TF, Marincek B, Hilfiker PR. Electrocardiographically gated multi-detector row CT for assessment of valvular morphology and calcification in aortic stenosis. Radiology. 2002;225(1):120–8.

Assessment of Aortic Stenosis Severity: Determining Timing to Surgery

8

Philippe Pibarot and Jean G. Dumesnil

Introduction

"Degenerative" or calcific aortic stenosis (AS) is a complex, multi-faceted, and systemic disease that may not be solely limited to the aortic valve but may also include reduced arterial compliance as well as alterations of LV geometry and function. This particular nature of the disease underlines the need for a more comprehensive assessment of AS severity going beyond the simple measurement of the conventional parameters of stenosis severity (i.e. peak aortic jet velocity, pressure gradients, valve effective orifice area) or LV function (i.e. LVEF). The present chapter thus proposes to review newer concepts to quantify the disease severity taking into account the interrelation between the different valvular, arterial, and ventricular variables that may be responsible for the appearance of symptoms or poorer prognosis in patients with AS.

Until recently the etiology of calcific aortic stenosis (AS), which is by far the most prevalent form of aortic valve disease, was thought to be degenerative as a result of wear and tear of the valve due to aging. There is now compelling epidemiological and histo-pathological data suggesting that "degenerative" calcific AS is, in fact, an active and multi-faceted disease that involves atherosclerotic- like processes (Rajamannan et al. 2007). In this context, it is thus not surprising that many patients with this disease also have manifestations of these pathologic processes in other target organs. In particular, a large proportion of patients with AS also present with concomitant systolic hypertension, which is related to increased rigidity of the arterial wall; as well, these patients may also have alterations of LV function which might not only be due to AS but also to concomitant hypertension or coronary artery disease and in varying proportions depending on the severity of each entity (Briand et al. 2005). In this context, it should be emphasized that the pathophysiology of adverse outcomes in AS is essentially due to an imbalance between the increase in LV hemodynamic load due to the valvular obstruction and/or concomitant arterial hypertension, and the capacity of the left ventricle to overcome this increase in load both at rest and during exercise. The present chapter thus proposes to review approaches to optimize the quantification of disease severity taking into account the inter-relation between the different valvular, arterial, and ventricular variables that may be responsible for the appearance of symptoms or poorer prognosis in patients with AS.

P. Pibarot, DVM, Ph.D. (✉)
Department of Medicine, Laval University, Quebec, QC, Canada

Canadian Institutes of Health research, Ottawa, Canada
e-mail: Philippe.pibarot@med.ulaval.ca

J.G. Dumesnil, M.D., FRCP(C)
Department of Medicine, Laval University, Quebec, QC, Canada

N.M. Rajamannan (ed.), *Cardiac Valvular Medicine*,
DOI 10.1007/978-1-4471-4132-7_8, © Springer-Verlag London 2013

Assessment of the Aortic Valve

Conventional Parameters of Stenosis Severity

The ACC/AHA and ESC guidelines generally recommend aortic valve replacement (AVR) in patients with severe AS who have symptoms, LV systolic dysfunction, and/or undergo coronary artery bypass graft surgery or other heart surgery (Fig. 8.1) (Bonow et al. 2006; Vahanian et al. 2007). Hemodynamic severity of AS is generally described by three basic parameters: peak aortic jet velocity, mean transvalvular pressure gradient, and aortic valve area (AVA). Peak aortic jet velocity is recorded with continuous wave Doppler from the window yielding the highest velocity signal, and obtaining a parallel intercept angle between the direction of blood flow and the ultrasound beam (Fig. 8.2). The ACC/AHA and ESC guidelines propose a peak aortic jet velocity >4.0 m/s, a mean gradient >40 mmHg and an AVA < 1.0 cm² as the criteria to be utilized to identify severe AS (Fig. 8.1 and Table 8.1) (Bonow et al. 2006; Vahanian et al. 2007). These guidelines have important inconsistencies which are critical for the management of AS: (i) The criteria used to define severe AS are derived from outcome studies based on catheterization data; yet the guidelines make no distinction between echo and catheterization data although, due to pressure recovery (see below and Chap. 1), gradients will always tend to be higher and AVA lower by echo than by catheterization. (ii) The severity criteria are inherently inconsistent with one another (Carabello 2002; Minners et al. 2008). In a patient with normal transvalvular flow rate, the mean gradient that theoretically corresponds to an AVA value of 1.0 cm² is closer to

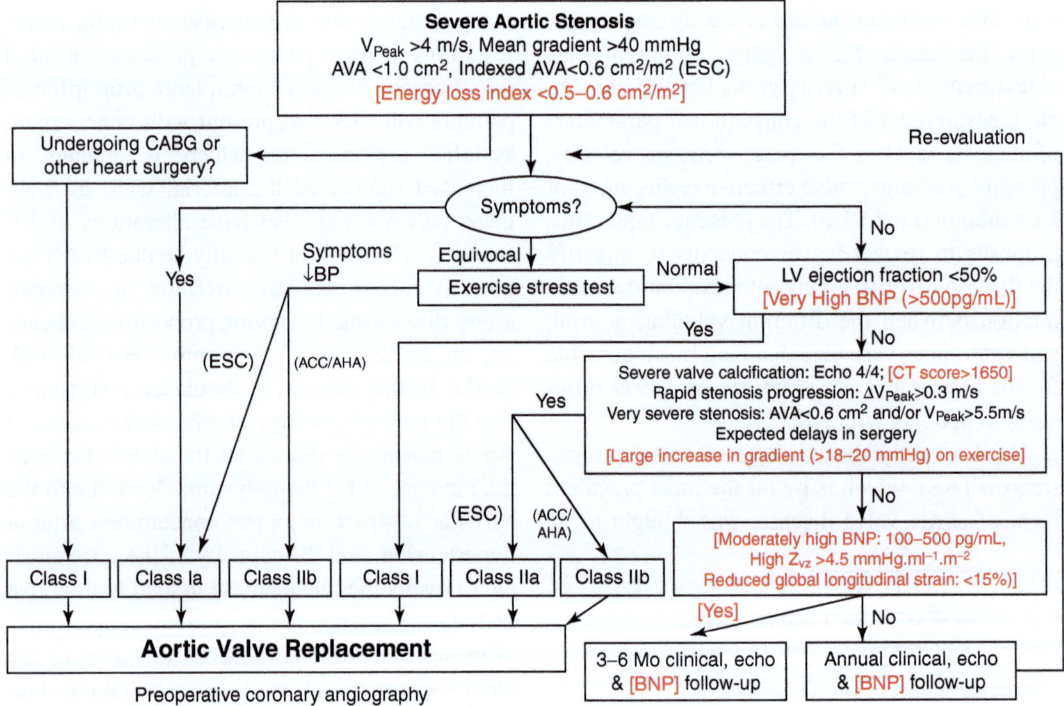

Fig. 8.1 Algorithm for the management of patients with aortic stenosis. This figure shows the algorithm for the management of severe AS. The text in *black* refers to the recommendations proposed in the ACC/AHA and ESC guidelines whereas the text in *red* and between [] represents the new emerging parameters that may eventually contribute improving the assessment and management of AS. However, these new parameters will need to be further validated in future studies. *AVA* aortic valve effective orifice area, *BP* blood pressure, V_{Peak} peak aortic jet velocity (Adapted with permission from (Pibarot and Dumesnil 2012a))

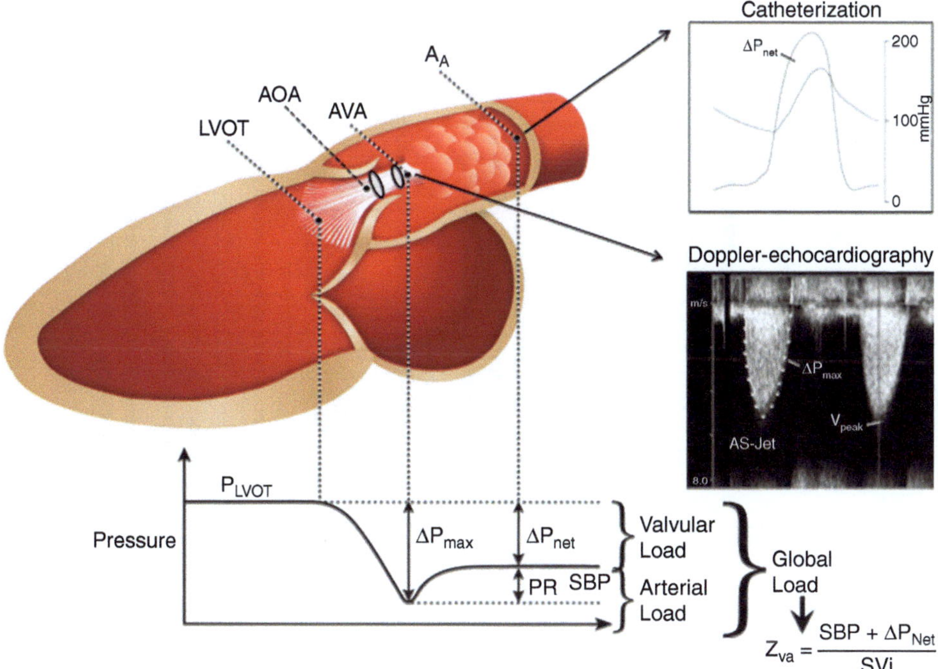

Fig. 8.2 Blood flow and pressure across the LV outflow tract, aortic valve, and ascending aorta during systole. When the blood flow contracts to pass through a stenotic orifice, a portion of the potential energy of the blood, i.e. pressure, is converted into kinetic energy, i.e. velocity, thus resulting in a pressure drop and acceleration of flow. Downstream of the vena contracta, a large part of the kinetic energy is irreversibly dissipated as heat because of flow turbulences. The remaining portion of the kinetic energy that is reconverted back to potential energy is called the "pressure recovery" (PR). The global hemodynamic load imposed on the LV results from the summation of the valvular load and the arterial load. This global load can be estimated by calculating the valvulo-arterial impedance. In patients with medium or large size ascending aorta, the impedance can be calculated with the standard Doppler mean gradient in place of the net mean gradient. *AOA* anatomic valve orifice area, *AVA* aortic valve effective orifice area, i.e. the cross-sectional area of the vena contracta of the transvalvular flow jet, A_A cross-sectional area of the aorta at the level of the sino-tubular junction, *LVOT* LV outflow tract, P_{LVOT} pressure in the LV outflow tract, V_{peak} peak aortic jet velocity, ΔP_{max} maximum transvalvular pressure gradient recorded at the level of vena contracta (i.e. mean gradient measured by Doppler), ΔP_{net} net transvalvular pressure gradient recorded after pressure recovery (i.e. mean gradient measured by catheterization), *SBP* systolic blood pressure, *SVi* stroke volume index, Z_{va} valvulo-arterial impedance (Reproduced with permission from Pibarot and Dumesnil (2012a))

30–35 mmHg rather than to the 40 mmHg cut-off value of proposed in the guidelines (Bonow et al. 2006; Vahanian et al. 2007). Chapter 1 provides results from metanalysis to show the variability in the techniques. Studies have suggested to lower down the cut-off value of AVA for severe AS from 1.0 to 0.8 cm^2 may be necessary (Minners et al. 2008). Other studies report that an AVA < 1.0 cm^2 does predict excess mortality and morbidity irrespective of the level of gradient and the presence of symptoms (Hachicha et al. 2007; Barasch et al. 2008; Pai et al. 2008; Dumesnil et al. 2010). Future studies are needed to determine the outcome of the particular subset of patients with an AVA between 0.8 and 1.0 cm^2, especially when treated conservatively.

The majority of patients with AS can be managed adequately with the use of conventional parameters of disease severity such as peak jet velocity, mean gradient, and AVA. However, in light of the above considerations, it becomes evident that the mode of presentation of many patients with calcific AS is more complex than previously believed and thus warrants more comprehensive evaluations that can include the following parameters.

Table 8.1 Clinical parameters for assessment of aortic stenosis (Pibarot and Dumesnil 2012a)

Parameter	Criteria for "severe"	Utility and advantages	Limitations
Quantification of valvular obstruction			
Peak aortic jet velocity[a,b] V_{Peak}	> 4 m/s	Easy to measure Low inter- intra- observer variability High specificity	Highly flow-dependent Overestimates LV energy loss in patients with small aortas May under- or over- estimate stenosis severity in presence of hypertension Underestimates stenosis severity in low flow states
Mean gradient[a,b] $\Delta P_{Mean}=4\times V_{Peak}{}^{2}$	> 40 mmHg	Same as peak aortic jet velocity	Same as peak aortic jet velocity
Valve effective orifice area[a,b] $AVA=SV_{LVOT}/VTI_{Ao}$	≤1.0 cm²	Less flow-dependent than gradient or peak velocity Reflects the intrinsic severity of valvular obstruction	Susceptible to measurements errors Overestimates LV energy loss in patients with small aortas May under- or over- estimate stenosis severity in presence of hypertension May overestimate stenosis severity in low flow states May overestimate severity in patients with small body size.
Indexed AVA[a] AVAI=AVA/BSA	≤0.6 cm²/m²	Same as AVA	May overestimate severity in obese patients
Energy loss index $ELI=[AVA\times A_A/A_A-AVA]/BSA$	≤0.5–0.6 cm²/m²	Less flow-dependent than gradient or peak velocity Takes into account pressure recovery and is ± equivalent to AVA measured by Gorlin Reflects the true LV energy loss caused by the stenosis Should be measured in patients with small aortas	Susceptible to measurements errors May under- or over- estimate stenosis severity in presence of hypertension May overestimate stenosis severity in low flow states
Stroke work loss $SWL=100\times(\Delta P_{Mean}/SBP+\Delta P_{Mean})$	>25 %	Less flow-dependent than gradient or peak velocity Takes into account pressure recovery	May underestimate stenosis severity and LV energy loss in presence of hypertension
Aortic valve calcification score[b]	Echo: ≥ 3/4[b] CT: >1650 AU	Can be estimated by echocardiography and quantitatively measured by multi-detector CT Correlates well with stenosis severity and predicts rapid stenosis progression Independent of hemodynamic conditions Useful in low flow states when echo assessment of stenosis hemodynamic severity is inconclusive	Echo: semi-quantitative assessment CT: exposure to radiation

Quantification of vascular load			
Systemic blood pressure[a] SBP/DBP	>140/90 mmHg	Easy to measure	Highly flow-dependent Underestimates severity of hypertension in low flow states
Systemic arterial compliance[a] SAC=SVI/SBP–DBP	≤0.6 ml · mmHg^{-1} · m^{-2}	Can be measured by Doppler-echocardiography Most frequent cause of increased arterial load in AS patients Can unmask hypertension in patients with pseudo-normalized blood pressure	Susceptible to measurements errors
Systemic vascular resistance[a] SVR=80×MBP/CO	>2000 dyn · s · cm^{-5}	Can be measured by Doppler-echocardiography Can unmask hypertension in patients with pseudo-normalized blood pressure	Susceptible to measurements errors
Quantification of global LV hemodynamic load			
Valvulo-arterial impedance[a] Z_{va}= SBP+ΔP_{Mean}/SVI	>4.5 mmHg · ml^{-1} · m^{2}	Can be measured by Doppler-echocardiography Reflects the global (valvular+arterial) load imposed on the LV Potentially superior to predict occurrence of symptoms and events	Susceptible to measurements errors Does not permit to discriminate the valvular vs. the arterial contribution to the global LV load
Quantification of LV systolic dysfunction			
LV ejection fraction[a,b]	<50 %	Widely used and validated with regards to outcome data	Susceptible to measurements errors Also influenced by LV geometry Underestimates the degree of myocardial systolic dysfunction in presence of LV concentric remodeling
Global longitudinal strain[a]	<14 %	Less influenced by LV geometry Superior to LVEF to assess intrinsic myocardial function	Cut-off values need to be further validated
Myocardial fibrosis		Can be measured by CMR Predicts poor outcomes after AVR	High cost and low availability of CMR

(continued)

Table 8.1 (continued)

Parameter	Criteria for "severe"	Utility and advantages	Limitations
Plasma natriuretic peptides[a]		Easy and inexpensive to measure Reflects the total burden of disease(s) on the myocardium Correlates well with myocardial systolic dysfunction and symptoms Predicts poor outcomes prior to and after AVR	High variability in the threshold values reported in the literature to predict poor outcomes Increase in BNP during serial follow-up may be superior to isolated measure Does not permit to discriminate the impact of the valvular stenosis vs. hypertension vs. other cardiovascular disease NT-ProBNP may be more sensitive to detect early LV systolic dysfunction but is more age-dependent.

Adapted with permission from Pibarot and Dumesnil (2012)

A_A cross-sectional area of the ascending aorta measured just downstream of the sino-tubular junction, *BSA* body surface area, *CO* cardiac output, *SBP*, *DBP*, *MBP* systolic, diastolic, and mean blood pressures, respectively, *SVI* stroke volume index

[a]Indicates the parameters we think should be part of the routine assessment of patients with AS

[b]Indicates the parameters that are included in the algorithms presented in the ACC/AHA and ESC guidelines for the management of AS

Pressure Recovery

The current guidelines (Bonow et al. 2006; Vahanian et al. 2007) make no distinction between catheterization and Doppler-echocardiographic measurements as if values for gradients and AVA measured by either technique were interchangeable (Fig. 8.1). Doppler estimates the maximal pressure drop through the valve from the maximal velocity recorded at that level whereas catheterization provides a measure of the net gradient between the left ventricle and the ascending aorta (Fig. 8.2). It is important to recognize as blood flow velocity decelerates between the valve and the ascending aorta, part of the kinetic energy is reconverted back to static energy due to a phenomenon called pressure recovery, and hence the net gradient recorded at catheterization is always less than the maximum pressure gradient measured by Doppler (Fig. 8.2) (Briand et al. 2005; Baumgartner et al. 1999; Garcia et al. 2000, 2003). The extent of pressure recovery is determined by the ratio between the AVA and the cross-sectional area of the ascending aorta, may lead to overestimation of severity (Briand et al. 2005; Baumgartner et al. 1999; Garcia et al. 2000, 2003). Conversely, patients with a large aneurysm of the ascending aorta or congenital bicuspid AS with a dilation of the ascending aorta will have less pressure recovery and therefore a more important energy loss for a given AVA.

The importance of pressure recovery can be accounted for by using the formula to estimate the net gradient from Doppler measurements (Baumgartner et al. 1999) as well as the formula to calculate the energy loss coefficient: $ELCo = (AVA \times A_A/A_A - AVA)$, where A_A is the cross-sectional area of the aorta measured at 1 cm downstream of the sino-tubular junction (Table 8.1) (Garcia et al. 2000). This parameter is more or less equivalent to the AVA obtained by catheterization with the use of the Gorlin formula (Garcia et al. 2000, 2003; Spevack et al. 2008; Bahlmann et al. 2010; Baumgartner et al. 2009; Rahimtoola 2010).

The stroke work loss, which is the ratio of the mean transvalvular gradient to the estimated LV systolic pressure (i.e. mean gradient/systolic blood pressure + mean gradient) is another index that indirectly accounts for the pressure recovery. And accordingly, this parameter has also been shown to be superior to the gradient or the AVA for predicting clinical outcomes (Bermejo et al. 2003). Both stroke work loss and the energy loss coefficient avoid incorrect estimation of stenosis severity due to pressure recovery, but these parameters only reflect the steady component of potential energy loss and do not account for kinetic energy, pulsatile flow, or downstream vascular compliance (Otto 2006).

Body Size

AVA and energy loss coefficient do not take into account cardiac output requirements in a given patient and hence, for a similar AVA the burden imposed by the stenosis on the ventricle will be higher in patients with a larger body size than in smaller patients. It thus follows that AS severity may be significantly overestimated in smaller patients and underestimated in larger patients when using un-indexed AVA or energy loss coefficient. Conversely the utilization of parameters indexed for body surface area may overestimate stenosis severity in obese patients. These caveats are important while evaluating the patient who may have confounding echo and or cath data as compared to the physical exam and symptom presentation.

Low Flow States

The chronic exposure to the high level of afterload from the stenotic valve may exceed the limit of LV compensatory mechanisms, and lead to an intrinsic impairment of myocardial function and a decrease in cardiac output which results in a decrease in transvalvular gradients. This situation is highly insidious because AS may appear less severe on the basis of the gradient, whereas, in fact, these patients are at a more advanced stage of their disease. Low-flow, low-gradient AS may occur with reduced or preserved LV ejection fraction (LVEF) and both situations are amongst the most challenging encountered clinical setting in patients with AS.

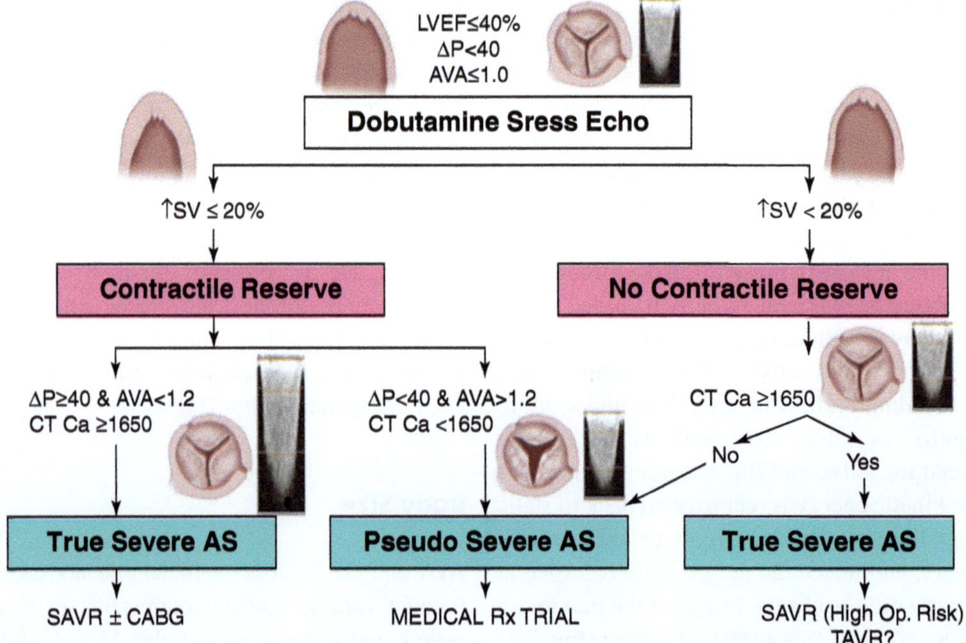

Fig. 8.3 Clinical decision making in low-LVEF, low-flow, low-gradient aortic stenosis. Dobutamine stress echocardiography (DSE) is useful to assess myocardial contractile reserve and to distinguish true- versus pseudo- severe aortic stenosis (AS). The quantification of valve calcification by multi-detector computed tomography (CT) may help to corroborate stenosis severity, especially in patients with no contractile reserve. This information aids decision making for therapeutic management. *AVA* aortic valve effective orifice area (in cm^2), *ΔP* mean transvalvular gradient (in mmHg), *Ca* calcium score (in Agatston Unit), *SV* stroke volume, *Op.* operative, *SAVR* surgical aortic valve replacement, *TAVR* transcatheter aortic valve replacement (Adapted with permission from Pibarot and Dumesnil (2012b))

The major challenge in patients with low-flow, low-gradient (<40 mmHg) AS and reduced LVEF (<40%), who represent approximately 5–10% of the AS population, is to distinguish true severe and "pseudo-severe" stenosis (de Filippi et al. 1995; Monin et al. 2003; Clavel et al. 2008). Pseudo-severe stenosis refers to the situation of a weakened ventricle that is not able to completely open a valve which otherwise would have been only mildly or moderately stenotic. Patients with low-LVEF, low-flow, low-gradient AS have a high operative mortality if treated surgically but an even poorer prognosis if treated medically (Monin et al. 2003; Clavel et al. 2008).

A low dose (up to 20 μg/kg/min) dobutamine stress echocardiography is thus helpful in these patients: (i) to assess the presence of myocardial contractile reserve, which provides information with regards to operative risk stratification; (ii) to differentiate a "pseudo-severe" from a true severe stenosis whereby, when the flow rate is increased by dobutamine, there is no or minimal change in AVA and a marked increase in gradient in the case of true severe AS as compared to a substantial increase in AVA and no or minimal increase in gradient in the case of pseudo-severe AS (de Filippi et al. 1995) (Fig. 8.3). Patients with true severe AS and contractile reserve are generally good candidates for AVR; patients with true severe AS but no contractile reserve may also benefit of AVR but they have a higher operative risk (Monin et al. 2003; Tribouilloy et al. 2009).

In these patients, transcatheter aortic valve replacement may be an alternative as it may reduce both the operative risk and the occurrence of prosthesis-patient mismatch (Clavel et al. 2010). Patients with pseudo-severe AS may not necessarily benefit from AVR but also have a poor prognosis if managed conservatively. Future studies are necessary to determine the optimal therapeutic strategy in this latter subset of patients.

Paradoxical Low-Flow, Low-Gradient AS

"Paradoxical low-flow, low-gradient AS" is a recently described entity whereby 10–25% of patients with severe AS on the basis of AVA (<1.0 cm^2, indexed AVA < 0.6 cm^2/m^2) have a low transvalvular flow rate (stroke volume index < 35 ml/m^2) and often a low gradient (<40 mmHg) despite the presence of a preserved LVEF (≥50%) (Hachicha et al. 2007; Barasch et al. 2008; Minners et al. 2010; Dumesnil and Shoucri 1991; Cramariuc et al. 2009a; Lancellotti et al. 2010a; Herrmann et al. 2011; Weidemann et al. 2009). Proper recognition of this entity is important since, due to the low gradients, these patients are often denied surgery when in fact they are often at a more advanced stage of the disease and have a worse prognosis if treated medically rather than surgically (Fig. 8.4).

Assessment of Vascular Load

Elderly patients with calcific AS may also have arterial atherosclerosis. Young subjects with a bicuspid aortic valve also commonly have reduced aortic elasticity as a result of structural abnormalities of the aortic wall and/or aortic dilation (Nistri et al. 2008). Hence, patients with calcific AS often have reduced compliance in the large arterial circulation and thereby resulting in systolic hypertension (Briand et al. 2005; Nistri et al. 2008). Briand et al. reported that total systemic arterial compliance estimated by dividing the stroke volume index as measured by echocardiography by pulse pressure (systolic minus diastolic blood pressures) as recorded by sphygmomanometer is severely reduced (<0.6 ml·m^{-2}·mmHg^{-1}) in about 40% of patients with AS (Briand et al. 2005) (Table 8.1). Furthermore, reduced arterial compliance and/or increased vascular resistance contribute to increase the LV afterload and thus the occurrence of myocardial dysfunction and adverse events (Briand et al. 2005; Antonini-Canterin et al. 2003). To this effect, Antonini-Canterin et al. have observed that symptoms of AS develop at a lower degree of stenosis severity in hypertensive patients, most likely because of the additional hemodynamic load due to hypertension (Antonini-Canterin et al. 2003). Finally, it should be emphasized that a normal blood pressure does not exclude an increase in vascular load since these pressures may be pseudo-normalized in up to 30% of patients with decreased systemic arterial compliance due to LV dysfunction and a concomitant decrease in cardiac output (Briand et al. 2005; Hachicha et al. 2007). Hence, blood pressure should be routinely recorded and systemic arterial compliance and vascular resistance should be calculated in patients evaluated for AS.

Assessment of Global Hemodynamic Load

To assess the global (valvular + arterial) LV hemodynamic load in AS patients, one can calculate the valvulo-arterial impedance (Z_{va}) (Fig. 8.2) by dividing the estimated LV systolic pressure (systolic arterial pressure + mean transvalvular gradient) by the stroke volume indexed for body surface area (Briand et al. 2005) (Table 8.1). This parameter provides an estimate of the cost in mmHg for each systemic ml of blood indexed for body size pumped by the left ventricle. Values of Z_{va} > 3.5 and 4.5 mmHg · ml^{-1} · m^2 indicate moderately and severely increased global LV hemodynamic load respectively (Hachicha et al. 2009). The Z_{va} has been shown to be superior to the standard parameters of AS severity (i.e. gradients and AVA) in predicting LV dysfunction and patient clinical outcomes (Briand et al. 2005; Hachicha et al. 2007, 2009; Cramariuc et al. 2009a; Lancellotti et al. 2010a, b; Herrmann et al. 2011). Calculation of Z_{va} can easily be done from measurements already performed during the routine examination. The parameter is useful with regards to prognosis but it remains important, from the standpoint of treatment, to delineate the relative contributions of the valvular and vascular components to the increased load.

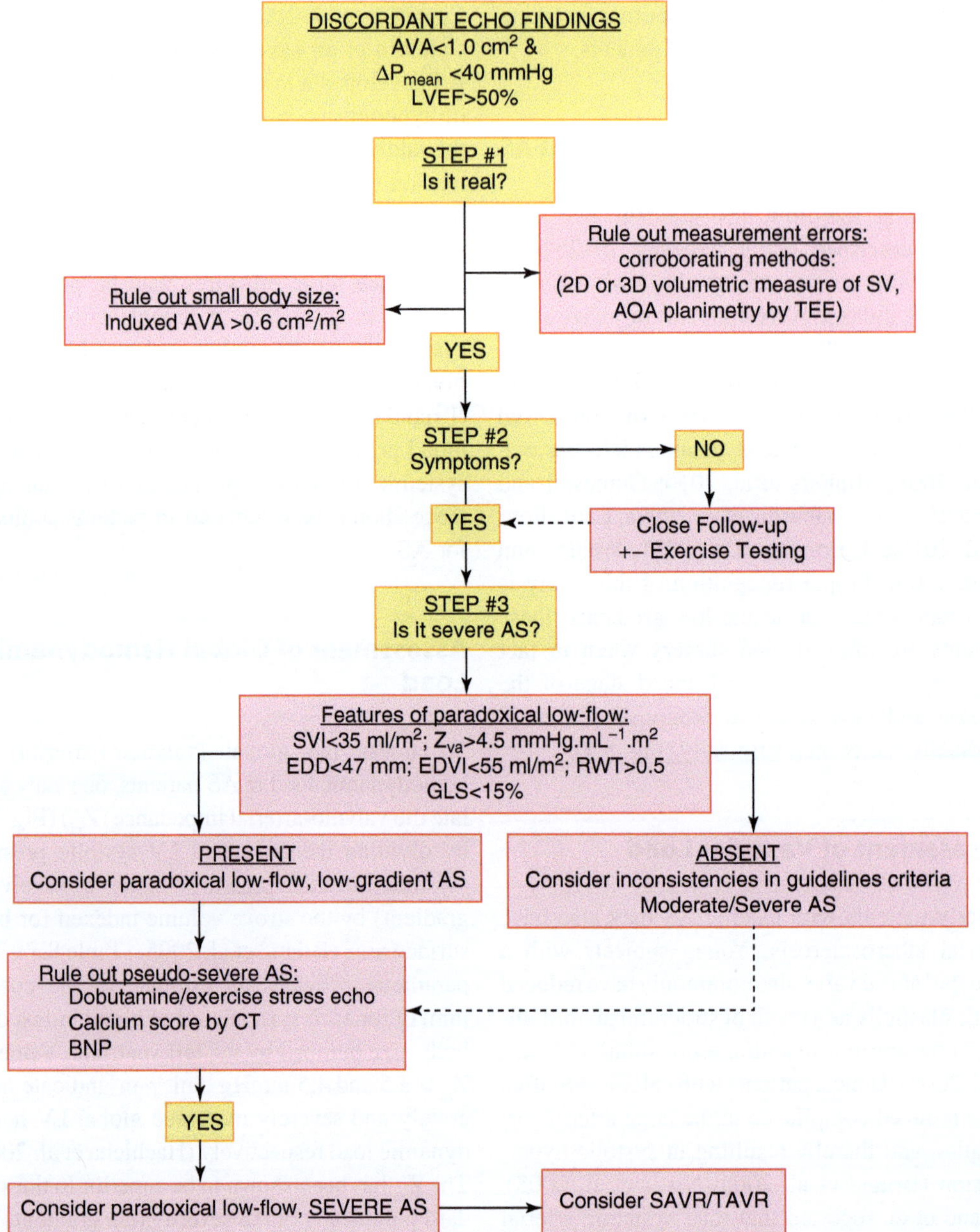

Fig. 8.4 Algorithm for differential diagnosis in patients with preserved LVEF presenting with a small aortic valve area but a low gradient. *AVA* aortic valve effective orifice area (in cm²), *AOA* aortic valve anatomic orifice area (in cm²), ΔP_{Mean} mean transvalvular gradient, *SV* stroke volume, *SVI* stroke volume index, Z_{va} valvulo-arterial impedance, *EDD* LV end-diastolic diameter, *EDVI* LV end-diastolic volume index, *RWT* relative wall thickness ratio, *GLS* global longitudinal strain, *TEE* transesophageal echocardiography, *SAVR* surgical aortic valve replacement, *TAVR* transcatheter aortic valve replacement

Assessment of Impact of Hemodynamic Load on the Myocardium

LV Remodeling and Hypertrophy

The pattern of the LV response to pressure overload in AS is highly heterogeneous and includes concentric remodeling, concentric hypertrophy, and eccentric hypertrophy (Carroll et al. 1992; Lund et al. 2010; Pagé et al. 2010). Hence, relative wall thickness ratio should be systematically measured in addition to LV mass because a large proportion of patients with AS have abnormal LV geometry (ratio>0.42; i.e. concentric remodeling) despite absence of LV hypertrophy defined as indexed LV mass >95 g/m^2 in women and >115 g/m^2 in men (Cramariuc et al. 2009a; Carroll et al. 1992; Lund et al. 2010; Pagé et al. 2010). More severe LV concentric remodeling or hypertrophy has been linked to worse myocardial function (Cramariuc et al. 2009a), increased risk of cardiovascular events (Cioffi et al. 2011), and increased operative and late mortality after aortic valve replacement (Orsinelli et al. 1993; Duncan et al. 2008). The pattern and magnitude of the LV adaptative response to AS is influenced by several factors including stenosis severity, age, gender, metabolic profile and also genetic factors (Carroll et al. 1992; Lund et al. 2010; Pagé et al. 2010). For the same degree of AS, women tend to predominantly develop concentric remodeling/hypertrophy, whereas men are more prone to develop eccentric hypertrophy (Carroll et al. 1992). Obesity and metabolic syndrome also predispose to the development of more concentric hypertrophy in presence of AS (Lund et al. 2010; Pagé et al. 2010).

LV Systolic Dysfunction

LV systolic dysfunction on the basis of LVEF is a class I indication for AVR in patients with severe AS irrespective of symptoms and LVEF is the only parameter of LV function included in the guidelines (Fig. 8.1) (Bonow et al. 2006; Vahanian et al. 2007). Yet, several studies report that up to one third of asymptomatic patients with preserved LVEF have a significant impairment of intrinsic myocardial systolic function (Cramariuc et al. 2009a; Lancellotti et al. 2010b; Dumesnil et al. 1979; Ng et al. 2011) and that the parameters of LV longitudinal kinetics are superior to other indices of LV systolic function to detect myocardial dysfunction and damage (Dumesnil and Shoucri 1991; Herrmann et al. 2011; Weidemann et al. 2009; Dumesnil et al. 1979; Ng et al. 2011; Cramariuc et al. 2009b; Poulsen et al. 2007; Van Pelt et al. 2007) as well as to predict symptoms, exercise tolerance and outcomes (Lancellotti et al. 2010b; Poulsen et al. 2007; Takeda et al. 2001; Tongue et al. 2003; Lafitte et al. 2009). From a pathophysiological standpoint, these data are consistent with an increase in wall stress and intramyocardial pressure as well as the reduction in myocardial blood flow in AS at the level of subendocardium. Hence, as hypothesized by Dumesnil et al. 30 years ago, the selective impairment in longitudinal LV shortening is likely the consequence of increased subendocardial wall stress and resulting subendocardial ischemia and fibrosis due to the longitudinal alignment of the subendocardial cells (Dumesnil et al. 1979). Global longitudinal myocardial strain measured by speckle tracking can now be measured routinely and reproducibly and has emerged as the most promising alternative to detect and quantify intrinsic myocardial systolic dysfunction (Ng et al. 2011; Cramariuc et al. 2009b; Poulsen et al. 2007; Van Pelt et al. 2007); pending further validation, a threshold value of <15% has been proposed for this purpose (Lancellotti et al. 2010b; Ng et al. 2011).

Myocardial Damage

Recent studies (Weidemann et al. 2009; Azevedo et al. 2010) have reported that about one third of patients undergoing AVR for severe AS have severe myocardial fibrosis documented by cardiac magnetic resonance (CMR) and intra-operative myocardial biopsies. Moreover, myocardial fibrosis is often not- or only partially-reversible and is associated with increased risk of cardiovascular events and mortality during follow-up as well as persistence of LV dysfunction and symptoms (Herrmann et al. 2011; Weidemann et al. 2009; Azevedo et al. 2010; Nazarian 2011). The non-reversibility of myocardial fibrosis and associated dysfunction after AVR most likely depends on the type (replacement vs. interstitial) and extent (severe vs. mild) of fibrosis. The quantification of myocardial fibrosis by CMR could potentially be useful to improve risk stratification and follow-up as well as to recommend AVR before extensive fibrosis and ensuing irreversible myocardial dysfunction have developed. The implementation of such a measure is however less feasible due to high cost and low availability. Investigators have shown that the parameters of LV longitudinal function correlate well with the degree of myocardial fibrosis (Herrmann et al. 2011; Weidemann et al. 2009; Dumesnil et al. 1979). Hence, an alternate approach could be to routinely measure global LV longitudinal strain during follow-up and to perform CMR in selected cases.

Recent studies also show that Brain Natriuretic Peptide (BNP) levels correlate better with myocardial abnormalities (i.e. LVEF, LV longitudinal shortening, degree of myocardial fibrosis) and clinical outcomes than the usual parameters of AS severity (Herrmann et al. 2011; Weidemann et al. 2009; Poulsen et al. 2007; Gerber et al. 2003, 2005; Vanderheyden et al. 2004; Lancellotti et al. 2010c; Bergler-Klein et al. 2004, 2007; Monin et al. 2009). These findings further corroborate the concept that myocardial damage and clinical outcomes are primarily determined by the total burden of disease on the ventricle rather than by AS severity alone (Table 8.1). BNP levels may also have an added advantage over the indices of global load such as Z_{va} in that they also likely reflect the impact of other associated conditions (e.g. coronary artery disease, cardiomyopathy, etc.) on the myocardium. With regards to the clinical utilization of BNP, there are however three caveats worth mentioning. First, as emphasized, BNP levels are not specific to AS severity alone but rather reflect the total burden of disease(s) on the left ventricle. They should thus be interpreted in light of the parameters more specifically reflecting AS severity as well as arterial and global loads (Table 8.1). Second, the threshold values for adverse events appear to vary considerably from one study to the other. Third, BNP response is also influenced by age and gender (Steadman et al. 2010). Hence, unless the value are unequivocally elevated (e.g. BNP>500 pg/ml) (Bergler-Klein et al. 2004, 2007; Weber et al. 2006), an individual result should not be interpreted in isolation but rather in light of other clinical variables as well as variations with time which may be superior to an individual measurement to predict development of symptoms (Gerber et al. 2005). For NT-proBNP which is influenced by age, reference values in relation to the different age strata also need to be established. Nonetheless, BNP remains a robust predictor of outcomes in AS and we believe it should be routinely measured and become an integral part of the clinical decision making process. Moreover, it may have added value from the standpoint of cost-benefit since the continued observation of low and stable levels in an asymptomatic patient might preclude the unnecessary use of more expensive investigations.

Assessment of Symptoms

The onset of symptoms is one of the cornerstones in the decision-making algorithm presented in the ACC/AHA and ESC guidelines for the indications of AVR (Fig. 8.1) (Bonow et al. 2006; Vahanian et al. 2007). However, the concept proposed 40 years ago of patients with AS remaining asymptomatic for a long time and then developing explicit symptoms portending poor outcomes (Ross and Braunwald 1968), is no longer congruent with the new face of the disease that we encounter nowadays. Indeed, elderly patients have more comorbidities and are less physically active, which renders the assessment of symptoms much more complex and unreliable. Patients may also reduce their level of physical activity to avoid or minimize symptoms and the overall presentation often predisposes to under-reporting and/or underestimation of symptoms. Several studies have now demonstrated that exercise testing can be done safely in patients without apparent symptoms (Picano et al. 2009) and that the results can be used to identify patients at high risk of adverse events over the next 1–2 years (Amato et al. 2001; Alborino et al. 2002; Das et al. 2005; Lancellotti et al. 2005; Maréchaux et al. 2010). Both the ACC/AHA and ESC guidelines now support the role of exercise testing in asymptomatic AS patients, with recommendations that AVR be considered in those with exercise-induced symptoms or abnormal blood pressure responses (Fig. 8.1). Chapter 6 addresses the specifics of exercise testing in the valvular heart disease.

Assesment of Risk of Rapid Disease Progression

Several factors have been identified as predisposing to more rapid disease progression (Fig. 8.1): (i) Patients with a more severe stenosis defined as an AVA < 0.6 cm^2 (Bonow et al. 2006) or peak aortic jet velocity >5.5 m/s (Otto et al. 1997; Rosenhek et al. 2000, 2010) have a more rapid progression to symptoms and LV systolic dysfunction. (ii) The degree of aortic valve calcification is a powerful predictor of rapid valvular stenosis progression (Rosenhek et al. 2000). Semi-quantitative scoring of valve calcification can be done by echocardiography but multidetector computed tomography (CT) allows more accurate and quantitative assessments (Cueff et al. 2010; Messika-Zeitoun et al. 2007). The concern of radiation exposure however limits the use of this procedure for routine follow-up. (iii) Previous studies report an association between several traditional cardiovascular risk factors (i.e. hypercholesterolemia, hypertension, obesity, smoking) and faster stenosis progression There is mounting evidence that the metabolic syndrome and the type-2 diabetes are also associated with faster progression of the disease and faster deterioration of LV function, with little evidence for medical therapy for this field (Pagé et al. 2010; Rossebo et al. 2008; Briand et al. 2006; Katz et al. 2009) but it also remains to be determined if the course of the disease can be altered by changes in lifestyle and/or therapies targeting the associated metabolic abnormalities.

Timing to Intervention in AS

Management of Patients with Asymptomatic Severe AS

The management of patients with asymptomatic severe AS remains a source of debate (Bonow et al. 2006; Vahanian et al. 2007) and recent studies have suggested that those treated surgically may have better survival than those treated medically (Brown et al. 2008; Mihaljevic et al. 2008; Kang et al. 2010). This difference may be related to underestimation of symptoms and/or stenosis severity, especially in the elderly sedentary patients (Hachicha et al. 2007; Barasch et al. 2008; Mihaljevic et al. 2008). A "wait for symptoms" strategy may result in some patients being operated too late i.e. at a stage of the disease when myocardial impairment has become, at least in part, irreversible (Fig. 8.4).

In the AHA-ACC/ESC guidelines, AVR is considered a class I indication in patients with severe AS only if they have symptoms and/or LVEF < 50% or if they undergo other cardiac surgery (Fig. 8.1). As emphasized in these guidelines, one important objective in asymptomatic patients with severe AS and normal LVEF is to ensure that the patient is truly asymptomatic to the extent of performing an exercise test if the symptomatic status is equivocal. Otherwise, earlier referral to AVR despite the absence of symptoms can also be considered (Class IIa or IIb indication in the guidelines) when the following markers of rapid disease progression are present (Fig. 8.1): (i) Severe aortic valve calcification (Echo calcium score: 4/4) (Rosenhek et al. 2000), (ii) Rapid hemodynamic progression of the stenosis at serial echocardiographic exams (>0.3 m/s progression of peak jet velocity) (Otto et al. 1997; Rosenhek et al. 2000), and/or (iii) Very severe AS (AVA < 0.6 cm^2 and/or peak jet velocity >5.5 m/s) (Bonow et al. 2006; Rosenhek et al. 2010).

Besides the conventional parameters (i.e. peak jet velocity, gradient, AVA, valve calcification and LVEF) proposed in the guidelines to assess disease severity, there are several other emerging parameters that may be useful to further enhance risk stratification and clinical decision making in asymptomatic severe AS, including the following: (i) Energy loss index to more precisely assess stenosis severity in patients with AVA between 0.8 and 1.0 cm^2 and small aorta diameter (<30 mm); (ii) Z_{va} to determine the global (valvular + arterial) LV hemodynamic load, (iii) Plasma BNP to assess the impact of this hemodynamic load (and of other potential concomitant cardiopathies) on the myocardium, and (iv) Global longitudinal strain to confirm that the myocardial systolic function is truly normal. If these parameters are abnormal (see Table 8.1), it may be preferable to follow the patients more closely with a clinical, BNP level and/or echocardiographic evaluation every 3–6 months. If the aforementioned parameters are normal or mildly/moderately abnormal, the same follow-up can be extended to 6–12 months (Otto 2006). These emerging parameters (Monin et al. 2009) as well as composite risk scores including several standard/emerging parameters will have to be further validated in future large prospective studies before being implemented in routine practice.

Management of Patients with Symptomatic Moderate AS

The approach in patients with moderate AS who nonetheless have symptoms is first to confirm that the stenosis is truly moderate and not severe and then to determine what is the cause(s) of the symptoms. In this context it is important to reiterate that adverse outcomes in AS are in fine determined by the imbalance between global LV load and LV myocardial reserve. Hence, a patient with moderate AS and concomitant arterial hypertension may have a global hemodynamic load that is equivalent or superior to that of a patient with severe AS and no hypertension, and thus be symptomatic on that basis (Antonini-Canterin et al. 2003). The calculation of Z_{va} may be helpful in these cases to reconcile the apparent discordance between moderate stenosis severity and symptomatic status (Hachicha et al. 2009). If Z_{va} is high, an optimal and prudent treatment of hypertension would appear reasonable. Future studies are necessary to determine if AVR should nonetheless be contemplated in patients with optimal treatment of hypertension and persistence of symptoms. If Z_{va} is low, associated conditions such as coronary artery disease, intrinsic cardiomyopathy, pulmonary disease, etc. should be considered.

Finally, AS severity may progress rapidly in a substantial proportion of patients with moderate AS even if asymptomatic. Hence, closer (6–12 months) follow-up would appear judicious in such patients if there is presence of severe valve calcification at echocardiography or CT, large increase in gradient on exercise stress echo, or increase in BNP since last echocardiographic exam.

Management of Patients with Discordant Echocardiographic Findings

The clinician is often confronted to patients with preserved LVEF having discordant findings: e.g. an AVA = 0.8 cm^2 consistent with the presence of a severe AS but a mean gradient = 30 mmHg rather indicating the presence of a moderate AS (Minners et al. 2008; Hachicha et al. 2007; Jander et al. 2011). This situation raises uncertainty regarding the actual severity of the stenosis as well as the potential indication of AVR if the patient is symptomatic. There are several potential causes of such discordance between AVA and gradient in the context of preserved LVEF (Hachicha et al. 2007; Dumesnil et al. 2010; Jander et al. 2011): (i) Measurement errors (i.e. underestimation of stroke volume and AVA); (ii) Small body size; (iii) Inconsistency in guidelines criteria; and (iv) Paradoxical low-flow AS. Hence, it is important to make the differential diagnosis between these four potential situations given they have markedly different implications in terms of therapeutic management. In the last situation AVR may be beneficial, whereas in the three others, it may not. This differential diagnosis can be achieved by: (i) using several different Doppler-echocardiographic methods (2D or 3D volumetric methods) or other imaging modalities (CMR) to corroborate the measurements of stroke volume and AVA, (ii) calculating the indexed AVA, (iii) identifying the typical features of paradoxical low-flow AS (small LV cavity size with pronounced concentric remodeling, reduced stroke volume, high Z_{va}, and reduced myocardial longitudinal shortening).

Conclusion

Calcific AS is a complex, multi-faceted disease that may not be solely limited to the aortic valve but may also be frequently associated with reduced systemic arterial compliance as well as alterations of LV geometry and function. This changing face of the disease underlines the need for a more comprehensive assessment of AS severity going beyond the simple measurement of the standard parameters of stenosis severity (i.e. peak jet velocity, pressure gradients, AVA) or LV function (i.e. LVEF) to include the following parameters: (i) the energy loss index for the assessment of valvular load, (ii) the systemic arterial compliance and valvular resistance for the assessment of arterial load and, (iii) the valvulo-arterial impedance and BNP to quantify the global LV hemodynamic load and its repercussion on the myocardium, and (iv) the global longitudinal strain to assess the presence and severity of intrinsic myocardial dysfunction. Moreover, exercise stress testing and exercise stress echocardiography provide important tools to unmask symptoms, lack of valve opening reserve, and/or latent myocardial systolic dysfunction unrevealed by assessment in the resting state. Dobutamine-stress echocardiography greatly aids risk stratification and clinical decision making in patients with low-flow, low-gradient AS. A comprehensive approach that integrates these novel parameters is key to appropriately assess the patients with AS whom we see nowadays and other imaging modalities such as CT and CMR are often needed to complement or confirm the information obtained by clinical, Doppler-echocardiographic, or blood biomarkers evaluations.

References

Alborino D, Hoffmann JL, Fournet PC, Bloch A. Value of exercise testing to evaluate the indication for surgery in asymptomatic patients with valvular aortic stenosis. J Heart Valve Dis. 2002;11:204–9.

Amato MC, Moffa PJ, Werner KE, Ramires JA. Treatment decision in asymptomatic aortic valve stenosis: role of exercise testing. Heart. 2001;86:381–6.

Antonini-Canterin F, Huang G, Cervesato E, et al. Symptomatic aortic stenosis: does systemic hypertension play an additional role? Hypertension. 2003;41:1268–72.

Azevedo CF, Nigri M, Higuchi ML, et al. Prognostic significance of myocardial fibrosis quantification by histopathology and magnetic resonance imaging in patients with severe aortic valve disease. J Am Coll Cardiol. 2010;56:278–87.

Bahlmann E, Cramariuc D, Gerdts E, et al. Impact of pressure recovery on echocardiographic assessment of asymptomatic aortic stenosis: a SEAS Substudy. JACC Cardiovasc Imaging. 2010;3:555–62.

Barasch E, Fan D, Chukwu EO, et al. Severe isolated aortic stenosis with normal left ventricular systolic function and low transvalvular gradients: pathophysiologic and prognostic insights. J Heart Valve Dis. 2008;17:81–8.

Baumgartner H, Steffenelli T, Niederberger J, Schima H, Maurer G. "Overestimation" of catheter gradients by Doppler ultrasound in patients with aortic stenosis: a predictable manifestation of pressure recovery. J Am Coll Cardiol. 1999;33:1655–61.

Baumgartner H, Hung J, Bermejo J, et al. Echocardiographic assessment of valve stenosis: EAE/ASE recommendations for clinical practice. J Am Soc Echocardiogr. 2009;22:1–23.

Bergler-Klein J, Klaar U, Heger M, et al. Natriuretic peptides predict symptom-free survival and postoperative outcome in severe aortic stenosis. Circulation. 2004;109:2302–8.

Bergler-Klein J, Mundigler G, Pibarot P, et al. B-type natriuretic peptide in low-flow, low-gradient aortic stenosis: relationship to hemodynamics and clinical outcome. Circulation. 2007;115:2848–55.

Bermejo J, Odreman R, Feijoo J, Moreno MM, Gomez-Moreno P, Garcia-Fernandez MA. Clinical efficacy of Doppler-echocardiographic indices of aortic valve stenosis:a comparative test-based analysis of outcome. J Am Coll Cardiol. 2003;41:142–51.

Bonow RO, Carabello BA, Kanu C, et al. ACC/AHA 2006 guidelines for the management of patients with valvular heart disease: a report of the American College of Cardiology/American Heart Association Task Force on Practice Guidelines (writing committee to revise the 1998 Guidelines for the Management of Patients With Valvular Heart Disease): developed in collaboration with the Society of Cardiovascular Anesthesiologists: endorsed by the Society for Cardiovascular Angiography and Interventions and the Society of Thoracic Surgeons. Circulation. 2006;114:e84–231.

Briand M, Dumesnil JG, Kadem L, et al. Reduced systemic arterial compliance impacts significantly on left ventricular afterload and function in aortic stenosis: Implications for diagnosis and treatment. J Am Coll Cardiol. 2005;46:291–8.

Briand M, Lemieux I, Dumesnil JG, et al. Metabolic syndrome negatively influences disease progression and prognosis in aortic stenosis. J Am Coll Cardiol. 2006;47:2229–36.

Brown ML, Pellikka PA, Schaff HV, et al. The benefits of early valve replacement in asymptomatic patients with severe aortic stenosis. J Thorac Cardiovasc Surg. 2008; 135:308–15.

Carabello BA. Aortic stenosis. N Engl J Med. 2002;346: 677–82.

Carroll JD, Carroll EP, Feldman T, et al. Sex-associated differences in left ventricular function in aortic stenosis of the elderly. Circulation. 1992;86:1099–107.

Cioffi G, Faggiano P, Vizzardi E, et al. Prognostic value of inappropriately high left ventricular mass in asymptomatic severe aortic stenosis. Heart. 2011;97:301–7.

Clavel MA, Fuchs C, Burwash IG, et al. Predictors of outcomes in low-flow, low-gradient aortic stenosis: results of the multicenter TOPAS Study. Circulation. 2008; 118:S234–42.

Clavel MA, Webb JG, Rodés-Cabau J, et al. Comparison between transcatheter and surgical prosthetic valve implantation in patients with severe aortic stenosis and reduced left ventricular ejection fraction. Circulation. 2010;122:1928–36.

Cramariuc D, Cioffi G, Rieck AE, et al. Low-flow aortic stenosis in asymptomatic patients: valvular arterial impedance and systolic function from the SEAS substudy. JAAC Cardiovasc Imaging. 2009a;2:390–9.

Cramariuc D, Gerdts E, Davidsen ES, Segadal L, Matre K. Myocardial deformation in aortic valve stenosis - relation to left ventricular geometry. Heart. 2009b;96: 106–12.

Cueff C, Serfaty JM, Cimadevilla C, et al. Measurement of aortic valve calcification using multislice computed tomography: correlation with haemodynamic severity of aortic stenosis and clinical implication for patients with low ejection fraction. Heart. 2011;97: 721–6.

Das P, Rimington H, Chambers J. Exercise testing to stratify risk in aortic stenosis. Eur Heart J. 2005;26:1309–13.

de Filippi CR, Willett DL, Brickner E, et al. Usefulness of dobutamine echocardiography in distinguishing severe from nonsevere valvular aortic stenosis in patients with depressed left ventricular function and low transvalvular gradients. Am J Cardiol. 1995;75:191–4.

Dumesnil JG, Shoucri RM. Quantitative relationships between left ventricular ejection and wall thickening and geometry. J Appl Physiol. 1991;70:48–54.

Dumesnil JG, Shoucri RM, Laurenceau JL, Turcot J. A mathematical model of the dynamic geometry of the intact left ventricle and its application to clinical data. Circulation. 1979;59:1024–34.

Dumesnil JG, Pibarot P, Carabello B. Paradoxical low flow and/or low gradient severe aortic stenosis despite preserved left ventricular ejection fraction: implications for diagnosis and treatment. Eur Heart J. 2010;31:281–9.

Duncan AI, Lowe BS, Garcia MJ, et al. Influence of concentric left ventricular remodeling on early mortality after aortic valve replacement. Ann Thorac Surg. 2008;85:2030–9.

Garcia D, Pibarot P, Dumesnil JG, Sakr F, Durand LG. Assessment of aortic valve stenosis severity: A new index based on the energy loss concept. Circulation. 2000;101:765–71.

Garcia D, Dumesnil JG, Durand LG, Kadem L, Pibarot P. Discrepancies between catheter and Doppler estimates of valve effective orifice area can be predicted from the pressure recovery phenomenon: practical implications with regard to quantification of aortic stenosis severity. J Am Coll Cardiol. 2003;41:435–42.

Gerber IL, Stewart RA, Legget ME, et al. Increased plasma natriuretic peptide levels reflect symptom onset in aortic stenosis. Circulation. 2003;107:1884–90.

Gerber IL, Legget ME, West TM, Richards AM, Stewart RA. Usefulness of serial measurement of N-terminal pro-brain natriuretic peptide plasma levels in asymptomatic patients with aortic stenosis to predict symptomatic deterioration. Am J Cardiol. 2005;95: 898–901.

Hachicha Z, Dumesnil JG, Bogaty P, Pibarot P. Paradoxical low flow, low gradient severe aortic stenosis despite preserved ejection fraction is associated with higher afterload and reduced survival. Circulation. 2007;115:2856–64.

Hachicha Z, Dumesnil JG, Pibarot P. Usefulness of the valvuloarterial impedance to predict adverse outcome in asymptomatic aortic stenosis. J Am Coll Cardiol. 2009;54:1003–11.

Herrmann S, Stork S, Niemann M, et al. Low-gradient aortic valve stenosis: myocardial fibrosis and its influence on function and outcome. J Am Coll Cardiol. 2011;58:402–12.

Higgins J, Jamieson WR, Benhameid O, et al. Influence of patient gender on mortality after aortic valve replacement for aortic stenosis. J Thorac Cardiovasc Surg. 2011;142:595–601. 601.

Jander N, Minners J, Holme I, et al. Outcome of patients with low-gradient "severe" aortic stenosis and preserved ejection fraction. Circulation. 2011;123:887–95.

Kang DH, Park SJ, Rim JH, et al. Early surgery versus conventional treatment in asymptomatic very severe aortic stenosis. Circulation. 2010;121:1502–9.

Katz R, Budoff MJ, Takasu J, et al. Relationship of metabolic syndrome to incident aortic valve calcium and aortic valve calcium progression: the multi-ethnic study of atherosclerosis (MESA). Diabetes. 2009;58: 813–9.

Lafitte S, Perlant M, Reant P, et al. Impact of impaired myocardial deformations on exercise tolerance and prognosis in patients with asymptomatic aortic stenosis. Eur J Echocardiogr. 2009;10:414–9.

Lancellotti P, Lebois F, Simon M, Tombeux C, Chauvel C, Pierard LA. Prognostic importance of quantitative exercise Doppler echocardiography in asymptomatic valvular aortic stenosis. Circulation. 2005;112:I377–82.

Lancellotti P, Donal E, Magne J, et al. Impact of global left ventricular afterload on left ventricular function in asymptomatic severe aortic stenosis: a two-dimensional speckle-tracking study. Eur J Echocardiogr. 2010a;11:537–43.

Lancellotti P, Donal E, Magne J, et al. Risk stratification in asymptomatic moderate to severe aortic stenosis: the importance of the valvular, arterial and ventricular interplay. Heart. 2010b;96:1364–71.

Lancellotti P, Moonen M, Magne J, et al. Prognostic effect of long-axis left ventricular dysfunction and B-type natriuretic peptide levels in asymptomatic aortic stenosis. Am J Cardiol. 2010c;105:383–8.

Lund BP, Gohlke-Barwolf C, Cramariuc D, Rossebo AB, Rieck AE, Gerdts E. Effect of obesity on left ventricular mass and systolic function in patients with asymptomatic aortic stenosis (a Simvastatin Ezetimibe in Aortic Stenosis [SEAS] substudy). Am J Cardiol. 2010;105:1456–60.

Maréchaux S, Hachicha Z, Bellouin A, et al. Usefulness of exercise stress echocardiography for risk stratification of true asymptomatic patients with aortic valve stenosis. Eur Heart J. 2010;31:1390–7.

Messika-Zeitoun D, Bielak LF, Peyser PA, et al. Aortic valve calcification: determinants and progression in the population. Arterioscler Thromb Vasc Biol. 2007;27:642–8.

Mihaljevic T, Nowicki ER, Rajeswaran J, et al. Survival after valve replacement for aortic stenosis: implications for decision making. J Thorac Cardiovasc Surg. 2008;135:1270–8.

Minners J, Allgeier M, Gohlke-Baerwolf C, Kienzle RP, Neumann FJ, Jander N. Inconsistencies of echocardiographic criteria for the grading of aortic valve stenosis. Eur Heart J. 2008;29:1043–8.

Minners J, Allgeier M, Gohlke-Baerwolf C, Kienzle RP, Neumann FJ, Jander N. Inconsistent grading of aortic valve stenosis by current guidelines: haemodynamic studies in patients with apparently normal left ventricular function. Heart. 2010;96:1463–8.

Monin JL, Quere JP, Monchi M, et al. Low-gradient aortic stenosis: operative risk stratification and predictors for long-term outcome: a multicenter study using dobutamine stress hemodynamics. Circulation. 2003;108:319–24.

Monin JL, Lancellotti P, Monchi M, et al. Risk score for predicting outcome in patients with asymptomatic aortic stenosis. Circulation. 2009;120:69–75.

Nazarian S. Is ventricular arrhythmia a possible mediator of the association between aortic stenosis-related midwall fibrosis and mortality? J Am Coll Cardiol. 2011;58:1280–2.

Ng AC, Delgado V, Bertini M, et al. Alterations in multidirectional myocardial functions in patients with aortic stenosis and preserved ejection fraction: a two-dimensional speckle tracking analysis. Eur Heart J. 2011;32:1542–50.

Nistri S, Grande-Allen J, Noale M, et al. Aortic elasticity and size in bicuspid aortic valve syndrome. Eur Heart J. 2008;29(4):472–9.

Orsinelli DA, Aurigemma GP, Battista S, Krendel S, Gaasch WH. Left ventricular hypertrophy and mortality after aortic valve replacement for aortic stenosis. A high risk subgroup identified by preoperative relative wall thickness. J Am Coll Cardiol. 1993;22:1679–83.

Otto CM. Valvular aortic stenosis: disease severity and timing of intervention. J Am Coll Cardiol. 2006;47:2141–51.

Otto CM, Burwash IG, Legget ME, et al. Prospective study of asymptomatic valvular aortic stenosis. Clinical, echocardiographic, and exercise predictors of outcome. Circulation. 1997;95:2262–70.

Pagé A, Dumesnil JG, Clavel MA, et al. Metabolic syndrome is associated with more pronounced impairment of LV geometry and function in patients with calcific aortic stenosis: a substudy of the ASTRONOMER trial. (Aortic Stenosis Progression Observation Measuring Effects of Rosuvastatin). J Am Coll Cardiol. 2010;55:1867–74.

Pai RG, Varadarajan P, Razzouk A. Survival benefit of aortic valve replacement in patients with severe aortic stenosis with low ejection fraction and low gradient with normal ejection fraction. Ann Thorac Surg. 2008;86:1781–9.

Pibarot P, Dumesnil JG. Improving assessment of aortic stenosis. J Am Coll Cardiol. 2012a (in press).

Pibarot P, Dumesnil JG. Low-flow, low-gradient aortic stenosis in normal and depressed LV ejection fraction. J Am Coll Cardiol. 2012b (in press).

Picano E, Pibarot P, Lancellotti P, Monin JL, Bonow RO. The emerging role of exercise testing and stress echocardiography in valvular heart disease. J Am Coll Cardiol. 2009;54:2251–60.

Poulsen SH, Sogaard P, Nielsen-Kudsk JE, Egeblad H. Recovery of left ventricular systolic longitudinal strain after valve replacement in aortic stenosis and relation to natriuretic peptides. J Am Soc Echocardiogr. 2007;20:877–84.

Rahimtoola SH. Determining that aortic valve stenosis is severe: back-to-the-future: physical examination and aortic valve area index/energy loss index 0.6 cm2/m2. JACC Cardiovasc Imaging. 2010;3:563–6.

Rajamannan NM, Bonow RO, Rahimtoola SH. Calcific aortic stenosis: an update. Nat Clin Pract Cardiovasc Med. 2007;4:254–62.

Rosenhek R, Binder T, Porenta G, et al. Predictors of outcome in severe, asymptomatic aortic stenosis. N Engl J Med. 2000;343:611–7.

Rosenhek R, Zilberszac R, Schemper M, et al. Natural history of very severe aortic stenosis. Circulation. 2010;121:151–6.

Ross Jr J, Braunwald E. Aortic stenosis. Circulation. 1968;38:61–7.

Rossebo AB, Pedersen TR, Boman K, et al. Intensive lipid lowering with simvastatin and ezetimibe in aortic stenosis. N Engl J Med. 2008;359:1343–56.

Spevack DM, Almuti K, Ostfeld R, Bello R, Gordon GM. Routine adjustment of doppler echocardiographically derived aortic valve area using a previously derived equation to account for the effect of pressure recovery. J Am Soc Echocardiogr. 2008;21:34–7.

Steadman CD, Ray S, Ng LL, McCann GP. Natriuretic peptides in common valvular heart disease. J Am Coll Cardiol. 2010;55:2034–48.

Takeda S, Rimington H, Smeeton N, Chambers J. Long axis excursion in aortic stenosis. Heart. 2001;86:52–6.

Tongue AG, Dumesnil JG, Laforest I, Thériault C, Durand LG, Pibarot P. Left ventricular longitudinal shortening in patients with aortic stenosis: relationship with symptomatic status. J Heart Valve Dis. 2003;12:142–9.

Tribouilloy C, Levy F, Rusinaru D, et al. Outcome after aortic valve replacement for low-flow/low-gradient aortic stenosis without contractile reserve on dobutamine stress echocardiography. J Am Coll Cardiol. 2009;53:1865–73.

Vahanian A, Baumgartner H, Bax J, et al. Guidelines on the management of valvular heart disease: the Task Force on the Management of Valvular Heart Disease of the European Society of Cardiology. Eur Heart J. 2007;28:230–68.

Van Pelt NC, Stewart RA, Legget ME, et al. Longitudinal left ventricular contractile dysfunction after exercise in aortic stenosis. Heart. 2007;93:732–8.

Vanderheyden M, Goethals M, Verstreken S. Wall stress modulates brain natriuretic peptide production in pressure overload cardiomyopathy. J Am Coll Cardiol. 2004;44:2349–54.

Weber M, Hausen M, Arnold R, et al. Prognostic value of N-terminal pro-B-type natriuretic peptide for conservatively and surgically treated patients with aortic valve stenosis. Heart. 2006;92:1639–44.

Weidemann F, Herrmann S, Stork S, et al. Impact of myocardial fibrosis in patients with symptomatic severe aortic stenosis. Circulation. 2009;120:577–84.

Balloon Aortic Valvuloplasty

9

M. Chrissoheris and K. Spargias

Introduction

Balloon aortic valvuloplasty (BAV) refers to transcatheter balloon dilatation of valvular aortic stenosis (AS) in order to alleviate the mechanical impediment to left ventricular outflow and provide relief from heart failure symptomatology. The procedure has been applied successfully in congenital aortic valve stenosis (Fratz et al. 2008) and has been studied extensively in calcific degenerative aortic stenosis in adults (Safian et al. 1988a; McKay et al. 1987; Cribier et al. 1986; Berland et al. 1989; Bernard et al. 1990; American Heart Association 1991; Kuntz et al. 1992) were its role is mostly palliative or as a bridge to more definitive surgical or interventional therapy. After initial enthusiasm following the introduction of the technique in 1985 when it was heralded as a possible viable alternative to surgical aortic valve replacement, BAV fell by the wayside due to recognition of transient improvement in aortic stenosis hemodynamics, associated morbidity and even mortality of the procedure, and failure to alter the natural history of symptomatic aortic stenosis (Lieberman et al. 1995). However after a long period of decline, BAV has had exponential growth in recent years in parallel with the advent of transcatheter aortic valve replacement (Dean 2009; Hara et al. 2007). Refinements in BAV technique have led to improved safety and reduced morbidity and novel applications (e.g. drug coated balloons (Spargias et al. 2009a)) are being developed.

M. Chrissoheris, M.D. (✉) • K. Spargias, M.D.
Transcatheter Heart Valve Department,
HYGEIA Hospital,
N. Attikis, Greece
e-mail: mchrissoheris@hotmail.com

Pathology of Aortic Stenosis and Restenosis Following BAV

The normal aortic valve leaflet consists of a 3-layer architecture (ventricularis, spongiosa, fibrosa) and the process of degenerative aortic stenosis has been shown in histologic studies to be rather similar to the process of atherosclerosis (Hara et al. 2007). Early valve lesions consist of subendothelial thickening on the aortic side with extracellular lipid (oxidized LDL, lipoprotein (a) and protein accumulation as well as extracellular mineralization (Dal-Bianco et al. 2008). In addition, a cellular infiltrate is also present consisting of macrophages and lipid laden foam cells as well as T lymphocytes. Initial endothelial injury is thought to be related mechanical forces from shear stress and abnormal flow patterns. Despite similarities with atherosclerosis, differences are noted including more prominent micromineralization in AS (Otto et al. 1994a). In all, degenerative AS is an active process, not an isolated "wear and tear" phenomenon. In addition to valve leaflet calcification, there is also extravalvular calcification of the aortic root that decreases the mobility of valve leaflets; finally,

N.M. Rajamannan (ed.), *Cardiac Valvular Medicine*,
DOI 10.1007/978-1-4471-4132-7_9, © Springer-Verlag London 2013

overall longitudinal remodeling of the aortic root has been described in patients with severe AS (Akhtar et al. 2009).

The mechanism of BAV is related to intraleaflet fractures within calcified nodular deposits, improved leaflet hinge point mobility within the aortic root, scattered leaflet microfractures and less commonly separation of fused leaflets (Hara et al. 2007; Ben-Dor et al. 2010; Dorros et al. 1990). Additionally, enhanced compliance of the rigidly calcified adjacent root may also contribute. Following successful BAV, the process of restenosis sets in with scar tissue filling up splits between commissures, small tears, lacerations in collagenous valve stroma and fractures in calcifications (Kuntz et al. 1992; Dorros et al. 1990; Feldman et al. 1993; van den Brand et al. 1992). Both the process of calcific aortic stenosis as well as restenosis following BAV are active, and thus potentially modifiable (Otto et al. 1994a).

In contrast to calcific AS, congenital aortic stenosis is caused by fusion of one or more commissures leading to a bicuspid or unicuspid valve. The mechanism of BAV in congenital AS is considered to be splitting of fused commissures leading to improved leaflet mobility but with the possibility of inducing variable degrees of aortic regurgitation.

Acute Hemodynamic and Functional Outcomes

The acute hemodynamic effects of BAV have been studied extensively especially in the early era when the procedure was first applied in calcific aortic stenosis. On average BAV increases the aortic valve area by 50% and decreases the peak transaortic gradient by 30–50% (Kuntz et al. 1992). In the NHLBI registry (American Heart Association 1991), effective aortic valve area (AVA) increased from 0.5 ± 02 to 0.8 ± 0.3 cm^2 with a reduction in peak to peak transaortic gradient from 65 ± 28 to 31 ± 18 mmHg and in the mean gradient from 55 ± 21 to 29 ± 13 mmHg. Similarly in the Mansfield registry (McKay 1991), AVA increased from 0.50 ± 0.18 to 0.82 ± 0.30 cm^2, with a reduction in mean gradient from 60 ± 23 to 30 ± 13 mmHg and an improvement in cardiac output from 3.86 ± 1.26 to 4.05 ± 1.31 lt/min. In the series from Mount Sinai Hospital (Agarwal et al. 2005), AVA increased from 0.61 ± 0.19 to 1.2 ± 0.3 cm^2, with a drop in peak pressure gradient from 55 ± 22 to 20 ± 11 mmHg and with an increase in cardiac output from 4 ± 1 to 5 ± 2 l/min. In a more contemporary series (n = 262) (Ben-Dor et al. 2010) that reflects refinements in the BAV technique the AVA as measured hemodynamically increased from 0.58 ± 0.3 to 0.96 ± 0.3 cm^2 and the mean gradient decreased from 46.3 ± 19.7 to 21.4 ± 12.4 mmHg. The average increase in AVA for de novo BAV was noted to be 0.41 ± 0.24 cm^2. For repeated BAV procedures the improvement in AVA was noted to be less than for first time BAV with a mean increase of 0.28 ± 0.24 cm^2. In aggregate, the BAV procedure leads to highly statistically significant but hemodynamically modest improvements in AVA and transvalvular gradients, that for most patients remain in the severe stenosis range (albeit less severe) (Otto et al. 1994b). Other parameters of hemodynamic interest include changes in left ventricular filling pressures, improvement in systolic and mean pulmonary artery pressure and overall increase in cardiac output (Ben-Dor et al. 2010; Agarwal et al. 2005).

It is important to point that during BAV a brief ischemic period develops due to drop in coronary perfusion pressure, increased wall stress, and rapid ventricular pacing. Following BAV, a drop in the afterload of the left ventricle occurs due to increase in AVA as well as due to reflex vasodilation from baroreceptor stimulation and release of humoral factors. In addition a decrease in preload may occur due to vasodilation and volume/blood loss that leads to decreased left ventricular (LV) filling pressures. These hemodynamic changes are reflected on a decrease in left ventricular peak systolic pressure, as well as in the left ventricular end-diastolic pressure and volume, and should be taken into account when assessing the acute effect of BAV (American Heart Association 1991).

Of particular interest is the group of patients with LV systolic dysfunction and severe aortic stenosis. BAV often leads to significant improvement in ejection fraction (EF) with corresponding clinical improvement (Berland et al. 1989; Safian et al. 1988b). In the study by Berland et al. (1989) of 55 patients with an EF < 40%, BAV resulted in increase of AVA from 0.47 ± 0.15 to 0.83 ± 0.27 cm^2, the peak gradient declined from 66 ± 24 to 28 ± 14 mmHg and the EF increased from 29 ± 7 to 34 ± 9 mmHg. In the study by Safian et al. (1988b) of 28 patients, with baseline EF 37 ± 11% that underwent valvuloplasty, AVA increased from 0.5 ± 0.1 cm^2 to 0.9 ± 0.2 cm^2, peak to peak gradient declined from 69 ± 25 mmHg to 35 ± 15mmHg and the cardiac output increased from 4.2 ± 1.1 l/min to 4.8 ± 1.6 l/min. More importantly the EF (measured by MUGA) improved in aggregate from 37 ± 11 to 44 ± 14% (at 48 h). However in both these studies and although on average there was improvement in EF, there was a subset of patients that showed no improvement in systolic function and these were patients that were characterized by adverse and advanced left ventricular remodeling with higher left ventricular end diastolic volumes and dimensions with corresponding higher wall stress. Furthermore, it has been shown that NT–pro-BNP levels decline in direct correlation to the decrease in the transvalvular pressure gradient after BAV in patients with AS at high surgical risk (Spargias et al. 2009b).

Intermediate-Long Term Hemodynamic and Functional Outcomes

Following successful BAV with the associated clinical and hemodynamic improvement, a significant number of patients develop restenosis, i.e. a loss of >50% of the gain in AVA from the original BAV (Kuntz et al. 1992). Repeat catheterization at 6 months in patients with recurrent symptoms reveals that AVA has returned to baseline levels in up to 80% (Otto et al. 1994b). Even in asymptomatic patients with sustained clinical improvement, cardiac catheterization shows a return to baseline AVA in up to 62% (American Heart Association 1991). In the NHLBI study (Otto et al. 1994b), although AVA and mean gradients had improved from 0.57 ± 0.21 to 0.78 ± 0.31 cm^2 and from 49 ± 16 to 38 ± 14 mmHg respectively following BAV, at 6 months AVA had decreased to 0.65 ± 0.15 cm^2 and mean gradients had risen to 43 ± 15 mmHg. The high overall restenosis rate reflects also on the inability of BAV to alter the natural history of symptomatic severe calcific aortic stenosis with lack of any significant difference in survival between patients undergoing valvuloplasty vs. no intervention at all (Cubeddu et al. 2009). Predictors of mortality post BAV have been identified as NYHA IV functional status, degree of LV systolic dysfunction, coronary artery disease, renal failure, pulmonary hypertension, systolic BP< 100 mmHg, low cardiac output (<3.0 l/min) (Otto et al. 1994b; O'Neill 1991) In all, 6-month mortality has been reported as high as 52.9% in a more contemporary series of patients, with worse outcomes for patients with final AVA post BAV of less than <1.0 cm^2 and patients that did not proceed to have TAVI or surgical AVR (Ben-Dor et al. 2010).

BAV Techniques

The procedure of BAV has been refined in recent years in order to enhance patient safety and outcomes.

Access

In the majority of patients treated, a retrograde (or "arterial") approach (Cubeddu et al. 2009) is utilized via the femoral artery (rarely from the brachial or axillary artery). If a double balloon technique (Dorros et al. 1990) is employed then access will need to be obtained from both femoral arteries. An alternative is the antegrade ("venous") approach (Cubeddu et al. 2009) which was initially developed in order to minimize complications at the arterial access site, and involves access through the femoral vein and transeptal puncture to gain access to the left side of the heart. Arterial access sheaths depend on choice of balloon and range between 7 and 14F. Vascular closure devices (suture based or collagen plug devices) are often employed to minimize bleeding and other vascular complications (Agarwal et al. 2005;

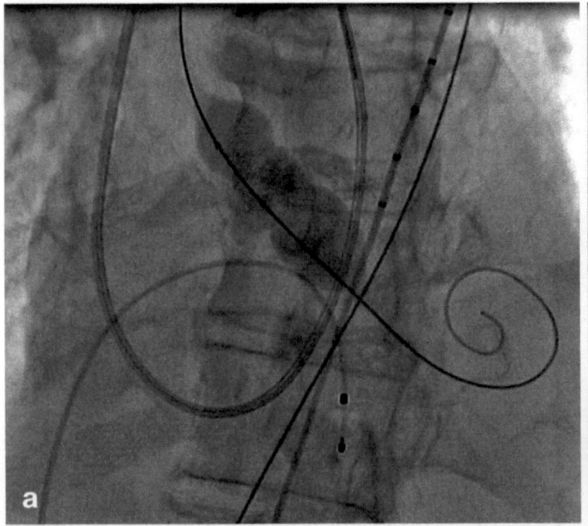

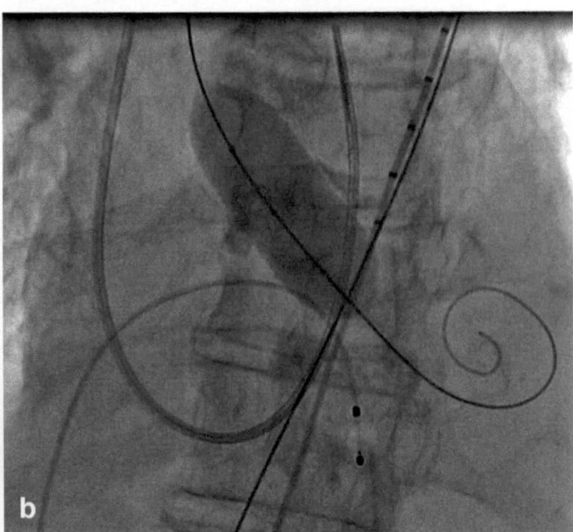

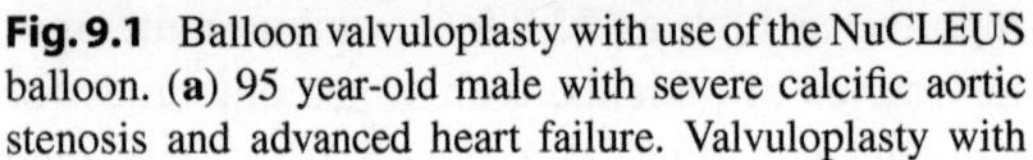

Fig. 9.1 Balloon valvuloplasty with use of the NuCLEUS balloon. (**a**) 95 year-old male with severe calcific aortic stenosis and advanced heart failure. Valvuloplasty with 20×40 mm NUCLEUS balloon. Note the hour-glass appearance that allows for improved stability during valvuloplasty. (**b**) Appearance at peak balloon inflation

Witzke et al. 2010). Antithrombotic therapy is usually administered with unfractionated heparin at a dose of 10–70 iu/kg after sheath insertion to the femoral arteries with a goal activated clotting time (ACT) ≥250 s (Witzke et al. 2010). A key point in the observed substantial decrease in vascular complications over the recent years is better understanding of vascular anatomy prior to BAV procedure as many patients (especially those destined to proceed to TAVI) have had imaging with MDCT, and the better of the two iliofemoral systems is chosen for the procedure. Additionally careful puncture of the femoral artery with micropuncture systems or with use of hydrophilic wires from the contralateral side to delineate the course of the artery have also led to substantial decrease in vascular complications.

Balloon Types

Single balloon is most commonly utilized, with double balloon technique less often employed. The length of the balloon is important as longer balloons up to 40 mm provide more reliable seating and more efficient BAV with less instances of rapid ventricular pacing. The diameter of the balloon is chosen not to exceed the diameter of the annulus as measured by transthoracic echocardiography to minimize risk of annulus rupture (Cubeddu et al. 2009). In the past the balloon diameter was chosen also to be less than the measured diameter of the sinotubular junction. A significant improvement in balloon design is the hour-glass design of the Nucleus balloon (NuMED) (Fig. 9.1) that enhances stability during inflation and may even preclude the use of rapid pacing in some patients (Hamid et al. 2010). The balloons are delivered over preshaped extra stiff Amplatz wires that form a wide loop in the left ventricle to minimize risk of ventricular rupture, and are inflated with a mixture of saline with contrast at a ratio of 8:1 to ensure rapid inflation-deflation times. (Table 9.1 provides list with commercially available valvuloplasty balloons).

Rapid Ventricular Pacing

The introduction of rapid ventricular pacing aims to transiently suppress mechanical contraction of the left ventricle and provide precise and stable balloon positioning during valvuloplasty (Witzke et al. 2010). Pacing at a rate between 180 and 200/min is performed with temporary pacemaker wire at the RV apex and once systolic blood pressure drops to below 50–60 mmHg and pulse pressure below 15 mmHg, valvuloplasty is performed for

Table 9.1 Currently available balloons for valvuloplasty

Balloon name	Company	Diameter (mm)	Length (cm)	Introducer size (F)	Rated burst (Atm)	Compliance
CRISTAL	BALT	15–40	4–6	8–10	3–6	Semi-compliant
VACS II	OSYPKA AG	4–30	2–6	7–10	1.5–6	Non-compliant
VACS III		5–25	2–5		4–15	
Z-MED	NuMED	2–40	2–8	6–16	1–10	Non-compliant
Z-MED X		8–30	2–6	7–13	2–10	
Z-MED II		4.0–30	2–10	5–16	3–15	
Z-MED IIX		8–30	2–6	7–16	3–15	
NuCLEUS		10–30	3–6	7–14	2–9	
NuCLEUS-X		18–30	4–6	10–14	2–4	
Transfemoral	EDWARDS	20–23	4	14	6	Non-compliant
Transapical		20	3	14	6	

5–10 s. Rapid pacing enhances the efficiency of the procedure minimizing the risk of balloon migration and hence fewer inflations are needed. Although concerns had been raised regarding the potential of rapid pacing to trigger myocardial ischemia and ventricular stunning, in practice no significant differences were seen in adverse events when compared to BAV without rapid pacing, and there were fewer balloon inflation requirements.

Balloon Inflation

In the era of rapid pacing, balloon inflation is performed for 5–10 s, whereas in the past prior to rapid pacing, balloon inflations were more prolonged (up to 60 s) if the systolic BP was maintained over 60 mmHg (Berland et al. 1989). Goals of adequate BAV were a decrease in mean pressure gradient of 30–40% or a visually assessed "optimal" balloon inflation (defined as visual decrease in the balloon waist within the aortic valve during maximal balloon inflation). If need for repeat balloon inflation, a minimum of 3 minutes for hemodynamic recovery is allowed between inflations.

BAV Complications

One of the main reasons that BAV fell by the wayside in the past was not only the lack of any substantial impact on the natural history of symptomatic calcific AS, but also its association with perioperative morbidity and mortality. In the NHLBI registry (American Heart Association 1991) of 674 patients from 1989, death occurred in 3% of treated patients within 24 h of the procedure and in up to 8% cumulative at discharge. Major morbidity occurred in 25% of patients with the majority being related to vascular complications with need for transfusion. Other important complications included stroke in 2%, coronary occlusion or dissection in 1%, persistent hypotension in 8%, moderate or severe aortic regurgitation (caused by leaflet avulsion or annulus rupture) in 1%, VT/VF requiring defibrillation in 3%, vascular surgery in 5%, systemic embolism in 2%, AV block requiring pacing in 4% and need for intubation in 4%. In a more contemporary patient series (Ben-Dor et al. 2010) (2000–2009) reflecting refinements in technique, complication rates were significantly less, with intraprocedural death in 1.6%, stroke in 1.99%, moderate or severe AR in 1.3%, profound hypotension requiring CPR in 1.6%, tamponade in 0.3%, permanent pacemaker in 0.99% and serious vascular complication requiring intervention in 6.9%. The decline in serious vascular complications was attributed to smaller size sheaths (8–10F vs. 12–14F), vascular closure devices, and the use of multidetector computed tomography (MDCT) for peripheral vascular imaging. In total, severe complication rate in this contemporary series was 16.2%, significantly less than the previously reported as high as 31%. In addition, length of hospital stay was a mean of 4 days, whereas in the NHLBI registry was 7.6 days.

BAV Current Indications: Newer Applications

Current Indications

BAV for calcific aortic stenosis has been given a class IIb recommendation ("might be reasonable") as a bridge to surgery in hemodynamically unstable adult patients who are at high risk for AVR, or as a palliative procedure in those unable to undergo AVR due to serious comorbid conditions (Bonow et al. 2008). For children and young adults with congenital aortic stenosis (due to commissural fusion rather than calcific degeneration) BAV has been given a class I indication for symptomatic patients with peak to peak gradients >50 mmHg (or >60 mmHg if otherwise asymptomatic) (Bonow et al. 2008).

Newer Applications

Transcatheter aortic valve implantation is an established treatment for symptomatic severe calcific aortic in patients considered inoperable (Leon et al. 2010) or at high (but not prohibitive) (Smith et al. 2011) surgical risk. Valvuloplasty is commonly performed in order to pave the way for the subsequent prosthetic valve implantation. There are several key information provided by BAV that include:

- Assessment of annulus size (Babaliaros et al. 2008, 2010): Annulus sizing most commonly is performed during transthoracic/transesophageal echocardiography. However, there is often uncertainty about the true size of the annulus and choice of the correct prosthesis size. A prosthesis that is "small" for the annulus may lead to more paravalvular regurgitation, patient-prosthesis mismatch, or device embolization. On the other hand, a prosthesis that is "big" for the annulus may lead to injury or even rupture of the aortic root with detrimental outcome. It has been shown that BAV may be used to size the annulus either by measuring for added external pressure applied to the balloon during inflation, or with performance of contrast injection (Fig. 9.2) within the aortic root during balloon inflation to assess for regurgitation that would indicate incomplete sealing.
- Efficacy of rapid ventricular pacing: Rapid pacing during deployment of the balloon expandable valves is critical to ensure stable positioning. It is not uncommon to see that rapid pacing may not be as effective in suppressing mechanical ventricular systole at a particular rate and that faster pacing may be needed. Additionally problems with capturing may be anticipated during BAV and repositioning of the temporary wire may be performed.
- Anticipation of possible complications (coronary occlusion, sigmoid septum, potential for aortic injury): During TAVI the thickened and calcified native aortic valve leaflets are pushed to the side and serve to support and anchor the prosthesis in place. However there should be enough space in the sinuses of Valsalva to accommodate for the native leaflets without risking occlusion of the coronary ostia. During BAV we can assess the motion pattern of the calcified cusps and during simultaneous contrast injection anticipate potential complications (proximity to coronary ostia, sinotubular junction etc.).

In addition to the above, BAV may be utilized for post-dilatation following deployment of the valve prosthesis when there is evidence of incomplete valve expansion or significant paravalvular regurgitation.

Balloon sizes used for BAV during TAVI procedures are selected based on estimated annulus sizing by echocardiography or other 3D techniques. For the Edwards 23 mm prosthesis a 20×40 mm balloon and for the 26 mm prosthesis a 23×40 mm balloon is provided within the valve kit, when the transfemoral route is chosen. When the transapical or transaortic approach is used, then a 20×30 mm balloon is provided for all prostheses sizes. For the self-expandable Core Valve prostheses, the diameter of the balloon is based on the annulus size and a variety of commercially available balloons may be used.

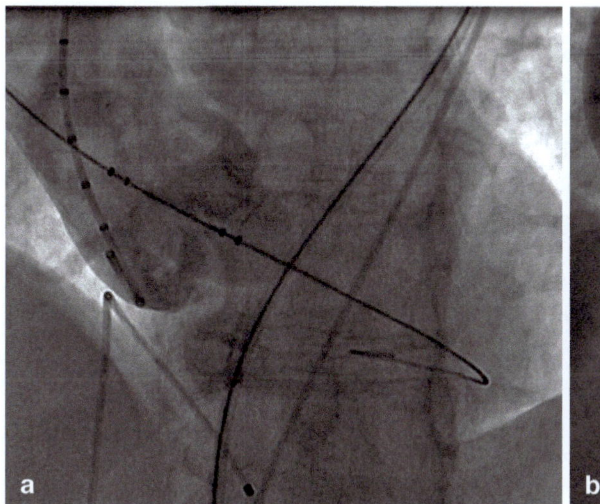

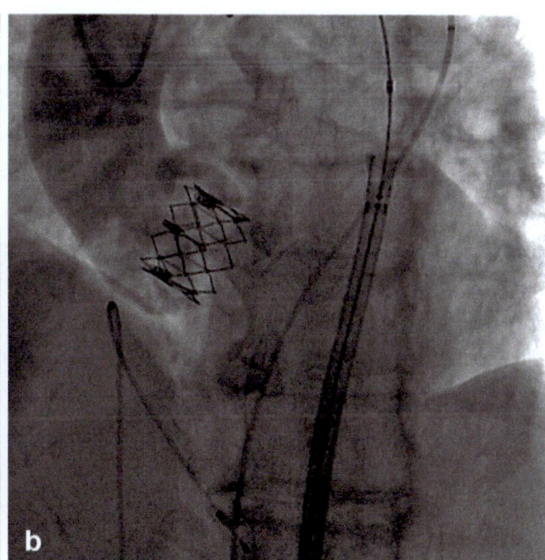

Fig. 9.2 In patients undergoing transcatheter aortic valve implantation, balloon valvuloplasty is useful for assessment of annulus size. During peak balloon inflation, an injection of contrast in the proximal ascending aorta allows for assessment of aortic regurgitation suggestive of annulus size larger than balloon diameter. Complete sealing, i.e. lack of aortic regurgitation suggests annulus size at most equal to balloon diameter. In addition, simultaneous contrast aortography and balloon valvuloplasty offers important information regarding patency of coronary ostia, and efficacy of rapid pacing, (**a**) Synchronous contrast aortography. Annulus by TEE measured at 24 mm. Balloon valvuloplasty with a 23×30 mm balloon. Lack of aortic regurgitation noted suggesting adequate sealing of the annulus. Flow was noted in both coronary arteries. (**b**) Subsequently a 26 mm Sapien XT valve was deployed without angiographic paravalvular regurgitation

Drug Coated Valvuloplasty Balloons

In general, the process of calcific aortic stenosis has been shown to be the final result of three interrelated events: (1) Classical cardiovascular risk factors, (2) Genetic factors (Bosse et al. 2008), and (3) Valve biology (Rajamannan 2009). Together these factors lead to the final common pathway, the development of the calcifying osteoblast phenotype. The Achilles tendon of BAV is restenosis which leads to recurrence of symptoms in the majority of patients treated. Restenosis following BAV has been attributed to elastic recoil and prolonged scaring of the valve leaflets with evidence of fusion of split commissures, myofibroblast cell proliferation, valve thickening and ossification (Feldman et al. 1993; van den Brand et al. 1992). Thus both the process of calcific aortic stenosis and the process of restenosis following balloon valvuloplasty are active processes and potentially amenable to pharmacologic intervention. Following successful application of antiproliferative medications (Herdeg et al. 2000) (e.g. paclitaxel, sirolimus, everolimus) in the treatment of coronary artery disease with both drug coated stents as well as drug coated balloons (Scheller et al. 2004), there is developing interest in the application of drug coated valvuloplasty balloons. Experimental data have shown that therapeutic levels of the antiproliferative drug paclitaxel can be successfully delivered to the aortic valve leaflets following balloon valvuloplasty with specialized drug coated balloons (Spargias et al. 2009a). Furthermore, in experimental animal models of aortic stenosis (Spargias et al. 2012), balloon aortic valvuloplasty with paclitaxel coated balloons led to amelioration of the otherwise inevitable restenotic process with evidence of reduced extracellular matrix synthesis, cell proliferation and calcification in the paclitaxel-balloon treated leaflets that culminated in the following cellular and hemodynamic findings: (1) decreased leaflet thickness, (2) larger aortic valve area, (3) diminished stroke work loss and (4) decreased aortic valve resistance. These observations suggest that local paclitaxel delivery attenuated the myofibroblast osteogenic differentiation driving the restenosis process and typically seen following BAV with a plain balloon. Future studies will be needed to further evaluate the clinical implications of these findings and the possibility to offer palliative improvement in AS patients with limited life expectancy who may not be candidates for more definitive surgical or transcatheter aortic valve implantation.

References

Agarwal A, Kini AS, Attanti S, et al. Results of repeat balloon valvuloplasty for treatment of aortic stenosis in patients aged 59 to 104 years. Am J Cardiol. 2005; 95(1):43–7.

Akhtar M, Tuzcu EM, Kapadia SR, et al. Aortic root morphology in patients undergoing percutaneous aortic valve replacement: evidence of aortic root remodeling. J Thorac Cardiovasc Surg. 2009;137(4):950–6.

Babaliaros VC, Liff D, Chen EP, et al. Can balloon aortic valvuloplasty help determine appropriate transcatheter aortic valve size? JACC Cardiovasc Interv. 2008; 1(5):580–6.

Babaliaros VC, Junagadhwalla Z, Lerakis S, et al. Use of balloon aortic valvuloplasty to size the aortic annulus before implantation of a balloon-expandable transcatheter heart valve. JACC Cardiovasc Interv. 2010; 3(1):114–8.

Ben-Dor I, Pichard AD, Satler LF. Complications and outcome of balloon aortic valvuloplasty in high-risk or inoperable patients. JACC Cardiovasc Interv. 2010; 3(11):1150–6.

Berland J, Cribier A, Savin T, Lefebvre E, Koning R, Letac B. Percutaneous balloon valvuloplasty in patients with severe aortic stenosis and low ejection fraction. Immediate results and 1-year follow-up. Circulation. 1989;79(6):1189–96.

Bernard Y, Bassand JP, Anguenot T. Aortic valve area evolution after percutaneous aortic valvuloplasty. A prospective trial using a combined Doppler echocardiographic and haemodynamic method. Eur Heart J. 1990;11(2):98–107.

Bonow RO, Carabello BA, Chatterjee K. 2008 focused update incorporated into the ACC/AHA 2006 guidelines for the management of patients with valvular heart disease: a report of the American College of Cardiology/American Heart Association Task Force on Practice Guidelines (Writing Committee to revise the 1998 guidelines for the management of patients with valvular heart disease). Endorsed by the Society of Cardiovascular Anesthesiologists, Society for Cardiovascular Angiography and Interventions, and Society of Thoracic Surgeons. J Am Coll Cardiol. 2008;52(13):e1–142.

Bosse Y, Mathieu P, Pibarot P. Genomics: the next step to elucidate the etiology of calcific aortic valve stenosis. J Am Coll Cardiol. 2008;51(14):1327–36.

Cribier A, Savin T, Saoudi N, Rocha P, Berland J, Letac B. Percutaneous transluminal valvuloplasty of acquired aortic stenosis in elderly patients: an alternative to valve replacement? Lancet. 1986;1(8472):63–7.

Cubeddu RJ, Jneid H, Don CW, et al. Retrograde versus antegrade percutaneous aortic balloon valvuloplasty: immediate, short- and long-term outcome at 2 years. Catheter Cardiovasc Interv. 2009;74(2):225–31.

Dal-Bianco JP, Khandheria BK, Mookadam F, Gentile F, Sengupta PP. Management of asymptomatic severe aortic stenosis. J Am Coll Cardiol. 2008;52(16):1279–92.

Dean LS. Percutaneous aortic valvuloplasty: resurrection of something old with something new. Catheter Cardiovasc Interv. 2009;74(2):232–3.

Dorros G, Lewin RF, Stertzer SH, et al. Percutaneous transluminal aortic valvuloplasty – the acute outcome and follow-up of 149 patients who underwent the double balloon technique. Eur Heart J. 1990;11(5):429–40.

Feldman T, Glagov S, Carroll JD. Restenosis following successful balloon valvuloplasty: bone formation in aortic valve leaflets. Cathet Cardiovasc Diagn. 1993; 29(1):1–7.

Fratz S, Gildein HP, Balling G. Aortic valvuloplasty in pediatric patients substantially postpones the need for aortic valve surgery: a single-center experience of 188 patients after up to 17.5 years of follow-up. Circulation. 2008;117(9):1201–6.

Hamid T, Eichhofer J, Clarke B, Mahadevan VS. Aortic balloon valvuloplasty: is there still a role in high-risk patients in the era of percutaneous aortic valve replacement? J Interv Cardiol. 2010;23(4):358–61.

Hara H, Pedersen WR, Ladich E, et al. Percutaneous balloon aortic valvuloplasty revisited: time for a renaissance? Circulation. 2007;115(12):e334–8.

Herdeg C, Oberhoff M, Baumbach A, et al. Local paclitaxel delivery for the prevention of restenosis: biological effects and efficacy in vivo. J Am Coll Cardiol. 2000;35(7):1969–76.

Kuntz RE, Tosteson AN, Maitland LA, et al. Immediate results and long-term follow-up after repeat balloon aortic valvuloplasty. Cathet Cardiovasc Diagn. 1992; 25(1):4–9.

Leon MB, Smith CR, Mack M, et al. Transcatheter aortic-valve implantation for aortic stenosis in patients who cannot undergo surgery. N Engl J Med. 2010;363(17): 1597–607.

Lieberman EB, Bashore TM, Hermiller JB, et al. Balloon aortic valvuloplasty in adults: failure of procedure to improve long-term survival. J Am Coll Cardiol. 1995; 26(6):1522–8.

McKay RG. The Mansfield scientific aortic valvuloplasty registry: overview of acute hemodynamic results and procedural complications. J Am Coll Cardiol. 1991; 17(2):485–91.

McKay RG, Safian RD, Lock JE. Assessment of left ventricular and aortic valve function after aortic balloon valvuloplasty in adult patients with critical aortic stenosis. Circulation. 1987;75(1):192–203.

O'Neill WW. Predictors of long-term survival after percutaneous aortic valvuloplasty: report of the mansfield scientific balloon aortic valvuloplasty registry. J Am Coll Cardiol. 1991;17(1):193–8.

Otto CM, Kuusisto J, Reichenbach DD, Gown AM, O'Brien KD. Characterization of the early lesion of 'degenerative' valvular aortic stenosis. Histological and immunohistochemical studies. Circulation. 1994a; 90(2):844–53.

Otto CM, Mickel MC, Kennedy JW, et al. Three-year outcome after balloon aortic valvuloplasty. Insights into prognosis of valvular aortic stenosis. Circulation. 1994b;89(2):642–50.

Percutaneous balloon aortic valvuloplasty. Acute and 30-day follow-up results in 674 patients from the NHLBI Balloon Valvuloplasty Registry. Circulation. 1991;84(6):2383–97.

Rajamannan NM. Calcific aortic stenosis: lessons learned from experimental and clinical studies. Arterioscler Thromb Vasc Biol. 2009;29(2):162–8.

Safian RD, Berman AD, Diver DJ, et al. Balloon aortic valvuloplasty in 170 consecutive patients. N Engl J Med. 1988a;319(3):125–30.

Safian RD, Warren SE, Berman AD, et al. Improvement in symptoms and left ventricular performance after balloon aortic valvuloplasty in patients with aortic stenosis and depressed left ventricular ejection fraction. Circulation. 1988b;78(5 Pt 1):1181–91.

Scheller B, Speck U, Abramjuk C, Bernhardt U, Bohm M, Nickenig G. Paclitaxel balloon coating, a novel method for prevention and therapy of restenosis. Circulation. 2004;110(7):810–4.

Smith CR, Leon MB, Mack MJ, et al. Transcatheter versus surgical aortic-valve replacement in high-risk patients. N Engl J Med. 2011;364(23):2187–98.

Spargias K, Milewski K, Debinski M, et al. Drug delivery at the aortic valve tissues of healthy domestic pigs with a paclitaxel-eluting valvuloplasty balloon. J Interv Cardiol. 2009a;22(3):291–8.

Spargias K, Alexopoulos E, Thomopoulou S, et al. Effect of balloon valvuloplasty in patients with severe aortic stenosis on levels of N-terminal pro-B-type natriuretic peptide. Am J Cardiol. 2009b;104(6):846–9.

Spargias KGM, Hemetsberger R, Posa A, Pavo I, Huber K, Petrasi Z, Petnehazy O, Glogar D, Rajamannan N. Valvuloplasty with a paclitaxel-eluting balloon prevents restenosis in an experimental model of aortic stenosis. EuroIntervention. 2012.

van den Brand M, Essed CE, Di Mario C, et al. Histological changes in the aortic valve after balloon dilatation: evidence for a delayed healing process. Br Heart J. 1992;67(6):445–9.

Witzke C, Don CW, Cubeddu RJ, et al. Impact of rapid ventricular pacing during percutaneous balloon aortic valvuloplasty in patients with critical aortic stenosis: should we be using it? Catheter Cardiovasc Interv. 2010;75(3):444–52.

McKay RG, Safian RD, Lock JE, Mandell VS, Thurer RL, [illegible] valvuloplasty [illegible] Circulation. 1986;74:[illegible]

[illegible]

[illegible] in an experimental model of aortic stenosis. [illegible]

van den Brand M, Essed CE, [illegible] Histological changes in the aortic valve after balloon dilatation: evidence for a delayed healing process. Br Heart J. 1992;67:445–9.

Witzke C, Don CW, Cubeddu RJ, [illegible] Impact of rapid ventricular pacing during percutaneous balloon aortic valvuloplasty in patients with critical aortic stenosis: should we be using it? Catheter Cardiovasc Interv. 2010;75:444–52.

[illegible] patients [illegible] aortic stenosis. Circulation. [illegible]

[illegible] aortic valvuloplasty. [illegible] follow-up results in [illegible] patients [illegible] NHLBI Balloon Valvuloplasty Registry. Circulation. [illegible];84(6):2383–97.

[illegible] aortic [illegible] experimental and clinical studies. [illegible]

Safian RD, Berman AD, Diver DJ, [illegible] Balloon aortic valvuloplasty in 170 consecutive patients. N Engl J Med. 1988;319(3):125–30.

Safian RD, Warren SE, Berman AD, [illegible] Improvement in symptoms and left ventricular performance after balloon aortic valvuloplasty in patients with aortic stenosis and depressed left ventricular ejection fraction. Circulation. 1988;78:1181–91.

Imaging for TAVI

10

Alexandra Gonçalves and José Luis Zamorano

Introduction

Transcatheter aortic valve implantation (TAVI) is a recent technique for the treatment of patients with severe symptomatic AS, who are at high risk for conventional aortic valve replacement or considered inoperable (Vahanian et al. 2008). It is a challenging procedure that requires a multidisciplinary team approach, involving interventional cardiologists, cardiac and vascular surgeons, anesthesiologists and imaging specialists. Currently the Edwards SAPIEN™ and CoreValve™ valve are the prosthesis approved for transcatheter aortic stenosis treatment, both with good clinical and hemodynamic results at short and midterm follow-up (Rodes-Cabau et al. 2010; Leon et al. 2010; Smith et al. 2011). Each valve has specific characteristics and different aortic anatomic requirements, in consequence, imaging plays an essential task for proper patient's selection, decision on procedure access route and also for procedure guidance and patients' follow-up.

Pre-procedure Evaluation

At the time of patients' evaluation for TAVI the assessment of the anatomy of the aortic valve, aorta, and peripheral vasculature will determine the feasibility of the procedure, its best access approach and the prosthesis kind and size.

The Edwards SAPIEN™ valve is a cylindrical stainless steel balloon-expandable stent with three symmetric leaflets, made of bovine pericardium mounted inside (Fig. 10.1a). The stent also has a polyethylene terephthalate fabric skirt that decreases paravalvular leaks and it may be deployed via transfemoral or transapical route. The CoreValve™ ReValving system is a prosthesis made of porcine pericardial tissue sewn to form a trileaflet valve mounted within an asymmetrical self-expanding nitinol frame (Fig. 10.1b). The lower portion of the frame affixes the valve to the left ventricle outflow tract (LVOT), the mid-portion has a constrained waist that must be deployed at the level of the sinuses of Valsalva and coronary ostia with the upper section designed to fix and stabilize the prosthesis in the ascending aorta. The Corevalve™ is designed for arterial access (femoral or subclavian), although there are case reports of deployment using a transapical route

A. Gonçalves, M.D.
Cardiology Department,
University Hospital Ramón y Cajal,
Madrid, Spain

Hospital S. João/University of Porto Medical School,
Porto, Portugal
e-mail: alexandra.mgsg@gmail.com

J.L. Zamorano, M.D., Ph.D., FESC (✉)
Cardiology Department,
University Hospital Ramón y Cajal,
Madrid, Spain
e-mail: zamorano@secardiologia.es

N.M. Rajamannan (ed.), *Cardiac Valvular Medicine*,
DOI 10.1007/978-1-4471-4132-7_10,

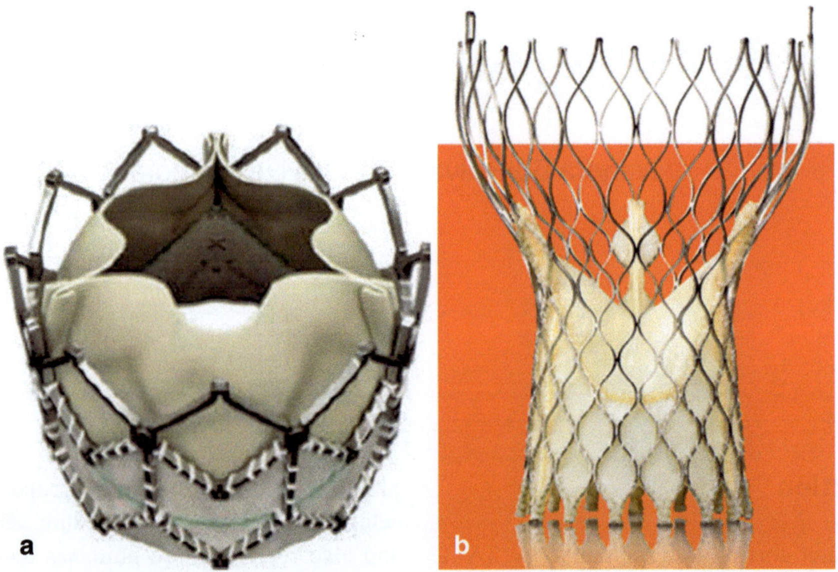

Fig. 10.1 (**a**) The Edward Sapien-XT™ valve (Courtesy from Edwards Lifesciences) and (**b**) The CoreValve™ system (Medtronic copyright, used with permission)

Table 10.1 Aortic anatomical requirements of contemporary transcatheter aortic valve prosthesis

	Prothesis size (mm)	AV annulus (mm)	S. valsalva (mm)	Sino tubular junction (mm)
Core valve	26	20–23	≥27	≤40
	29	23–27	≥28	≤43
	31	26–29	≥28	≤43
Edwards-Sapien	23	18–22	–	–
	26	21–25	–	–
	29	24–27		

(Lange et al. 2007). Both valves are currently available in three sizes, as presented in Table 10.1.

Transthoracic Echocardiography

The transthoracic echocardiography (TTE) evaluation provides anatomic and hemodynamic information. It establishes the presence of severe AS, which is defined by an AVA of ≤1 cm^2 (<0.6 cm^2/m^2) or a mean aortic valve gradient of ≥40 mmHg (Bonow et al. 2008; Vahanian et al. 2007). The left and right ventricular dimensions, morphology and function are also evaluated by TTE. The presence of LV thrombus or a haemodynamically significant LVOT obstruction, due to basal septal hypertrophy should be excluded, as they represent contraindications for the procedure. Subaortic septal bulge may also create an obstacle to proper seating of the aortic prosthesis (Piazza et al. 2008). The existence of a patch in the LV as well as significant pericardial calcification is a contraindication for TAVI using the transapical approach. (Vahanian et al. 2008) In addition, the presence of aortic regurgitation and the structure and function of the other valves should be evaluated and described.

TTE is the first assessment of the aortic annular dimension and anatomic characteristics of the aortic valve. It can be used to describe the number of cusps, mobility, thickness and calcification.

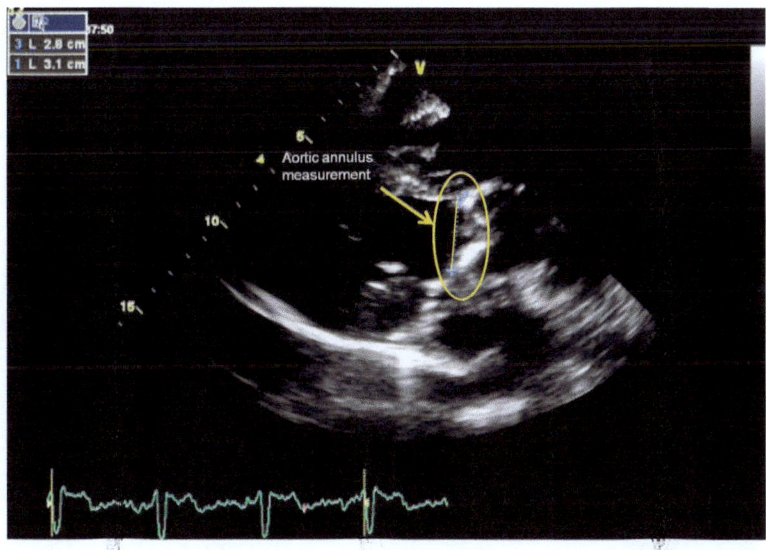

Fig. 10.2 Transthoracic echocardiography parasternal long-axis view for measurement of aortic annular dimension

The presence of a bicuspid aortic valve is still a contra-indication for TAVI because of the risk of spontaneous aortic dissection or incorrect deployment of the aortic prosthesis due to the elliptical valvular orifice. However, successful TAVI in bicuspid AS has already been reported (Delgado et al. 2009).

As presented in Table 10.1 the aortic annulus dimension dictates the eligibility for TAVI and prosthesis size, which is determinant to the procedural success. Using TTE the aortic annular dimension is measured in systole, in a parasternal long-axis view, zoomed on the LVOT, at the point of insertion of the aortic valve cusps, from tissue–blood interface to blood–tissue interface—trailing edge to leading edge (Fig. 10.2) (Zamorano et al. 2011). When TTE measurements of the annulus are doubtful, particularly if measurements are near critical cut-offs for valve selection or if the calcification extends from the aortic valve onto the anterior mitral leaflet or the septum, 2D Transesophageal echocardiography (TEE) and even 3D TEE evaluation may be necessary.

Transesophageal Echocardiography

TEE is recommended prior to TAVI to a better evaluation of the aortic root anatomy, particularly if there are any concerns about the assessment of the aortic annular size and the number of cusps.

The annular diameter at the level of the basal attachment of the aortic valve cusps, measured in systole determines the size of the prosthesis, irrespective of the type of the valve inserted (Table 10.1). There is a good correlation between TEE aortic annular measurements and TTE results; however TTE to some extent underestimates aortic annular size (Messika-Zeitoun et al. 2010).

When measuring the annular diameter with 2D TEE, there is an assumption of annular circularity, which may result in erroneous measurements in patients whose annuli are more oval shaped. This limitation can be overcome using multiplanar tools of 3D TEE (Fig. 10.3) (Zamorano et al. 2011) or multidetector computed tomography (MDCT). The later will be described in detail underneath in MDCT proper section. The final decision for the appropriate valve size mainly considers the annulus diameter, but in cases of borderline size decisions, the existence of large calcification in the native valve, may require a smaller prosthesis than the annular dimension alone would advise. Up to now there is no gold standard imaging technique for annular sizing for TAVI, but from the practical point of view TTE complemented with TEE accomplishes good results in most patients.

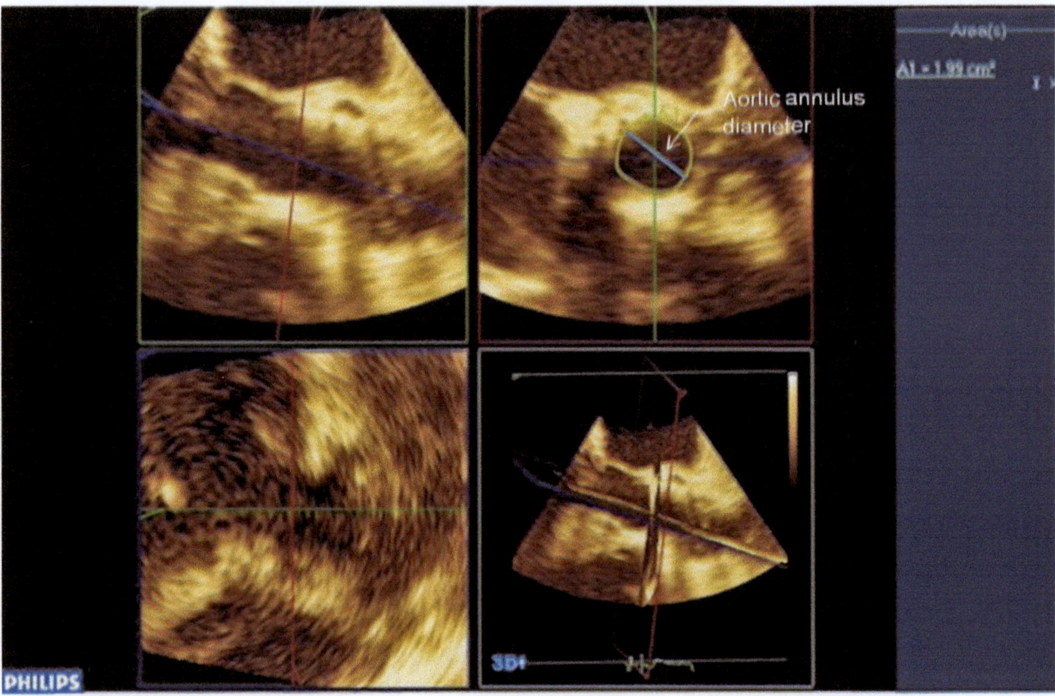

Fig. 10.3 3D Transesophageal echocardiography assessing shape and measurements of the aortic annulus

Using short-axis views of the aortic valve the number of cusps can be precisely illustrated and its opening classified as central or eccentric. It is relevant to describe the severity and eventual asymmetry of calcification, as the differences in the tension–force across the valve may cause asymmetric deployment of the prosthesis and increase the risk of compression of the coronary arteries. However TEE presents constrains at the time of calcification evaluation, being MDCT the best method available. (Schultz et al. 2011a) The distance from the aortic annulus to the ostia of the coronary arteries should be measured, because patients with cusps length larger than annular-ostial distances are at risk of ostial coronary occlusion at time of valve deployment, as the native cusps will be crushed to the side. Only the right coronary annular-ostial distance is possible to measure with 2D TEE, as the left coronary annular-ostial distance requires 3D TEE or MDCT.

Using TEE the characteristics of the ascending aorta, the aortic arch, and the descending thoracic aorta should be considered as the presence of large atheromas may increase the risk of peri-procedural embolization at the time of transfemoral approach.

Multidetector Computed Tomography (MDCT)

MDCT has a complementary role to echocardiography and angiography at the time of evaluation of patients before TAVI (Schwartz et al. 2011). It provides detailed anatomic visualization of the aortic root, thoraco-abdominal aorta and the iliofemoral access. Nevertheless, MDCT imaging is associated with the administration of iodinated contrast and exposure to ionizing radiation exposure, thus its use should be considered for individual patients based on risk and benefit.

Three-dimensional (3D) derived MDCT measurements provide precise dimensions for best prosthesis selection and sizing. Anatomically, the annulus is a crown-shaped 3-dimensional structure rather than a circular plane. As previously described, 2D echocardiography and aortic angiography give the extent of a single diameter, making

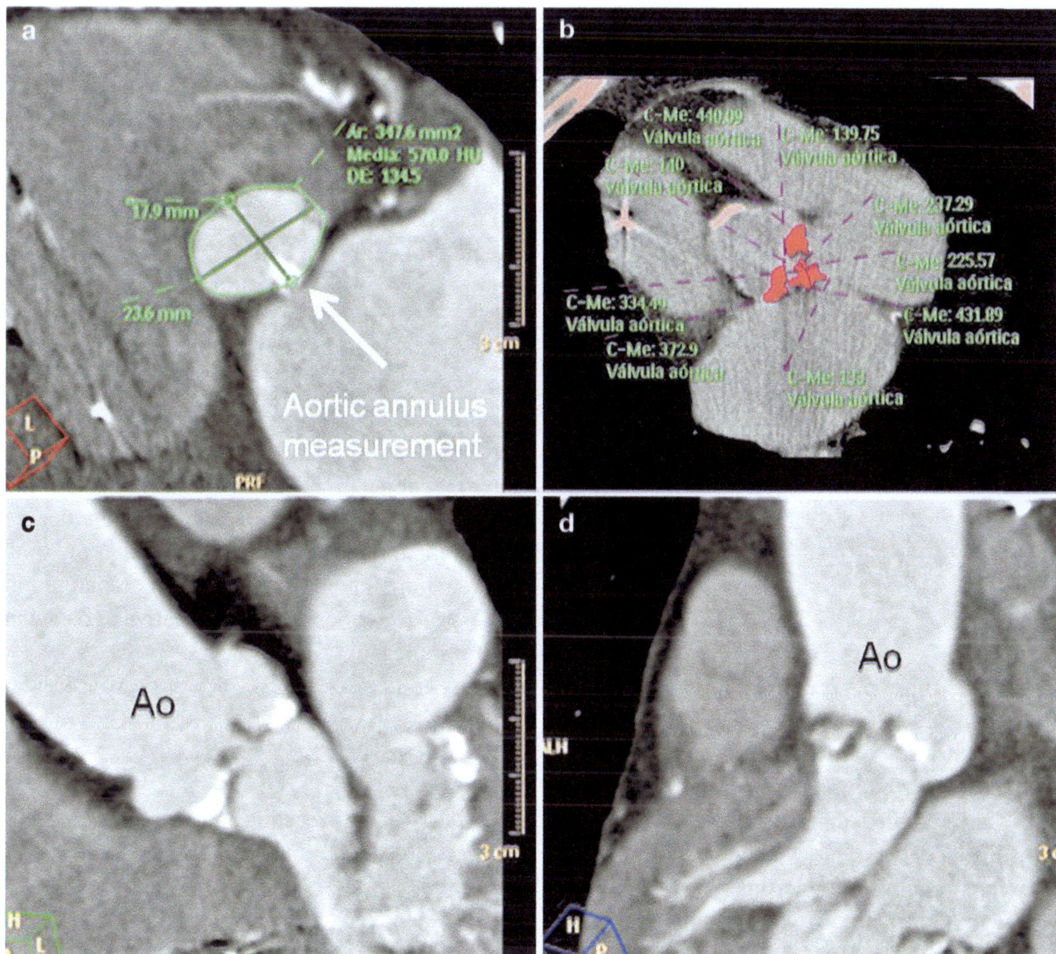

Fig. 10.4 Multidetector computed tomography assessing aortic valve calcification (**b**) and reconstruction of the aortic root (**a**, **c** and **d**) measuring minimal and maximal diameters, circumference and area at the level of aortic annulus (**a**). *Ao* aorta (Courtesy of Dr. Pedro Marcos-Alberca)

the assumption of annular orifice circularity. In contrast, 3D MDCT reconstruction of the annulus, orthogonal to the centre-axis of the LVOT, allows the assessment of minimal and maximal diameters, circumference and area measurements (Fig. 10.4). Although the use of 3D MDCT measurements for best prosthesis sizing may reduce the probability of error and present a more comprehensive definition of the annular size and shape, the mean of the maximum and minimum diameter measurements is comparable to 2D TEE measurement, remaining 2D TEE the most used technique (Messika-Zeitoun et al. 2010).

Moreover, the aortic valve can be assessed in detail, and its morphology precisely described, regarding the number of cusps and the aortic valve area, measured by planimetry. In comparison with echocardiography, MDCT has the ability to provide precise description of localization and extent of aortic cusps calcification. The relation between aortic valve calcification and pos TAVI paravalvular aortic regurgitation have been described, being paravalvular aortic regurgitation associated with a larger aortic annulus and with more severe aortic root calcification (Schultz et al. 2011a). Furthermore, dense aortic leaflet calcification measured on contrast MDCT discerned the need for an additional balloon post-dilatation, when using CoreValve™, for significant paravalvular regurgitation reduction (Schultz et al. 2011b).

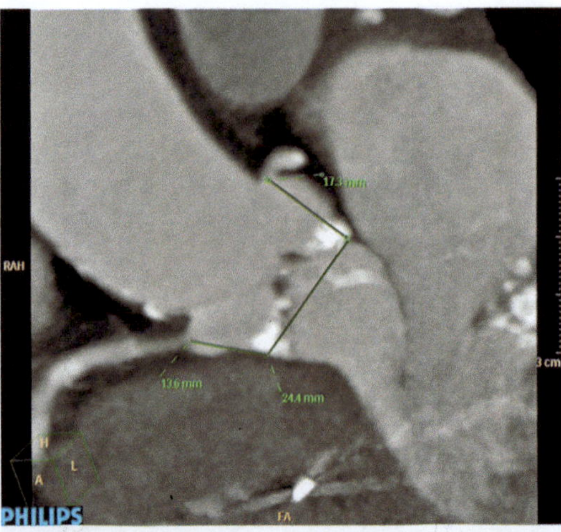

Fig. 10.5 Multidetector computed tomography measuring the distance between annulus and coronary ostia (Courtesy of Dr. Pedro Marcos-Alberca)

At the time of pre-procedural evaluation, MDCT includes a complete assessment of coronary anatomy with conventional coronary angiography, which generally is limited by the advanced calcified disease. However, the relationship between leaflet height and distance between annulus and coronary ostia, can be accurately measured, identifying patients at higher risk for coronary occlusion during the procedure, when the annulus- coronary ostia distance is <11 mm (Fig. 10.5).

The thoracic aorta evaluation is completed by the measurement of the aortic sinus diameter, sinotubular junction and ascending and descending aorta, using centerline reconstructions. The presence of significant aneurismal dilatation is considered a contraindication for the use of CoreValve (Table 10.1). Precise coaxial alignment of the prosthesis along the centerline of the aortic valve and aortic root is important during positioning to decrease the likelihood of complications as prosthesis embolization. MDCT offers the assessment of the aortic root in relation to the body axis and its pre-procedural angle prediction may decrease the number of aortograms required during the procedure, therefore shortening procedure time and contrast usage (Gurvitch et al. 2010).

Finally, MDCT allows the assessment of peripheral vasculature, considering caliber, tortuosity and calcification, being the minimum caliber of the common femoral artery dependent on the size of the prosthesis valve chosen. Using the previous Edward Sapien™ valve it was necessary a common femoral artery with a minimum of 8 mm of diameter, currently a minimum of 6 mm is required for both Edwards-XT™ and CoreValve™. Tortuosity and calcification are not prohibitive factors, but its combination is an adverse feature for site complications and central embolization. In addition the location of the bifurcation of the femoral artery and the degree of calcification have to be considered at the time of deciding the feasibility of the transfemoral access or for choosing the alternative subclavian or transapical approach.

Angiography

Previously to the procedure, aortography produces images of the coronary arteries, thoracic and abdominal aorta. It allows the measurement of vessel diameters, tortuosity and excludes the presence of aorta aneurism. Nevertheless, at time of measuring vessels calcification, angiography presents limitations, being MDCT the best method.

Fluoroscopy is used for measurement of aortic annulus, at the time of definitive prosthesis sizing decision and to guide the procedure. The alignment of the three aortic sinuses in the same plane defines the optimal plane and angiography projection for TAVI.

Peri-procedural Echocardiography During Transcatheter Aortic Valve Implantation

Peri-procedural 2D and 3D TEE can contribute for balloon and prosthesis positioning, to confirm prosthesis function immediately after

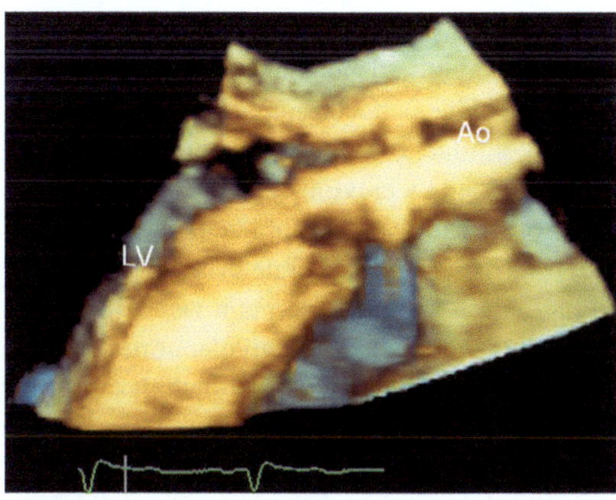

Fig. 10.6 3D Transesophageal echocardiography showing the catheter and the balloon through the native aortic valve. *Ao* aorta, *LV* left ventricle

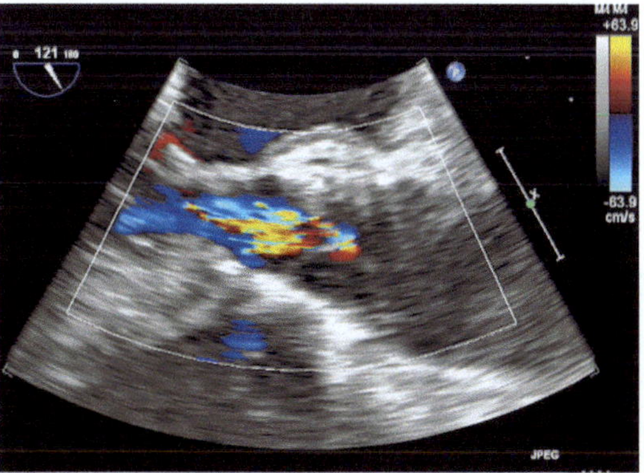

Fig. 10.7 2D transesophageal echocardiography showing aortic prosthesis central regurgitation

implantation and to rapidly detect complications. As in other intervention TEE guided procedures, the use of 3D, by its larger special resolution, presents advantages over 2D. It allows a better visualization of the guide wire path through the LV and around the mitral valve and subvalvular apparatus and permits a better evaluation of the prosthesis position on the balloon, relative to the native valve annulus and surrounding structures (Fig. 10.6).

At the time of valvuloplasty, TEE guidance is especially useful when the valve is not very calcified, as those valves are difficult to image on fluoroscopy and easy observed by TEE. The balloon inflation is performed during rapid right ventricular pacing, though the balloon may accidentally migrate during inflation. TEE can be used to confirm a secure position during inflation and to monitor the behaviour of the balloon and its effect on the calcified aortic cusps during inflation. During deployment of the prosthesis, 2D and 3D TEE aid to confirm the correct position of the valve and it is usually used in conjunction with fluoroscopy. The optimal position for the Edwards SAPIEN™ valve is with the ventricular side of the prosthesis positioned 2–4 mm below the annulus and for the CoreValve™, the ventricular edge of the prosthesis should be placed 5–10 mm below the aortic valve annular plane. After the deployment it is important to confirm that all the prosthetic cusps are moving well, that the valve stent has a circular configuration and to exclude significant valvular or paravalvular aortic regurgitation. Mild aortic regurgitation through the prosthesis, until the guidewire is removed and at the next few minutes after deployment is common. Small jets of paravalvular aortic regurgitation are frequent and it may occur even in a successful procedure, however severe aortic regurgitation is a serious complication and additional balloon inflation may be required.

Assessment of Complications

Among the various complications assessable by TEE, aortic regurgitation is the most common (Fig. 10.7) (Rodes-Cabau et al. 2010; Smith et al. 2011). It may occur as a consequence of incomplete expansion, incorrect positioning, restricted cusp motion, or inappropriate prosthetic size (Détaint et al. 2009). An undersized prosthesis may result in paravalvular aortic regurgitation. On the opposite, an oversized prosthesis has the risk of suboptimal stent expansion and central aortic regurgitation. Other mechanisms eventually responsible for aortic regurgitation are the presence of severe asymmetric calcification, causing paravalvular aortic leaks, or it may happen as a consequence of residual native aortic valve leaflet tissue prolapsing into the prosthesis, interfering with cusp motion and coaptation. The aortic regurgitation severity should be evaluated by the International recommended criteria (Zamorano et al. 2011).

Furthermore, in result of prosthesis mismatch, or failed pacing capture, prosthetic embolism may occur. If the embolization happens towards the aorta, it might be resolved through successful transcatheter repositioning, but if it happens towards the LV, surgical removal is usually the only option (Tuzcu 2008).

Other possible complications detectable by TEE are cardiac tamponade, secondary to wire perforation of the left or right ventricle and new LV dysfunction, which may be secondary to ostial occlusion by fragment embolization or by an obstructive portion of the valve frame, sealing cuff or by native cusp (Webb et al. 2006).

Moreover, sudden worsening of mitral regurgitation may occur due to right ventricular pacing, causing LV asynchrony, or as a consequence of prosthetic misplacement, towards the left ventricle outflow tract, with pressure exerted on the anterior mitral leaflet or by direct damage or distortion of the subvalvular apparatus. (Goncalves et al. 2010) A tear or rupture of the aortic root have been also observed during the procedure after balloon valvuloplasty or prosthesis deployment, especially in the presence of extensive annular calcification or prosthesis oversizing (Masson et al. 2009).

TEE is not mandatory during TAVI, as it usually requires general anesthesia and the probe may also partially obstruct the optimal fluoroscopic view, however it may be the main technique used for procedure guidance, particularly in patients with limited native valve calcification, (Zamorano et al. 2011) providing the best guidance and rapid assessment of complications.

Post-implantation Follow-Up

The imaging follow-up evaluation of patients with transcatheter aortic valves is mainly based on TTE. It is usually performed at the time of hospital discharge, at 1 month follow-up and at 6 or 12 months, depending on each institution protocol. The echocardiographic evaluation is mostly similar to surgically implanted prostheses, as guided by previously published guidelines for prosthetic valves (Zoghbi et al. 2009).

Nevertheless, the accurate evaluation of aortic regurgitation severity is a main issue, as it may consist of central and paravalvular aortic regurgitation and the latter frequently includes multiple small jets. Colour flow qualitative evaluation is the method most commonly used for the assessment of the regurgitant jet size. The guidelines suggest using the following criteria for jet width based on the % LVOT diameter occupied: ≤25% suggests mild, 26–64% suggests moderate, and >65% suggests severe. These methods are limited in the setting of paravalvular jets which are frequently eccentric and irregular in shape. The ASE/EAE guidelines suggest that for paravalvular jets, the proportion of the circumference of the sewing ring occupied by the jet gives a semi-quantitative guide to severity: <10% of the sewing ring suggests mild, 10–20% suggests moderate, and >20% suggests severe (Zoghbi et al. 2009). However, this concept assumes jet continuity, which may not be the case for transcatheter valves and therefore may overestimate the severity in presence of multiple small jets. For the quantitative approach the width of the vena contracta is an estimate of regurgitant severity, but in the setting of prostheses, portions of the sewing ring may not be imaged due to acoustic shadowing. In addition, there has been no validation for adding the vena contracta widths of multiple jets as it may be encountered post-TAVI. A new method using 3D TTE vena contracta planimetry has been recently described, showing an accurate alternative for quantitative evaluation and moderate AR recognition of paravalvular aortic regurgitation after TAVI (Goncalves et al. 2011). The quantitative methods for calculating regurgitant volume and effective regurgitant orifice area that rely on the comparison of stroke volumes across the aortic valve and a nonregurgitant valve may be also used for prosthetic valves evaluation (Zoghbi et al. 2009). However, the final interpretation should follow the principle of comprehensive evaluation and integrated approach.

At the time of effective orifice area calculation, it is essential that the pre-valvular velocity is recorded proximal to the stent and the post-valvular velocity (typically recorded with continuous-wave Doppler) distal to the stented valve. If the LVOT velocity used in calculations is erroneously recorded within the stent but proximal to the cusps, the result will be an overestimation of valve area (Zamorano et al. 2011). Similarly the LVOT diameter should be measured immediately proximal to the stent (Clavel et al. 2011).

In selected cases with suspicion of complications such as prosthesis malposition, MDCT by its higher spatial resolution is an appropriate technique, providing accurate information on the position and deployment of prosthesis.

Conclusion

The multimodality imaging approach optimizes the procedure and increases TAVI success. Using echocardiography, MDCT and angiography, an accurate evaluation of aortic stenosis severity, annulus sizing, aortic morphology and peripheral vascular anatomy are performed. These steps are decisive for appropriate patient selection. During TAVI procedure, TEE along with fluoroscopy can be used for guidance, to evaluate possible complications and the final result. At time of patients' short and long-term follow-up, echocardiography represents the ideal technique for prosthesis hemodynamic characterization, leaving MDCT reserved for particularly complex conditions.

References

Bonow RO, Carabello BA, Chatterjee K, de Leon Jr AC, Faxon DP, Freed MD, Gaasch WH, Lytle BW, Nishimura RA, O'Gara PT, O'Rourke RA, Otto CM, Shah PM, Shanewise JS. 2008 focused update incorporated into the ACC/AHA 2006 guidelines for the management of patients with valvular heart disease: a report of the American College of Cardiology/American Heart Association Task Force on Practice Guidelines (Writing Committee to revise the 1998 guidelines for the management of patients with valvular heart disease). Endorsed by the Society of Cardiovascular Anesthesiologists, Society for Cardiovascular Angiography and Interventions, and Society of Thoracic Surgeons. J Am Coll Cardiol. 2008;52:e1–142.

Clavel MA, Rodes-Cabau J, Dumont E, Bagur R, Bergeron S, De Larochelliere R, Doyle D, Larose E, Dumesnil JG, Pibarot P. Validation and characterization of transcatheter aortic valve effective orifice area measured by doppler echocardiography. JACC Cardiovasc Imaging. 2011;4:1053–62.

Delgado V, Tops LF, Schuijf JD, van der Kley F, van de Veire NR, Schalij MJ, Bax JJ. Successful deployment of a transcatheter aortic valve in bicuspid aortic stenosis: role of imaging with multislice computed tomography. Circ Cardiovasc Imaging. 2009;2:e12–3.

Détaint D, Lepage L, Himbert D, Brochet E, Messika-Zeitoun D, Iung B, Vahanian A. Determinants of significant paravalvular regurgitation after transcatheter aortic valve implantation: impact of device and annulus discongruence. JACC Cardiovasc Interv. 2009;2:821–7.

Goncalves A, Marcos-Alberca P, Zamorano JL. Echocardiography: guidance during valve implantation. EuroIntervention. 2010;6(Suppl G):G14–9.

Goncalves A, Almeria C, Marcos-Alberca P, Feltes G, Hernandez-Antolin R, Rodriguez E, Silva Cardoso JC, Macaya C, Zamorano JL. Three dimensional echocardiography in paravalvular aortic regurgitation assessment after transcatheter aortic valve implantation. J Am Soc Echocardiogr. 2011;25(1):47–55.

Gurvitch R, Wood DA, Leipsic J, Tay E, Johnson M, Ye J, Nietlispach F, Wijesinghe N, Cheung A, Webb JG. Multislice computed tomography for prediction of optimal angiographic deployment projections during transcatheter aortic valve implantation. JACC Cardiovasc Interv. 2010;3:1157–65.

Lange R, Schreiber C, Gotz W, Hettich I, Will A, Libera P, Laborde JC, Bauernschmitt R. First successful transapical aortic valve implantation with the corevalve revalving system: a case report. Heart Surg Forum. 2007;10:E478–9.

Leon MB, Smith CR, Mack M, Miller DC, Moses JW, Svensson LG, Tuzcu EM, Webb JG, Fontana GP, Makkar RR, Brown DL, Block PC, Guyton RA, Pichard AD, Bavaria JE, Herrmann HC, Douglas PS, Petersen JL, Akin JJ, Anderson WN, Wang D, Pocock S. Transcatheter aortic-valve implantation for aortic stenosis in patients who cannot undergo surgery. N Engl J Med. 2010;363:1597–607.

Masson JB, Kovac J, Schuler G, Ye J, Cheung A, Kapadia S, Tuzcu ME, Kodali S, Leon MB, Webb JG. Transcatheter aortic valve implantation: review of the nature, management, and avoidance of procedural complications. JACC Cardiovasc Interv. 2009;2:811–20.

Messika-Zeitoun D, Serfaty JM, Brochet E, Ducrocq G, Lepage L, Detaint D, Hyafil F, Himbert D, Pasi N, Laissy JP, Iung B, Vahanian A. Multimodal assessment of the aortic annulus diameter: implications for transcatheter aortic valve implantation. J Am Coll Cardiol. 2010;55:186–94.

Piazza N, de Jaegere P, Schultz C, Becker AE, Serruys PW, Anderson RH. Anatomy of the aortic valvar complex and its implications for transcatheter implantation of the aortic valve. Circ Cardiovasc Interv. 2008;1:74–81.

Rodes-Cabau J, Webb JG, Cheung A, Ye J, Dumont E, Feindel CM, Osten M, Natarajan MK, Velianou JL, Martucci G, DeVarennes B, Chisholm R, Peterson MD, Lichtenstein SV, Nietlispach F, Doyle D, DeLarochelliere R, Teoh K, Chu V, Dancea A, Lachapelle K, Cheema A, Latter D, Horlick E. Transcatheter aortic valve implantation for the treatment of severe symptomatic aortic stenosis in patients at very high or prohibitive surgical risk: acute and late outcomes of the multicenter canadian experience. J Am Coll Cardiol. 2010;55:1080–90.

Schultz CJ, Tzikas A, Moelker A, Rossi A, Nuis RJ, Geleijnse MM, van Mieghem N, Krestin GP, de Feyter P, Serruys PW, de Jaegere PP. Correlates on MSCT of paravalvular aortic regurgitation after transcatheter aortic valve implantation using the medtronic corevalve prosthesis. Catheter Cardiovasc Interv. 2011a;78: 446–55.

Schultz C, Rossi A, van Mieghem N, van der Boon R, Papadopoulou SL, van Domburg R, Moelker A, Mollet N, Krestin G, van Geuns RJ, Nieman K, de Feyter P, Serruys PW, de Jaegere P. Aortic annulus dimensions and leaflet calcification from contrast MSCT predict the need for balloon post-dilatation after TAVI with the medtronic corevalve prosthesis. EuroIntervention. 2011b;7:564–72.

Schwartz JG, Neubauer AM, Fagan TE, Noordhoek NJ, Grass M, Carroll JD. Potential role of three-dimensional rotational angiography and C-arm CT for valvular repair and implantation. Int J Cardiovasc Imaging. 2011;27(8):1205–22.

Smith CR, Leon MB, Mack MJ, Miller DC, Moses JW, Svensson LG, Tuzcu EM, Webb JG, Fontana GP, Makkar RR, Williams M, Dewey T, Kapadia S, Babaliaros V, Thourani VH, Corso P, Pichard AD, Bavaria JE, Herrmann HC, Akin JJ, Anderson WN, Wang D, Pocock SJ. Transcatheter versus surgical aortic-valve replacement in high-risk patients. N Engl J Med. 2011;364:2187–98.

Tuzcu EM. Transcatheter aortic valve replacement malposition and embolization: innovation brings solutions also new challenges. Catheter Cardiovasc Interv. 2008;72:579–80.

Vahanian A, Baumgartner H, Bax J, Butchart E, Dion R, Filippatos G, Flachskampf F, Hall R, Iung B, Kasprzak J, Nataf P, Tornos P, Torracca L, Wenink A. Guidelines on the management of valvular heart disease: the task force on the management of valvular heart disease of the European society of cardiology. Eur Heart J. 2007;28:230–68.

Vahanian A, Alfieri O, Al-Attar N, Antunes M, Bax J, Cormier B, Cribier A, De Jaegere P, Fournial G, Kappetein AP, Kovac J, Ludgate S, Maisano F, Moat N, Mohr F, Nataf P, Pierard L, Pomar JL, Schofer J, Tornos P, Tuzcu M, van Hout B, von Segesser LK, Walther T. Transcatheter valve implantation for patients with aortic stenosis: a position statement from the European association of cardio-thoracic surgery (EACTS) and the EUROPEAN society of cardiology (ESC), in collaboration with the European association of percutaneous cardiovascular interventions (EAPCI). Eur Heart J. 2008;29:1463–70.

Webb JG, Chandavimol M, Thompson CR, Ricci DR, Carere RG, Munt BI, Buller CE, Pasupati S, Lichtenstein S. Percutaneous aortic valve implantation retrograde from the femoral artery. Circulation. 2006; 113:842–50.

Zamorano JL, Badano LP, Bruce C, Chan KL, Goncalves A, Hahn RT, Keane MG, La Canna G, Monaghan MJ, Nihoyannopoulos P, Silvestry FE, Vanoverschelde JL, Gillam LD. EAE/ASE recommendations for the use of echocardiography in new transcatheter interventions for valvular heart disease. Eur Heart J. 2011;32: 2189–214.

Zoghbi WA, Chambers JB, Dumesnil JG, Foster E, Gottdiener JS, Grayburn PA, Khandheria BK, Levine RA, Marx GR, Miller Jr FA, Nakatani S, Quinones MA, Rakowski H, Rodriguez LL, Swaminathan M, Waggoner AD, Weissman NJ, Zabalgoitia M. Recommendations for evaluation of prosthetic valves with echocardiography and doppler ultrasound: a report From the American Society of Echocardiography's Guidelines and Standards Committee and the Task Force on Prosthetic Valves, developed in conjunction with the American College of Cardiology Cardiovascular Imaging Committee, Cardiac Imaging Committee of the American Heart Association, the European Association of Echocardiography, a registered branch of the European Society of Cardiology, the Japanese Society of Echocardiography and the Canadian Society of Echocardiography, endorsed by the American College of Cardiology Foundation, American Heart Association, European Association of Echocardiography, a registered branch of the European Society of Cardiology, the Japanese Society of Echocardiography, and Canadian Society of Echocardiography. J Am Soc Echocardiogr. 2009;22: 975–1014, quiz 1082–4.

Transcutaneous Aortic Valve Implantation

11

Margaret A. Lloyd and Charanjit S. Rihal

Introduction

Non-rheumatic, degenerative aortic stenosis is overwhelmingly a disease of the elderly. As many as 300,000 individuals in the United States have symptomatic aortic stenosis (AS). Prior studies suggest that patients with asymptomatic but hemodynamically significant AS have a high risk of dying or developing symptoms. A Mayo Clinic study demonstrated that the 1, 2, and 5 year probabilities of remaining free from operation or death were 80%, 63%, and 25% respectively in a cohort of 622 patients (Pellikka et al. 2005). The development of symptoms portends a high risk of death (Carabello 2002). Surgical intervention with mechanical or tissue prosthetic valves has long been the gold standard for treatment. Improved operative techniques and more durable valvular prostheses have resulted in excellent functional status and patient survival. While operative mortality at experienced centers with careful patient selection is low, frequently patients with calcific AS have increased operative risk (O'Brien et al. 2009). As such, a third to half of elderly patients with symptomatic AS are not candidates for operative intervention due to advanced age or severe co-morbidities (Bouma et al. 1999). Percutaneous aortic balloon valvuloplasty has not resulted in long-term relief, with early restenosis the rule.

Two transcutaneous aortic valve prostheses are undergoing evaluation in the United States, the Edwards SAPIEN heart valve system (Edwards Life sciences LLC, Irvine CA), a balloon expandable stainless steel prosthesis, and the Medtronic CoreValve (Medtronic Inc., Minneapolis MN), a self-expanding nitinol prosthesis. Both have had extensive use in Europe where CE Mark has been available for some time. At least four valves are currently approved or in clinical trials worldwide.

Transcutaneous Aortic Valve Implantation (TAVI): The PARTNER Trial

Since Cribier performed the first human TAVI in 2002, development of the technique has proceeded rapidly, with over 15,000 valves implanted in 43 countries at the end of 2011 (Cribier et al. 2002; Taylor 2011).

In November 2011 the U.S. Food and Drug Administration approved Edwards SAPIEN heart valve system after publication of the PARTNER (Placement of Aortic Transcatheter Valve) trial. The PARTNER trial was a multicenter, prospective, randomized trial evaluating a balloon-expandable stented valve prosthesis placed via the transapical or transfemoral route. Two parallel arms of the trial compared TAVI

M.A. Lloyd, M.D. (✉)
Department of Cardiology, Mayo Clinic, Rochester, MN, USA
e-mail: lloyd.margaret@mayo.edu

C.S. Rihal, M.D.
Division of Cardiovascular Diseases, Mayo Clinic, Rochester, MN, USA

N.M. Rajamannan (ed.), *Cardiac Valvular Medicine*,
DOI 10.1007/978-1-4471-4132-7_11, © Springer-Verlag London 2013

versus standard open surgical replacement (cohort A) and TAVI versus best medical care (including balloon valvuloplasty) in patients with symptomatic AS determined to be ineligible for open surgical intervention (cohort B). The trial was conducted in 21 centers in the United States, Canada, and Germany. The surgical arm (cohort A) included 699 patients (348 randomized to TAVI, 352 randomized to conventional surgery) (Smith et al. 2011); the medical arm (cohort B) included 358 patients (179 randomized to TAVI, 179 randomized to standard medical therapy) (Leon et al. 2010).

Medical Therapy Versus TAVI in Inoperable Patients

Enrollment into PARTNER Cohort B was suspended early due to marked improvement in outcomes in patients in the TAVI group. By design, a high-risk group of patients were enrolled, with a mean age of 83 years and a mean Society of Thoracic Surgeons score of 11–12, indicative of high surgical risk. Patients in this group had a high prevalence of comorbidities, including coronary disease and pulmonary conditions. At 1 year, 50.7% of patients treated medically had died, compared with 30.7% of those patients treated with TAVI (Table 11.1). This represented an absolute risk reduction of 20%, a need-to-treat ratio of five patients per life saved, and equates to 200 lives saved per thousand patients treated, an extraordinarily high figure. The combined endpoint of mortality or repeat hospitalizations was even more markedly reduced among TAVI treated patients.

The results of Cohort B overwhelmingly demonstrated increased survival and fewer cardiac symptoms in those survivors treated with TAVI compared to those treated with standard medical therapy (Table 11.2). These findings represent the first effective non-operative treatment for symptomatic AS, even more impressive in that the patients were not candidates for surgery. Importantly, 58% of surviving patients treated with standard therapy at 1 year had cardiac symptoms, compared to 25.2% of TAVI patients. This survival increase in the TAVI group was tempered by higher incidence of stroke, vascular complications, and major bleeding complications in this group compared to standard medical therapy. It is notable that the baseline prevalence of atrial fibrillation was significantly lower in the TAVI group versus the standard therapy group (32.9% vs. 48.8%).

Table 11.1 TAVI versus standard medical therapy (cohort B): primary endpoints

Endpoint	TAVI (%)	Standard (%)	p value
1 year all cause death	30.7	50.7	<0.001
1 year all cause death or repeat hospitalization	42.5	71.6	<0.001

Table 11.2 TAVI versus standard medical therapy (cohort B): secondary end points

Endpoint	TAVI (%)	Standard (%)	p value
30 day major stroke	5	1.1	0.06
30 day vascular complications	16.2	1.1	<0.001
1 year cardiac death	19.6	41.9	<0.001
1 year major bleeding	22.3	11.2	0.007
1 year survivors cardiac symptoms	25.2	58	<0.001

Standard Surgical Therapy Versus TAVI in High-Risk Patients

Patients in cohort A were randomized to either TAVI or conventional aortic valve replacement (AVR) surgery. Like those in cohort B, these patients were elderly, with a mean age of 84 years and STS scores between 11 and 12. Baseline prevalence of atrial fibrillation was the same in both groups (40.8% in the TAVI arm vs. 42.7% in the standard AVR arm). Approximately two-thirds of the patients in the TAVI arm had valves implanted via the femoral route, and approximately one-third were implanted transapically. One year mortality was similar between the two groups, demonstrating non-inferiority of TAVI compared to operative AVR (Table 11.3). As in the cohort B, the stroke was significantly higher in the TAVI group at year one (Table 11.4); however, the likelihood of being alive and free of stroke was similar between the two groups at 30 days and at 1 year (Table 11.5).

Table 11.3 TAVI versus standard AVR (cohort A): primary end point

Endpoint	TAVI (%)	Standard AVR (%)	p value
1 year all cause death	24.2	26.8	0.44

Table 11.4 TAVI versus standard AVR (cohort A): secondary end points

Endpoint	TAVI (%)	Standard AVR (%)	p value
30 day all cause death	3.4	6.5	0.07
30 day major stroke	3.8	2.1	0.2
30 day vascular complications	11.0	3.2	<0.001
1 year cardiac death	14.3	13.0	<0.001
1 year major bleeding	14.7	25.7	<0.001

Table 11.5 Combined event rate (cohort A): death and major stroke

Total endpoint	TAVI (%)	Standard AVR (%)	p value
30 day	6.9	8.2	0.52
1 year	26.5	28.0	0.68

Implantation Procedure

Procedural technique varies depending on the device being utilized. Baseline assessment consists of a thorough history and physical examination. In addition to the standard symptoms and signs of AS, particular attention should be paid to medical co-morbidity, degree of debility, frailty, and recovery potential. Frailty can be assessed quantitatively by using simple measures such as grip strength and walking times. Echocardiography, pulmonary function testing, and serum creatinine are key baseline tests. Transesophageal echocardiography is frequently necessary to assess left ventricular outflow track diameter and anatomy. Cardiac and vascular computed tomography is performed to examine the outflow tract, coronary artery position relative to the aortic annulus, degree of calcification of the ascending aorta, intimal atheroma, and to determine the suitability of the peripheral vasculature to accommodate an appropriately sized delivery system. If the iliofemoral system is inadequate (small lumen, excessive calcification, or tortuosity) then an alternate approach such as transapical access is used.

The size of the vascular sheath and delivery system required is determined by the size of the valve. The TAVI procedure is performed using sterile procedure with the patient under general anesthesia. The prosthetic heart valve is mounted onto a balloon catheter. Vascular access is obtained either by surgical cut down or percutaneous suture "preclose," aortography to determine optimal deployment angle is performed, and a temporary pacemaker is inserted. After standard aortic balloon valvuloplasty, the valve delivery system is advanced over a stiff guide wire across the native aortic valve and positioned (Fig. 11.1). The delivery system is flexible and can usually be advanced across the stenotic aortic valve without difficulty. During rapid right ventricular pacing to still cardiac motion, the balloon is expanded, deploying the valve. Under-expansion of the prosthetic valve during deployment or selection of a too-small valve can result in paravalvular aortic regurgitation, and increase the risk of embolization.

The Medtronic CoreValve system differs fundamentally from the Edwards SAPIEN valve system in that the valve is "unsheathed" after careful placement, allowing self-expansion of the valve. The lack of a deployment balloon allows for a smaller diameter delivery system which is a significant advantage.

Transapical placement is performed through an intercostal incision over the left ventricular apex with a dedicated delivery system. All patients receive peri-procedural heparin and anti-platelet therapy.

Unresolved Issues

The findings of this important trial indicate TAVI is a suitable therapeutic option for many patients with AS. Nevertheless, important questions remain:

Risk of Complications

Serious injury to the vasculature may occur during insertion or removal of the delivery system, and extreme care must be undertaken to avoid vascular injury as it is associated with a very poor

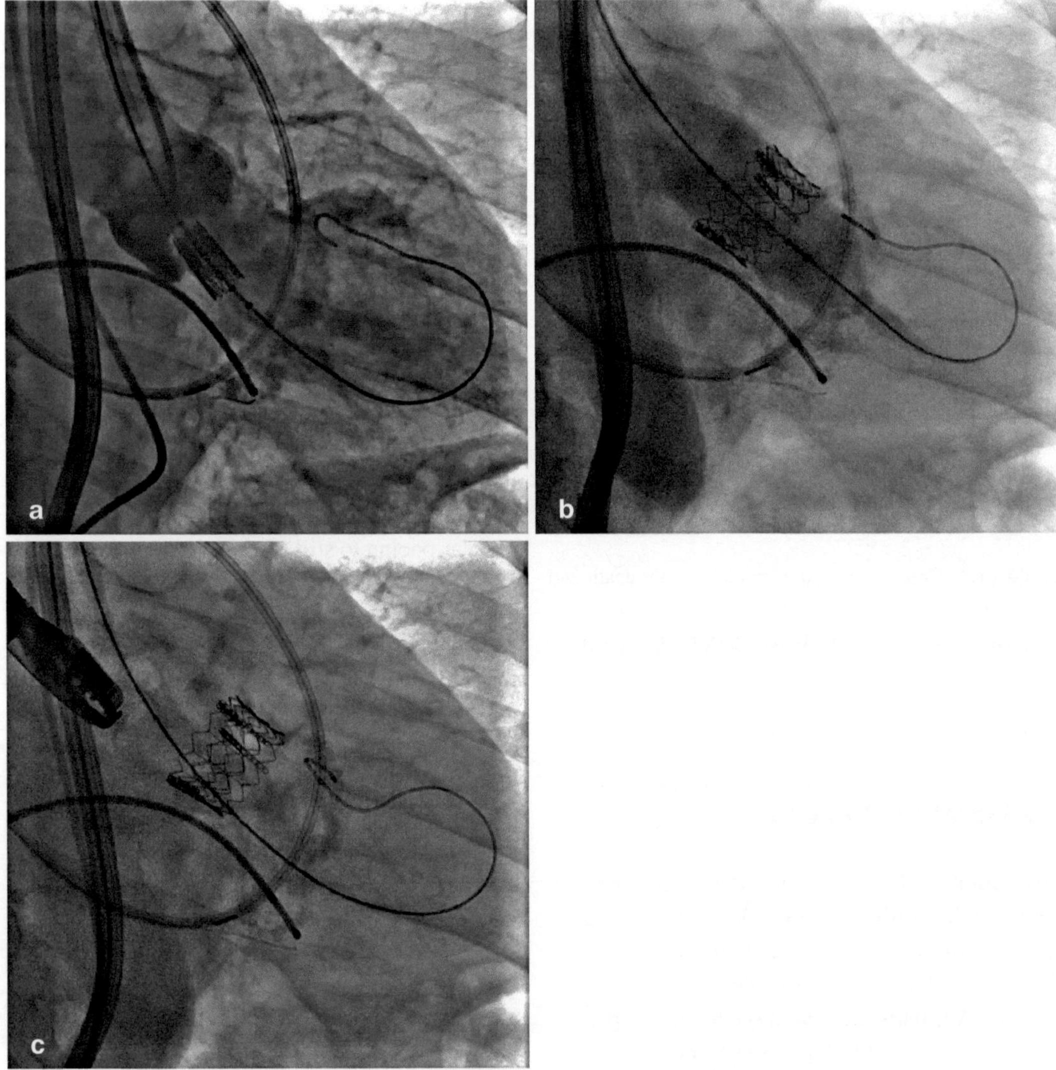

Fig. 11.1 Deploying Edwards-SAPIEN transcutaneous aortic valve via femoral access: (**a**) Positioning the balloon mounted valve across stenotic aortic valve. (**b**) Deploying the prosthetic valve with balloon inflation during rapid right ventricular pacing. (**c**) Deployed valve prosthesis after balloon withdrawal

prognosis. Operators performing the procedure must have expertise in management of vascular complications, including placement of bail-out devices such as covered stents. Valve embolization may occur, and is usually managed by carefully withdrawing the valve to the descending aorta and deploying it in that position. Coronary artery occlusion is a rare complication (approximately 3 per 1,000 procedures) and is related to sinus effacement and a short annulus-to-left main distance.

The stroke risk is clearly the most troubling aspect of TAVI. The etiology of periprocedural stroke may be due to embolic material dislodged from the stenotic valve or the aorta during the procedure and/or hypotension. Transcranial doppler study has suggested that most embolic events during transapical TAVI occur during balloon valvuloplasty and valve deployment (Drews et al. 2011). Newer generation devices provide smaller delivery catheters and will facilitate implantation with less mechanical trauma to vessel walls, hopefully reducing the risk of embolic stroke, vascular damage, and bleeding. Distal embolic protection devices are being evaluated, and may reduce the risk of embolic stroke. The mechanism of late stroke is likewise not clear, nor does the stroke rate differ between transfemoral and transapical implantation routes (Thuesen et al. 2011).

It is difficult to compare cerebral embolic event incidence in the PARTNER trial against historical investigations as most studies are observational, and stroke and transient ischemic attack not consistently defined or evaluated. When specifically comparing the incidence of complications between the two groups in the PARTNER Cohort A, it should also be noted that the operators in the TAVI arm were by definition "inexperienced," while experienced cardiovascular surgeons were performing surgical AVR, a mature procedure that has undergone five decades of refinement.

Durability

It is too early to determine the durability of aortic valves placed transcutaneously. Current mechanical and bioprosthetic valves have excellent long term but not indefinite functional and structural durability. However, over the past five decades of experience with standard prosthetic valves, some designs have performed well, while others developed late failure. Mechanical valves require lifelong anticoagulation, which presents its own set of risks.

The United Kingdom TAVI Registry provides the best performance estimate at this time (Moat et al. 2011). This registry was established in 2007, and captured all implants of both approved devices (Edwards SAPIEN and Medtronic CoreValve) in England and Wales through 2010. 870 patients were followed; 30 day survival was 92.9%, 1 year survival 78.6%, and 2 year survival 73.7%. Patients were deemed high-risk for surgery, resulting in a highly selected population. In multivariate analysis, left ventricular dysfunction, moderate/severe aortic regurgitation, and chronic obstructive pulmonary disease were independent predictors of mortality.

Ongoing trials are attempting to define appropriate patient populations for each approach. Given current understanding, individual clinical circumstances should be thoughtfully evaluated. For an elderly patient with a statistically limited expected lifespan, durability may not be a significant factor. For an otherwise healthy young adult, performance should be strongly considered when considering treatment approaches.

Transapical TAVI

The STACCATO trial was initiated to compare transapical TAVI versus conventional AVR; as reported at TCT 2011, the trial was stopped early due to adverse events in the TAVI arm of the trial (Thuesen et al. 2011). Events included severe paravalvular leakage, renal failure, major strokes, and myocardial infarction, resulting in termination of the trial after enrollment of 70 of an anticipated 200 patients. Further analysis and peer-reviewed publication of the data are needed before conclusions can be drawn.

It should be noted that the trial was initiated in 2008, when transcutaneous devices and delivery systems were still relatively crude, and operators were much less experienced. Additionally, some have criticized the trial design in being inadequately powered to detect true differences between the two groups.

Cost

A retrospective cost analysis of the PARTNER Cohort A patients has demonstrated that percutaneous TAVI via peripheral vascular access is economically superior to standard AVR (Reynolds et al. 2011; Cohen et al. 2011). Procedural costs were significantly higher with TAVI, but non-procedural costs were significantly lower with TAVI (Table 11.6). This overall reduction in cost associated with TAVI was primarily due to reduced length of hospital stay. This advantage was not seen in those who had TAVI via the transapical approach; hospital length of stay for this group was comparable to the standard AVR

Table 11.6 Cost analysis: cohort A

	Access site			
	Transfemoral		Transapical	
Cost element	TAVI ($)	Standard AVR ($)	TAVI ($)	Standard AVR ($)
Implant cost:				
Procedural	34,863	14,451	39,992	15,271
Non-procedural	31,192	54,228	44,940	58,139
Total implant cost	**66,055**	**68,679**	**84,932**	**73,410**
1 year follow-up	22,251	21,965	17,231	18,643
Total first year cost	**88,306**	**90,644**	**102,163**	**92,053**

group, and costs were approximately $10,000 more than the surgical group. Both transfemoral and transapical TAVI had fewer ICU days than their respective surgical groups, and lower or equivalent follow-up costs. Percutaneous TAVI was associated with a favorable cost of approximately $2,000/QALY.

At present costs associated with TAVI seem to be comparable to standard AVR. However, evaluation, treatment, and follow-up are currently dictated by trial protocols and do not necessarily reflect real-life clinical practice. Calculation of the true cost of each method needs to consider not only costs associated with valve implantation (whether transcutaneously or via standard operative approach), but costs associated with treatment of complications and follow-up procedures normalized for the effective lifespan of each device, and follow-up costs. Additional considerations are the social costs, i.e. patient time lost from work, limitations on activities, persistent symptoms, and quality of life after intervention. Finally, the costs of building hybrid facilities and training of operators and other medical personnel need to be factored into any cost calculation. While it is too early in the TAVI experience to accurately determine these costs, in the current healthcare environment absolute and relative cost will guide practice and reimbursement.

Other Considerations

Ideal antithrombotic regimens have not yet been determined, nor is it known if different valve designs will differ in thrombotic potential. Most clinical trials have emperically utilized dual anti-platelet regimens. It is not yet known if long-term antithrombotic treatment will be necessary.

The risk of endocarditis in TAVI and appropriate treatment should it occur are unknown. There was no difference in the need for post-treatment pacemaker between any of the arms of both cohorts in the PARTNER trial, although others have reported a higher incidence of permanent pacemaker implantation after TAVI compared to standard AVR (Wenaweser et al. 2011). Over a third of 243 patients in the United Kingdom required permanent pacing within 30 days after receiving the Medtronic CoreValve in one report – likely related to the longer device and impingement upon the conduction system – while the need for permanent pacing after standard AVR is generally less than 10% (Khawaja et al. 2011; Dawkins et al. 2008).

The ease of implantation, durability, associated complication rate, and cost will all be factors in gaining approval of regulatory agencies and market share. Some models and delivery systems may be preferable to others in certain clinical settings. The safety and efficacy profile of each unique device will need to be studied.

Valve-in-Valve TAVI

Case reports document at least 50 transcutaneous valves implanted world-wide to treat bioprosthetic aortic valvular stenosis (Gurvitch et al. 2011). This technique may be especially useful in selected patients given the higher risk associated with re-do AVR. Considerations include internal bioprosthetic diameter, whether the failed valve is stented or stentless, and the mechanism of bioprosthetic failure.

Position Statement by Professional Societies

TAVI is a developing, transformational technology which is radically changing the approach to the treatment of valvular and structural heart disease. The American College of Cardiology and Society of Thoracic Surgeons have published recommendations to facilitate the successful integration of this procedure into clinical practice for the ultimate benefit to patients (Holmes & Mack 2011). Those recommendations include:

Implantation at Specialized Heart Centers, with Trained, Experienced Personnel

The multidisciplinary team should include the primary cardiologist, cardiovascular surgeons, interventional cardiologists, heart failure specialists, and imaging specialists. Facilities should include hybrid operating rooms and cardiac laboratories. The centers should participate in clinical trials and registries, and follow standardized clinical protocols. The recent consensus document for TAVI (Tommaso et al. 2012) and the minimal number to proficiency (Alli et al. 2012) will help to continue to improve outcomes for operators performing these procedures in the future.

Formal Operator Training Programs

The implant volume in the U.S. has been limited by availability of TAVI only through clinical trials until the recent approval of the Edwards Sapien valve. Practicing interventional cardiologists and cardiovascular surgeons are getting early experience, limiting trainee exposure. Formal guidelines for trainee certification (case volume, performace, duration of training) need to be developed.

Outcome Assessment

Both societies recommend ongoing clinical trials to better define indications for TAVI, assess risk of complications, and identify unique safety and efficacy features of various devices. They also recommend linked clinical and administrative databases to facilitate post-market surveillance, comparative effectiveness, and cost data.

Conclusion

As life spans have increased, so has the incidence of significant AS. Many patients do not require intervention until later in life, when unfortunately comorbidities and age may render operative risk prohibitive. Medical management and percutaneous balloon valvuloplasty are not effective treatments and until recently surgical replacement was the only option for critical, symptomatic AS.

The development of TAVI is an extremely important milestone in the treatment of valvular heart disease. The data have clearly demonstrated that TAVI is superior to medical management and balloon valvuloplasty for inoperable severe AS. The data also suggest that TAVI is equivalent to standard AVR in this population. As technology improves, operators gain experience, and patient selection criteria are identified, ease of implant should improve and the risk of complications and adverse events is expected to decrease.

Ongoing studies are needed to assess efficacy and complication risk in newer devices, especially as this new technology is utilized in other patient populations and as operators gain experience. Longitudinal studies, active post-market surveillance, and clinical databases should be developed to assess long-term durability and performance.

References

Alli OO, Booker JD, Lennon RJ, Greason KL, Rihal CS, Holmes Jr DR. Transcatheter aortic valve implantation: assessing the learning curve. JACC Cardiovasc Interv. 2012;5:72–9.

Bouma BJ, van den Brink RBA, van der Meulen JHP, et al. To operate or not on elderly patients with aortic stenosis: the decision and its consequences. Heart. 1999;82:143–8.

Carabello BA. Clinician update: evaluation and management of patients with aortic stenosis. Circulation. 2002;105:1746–50.

Cohen DJ, Reynolds MR, Magnuson EA. Quality of life after transcatheter vs. surgical aortic valve replacement: results from the PARTNER trial (cohort A). J Am Coll Cardiol. 2011;58(Suppl B):xiii.

Cribier A, Eltchaninoff H, Bash A, et al. Percutaneous transcatheter implantation of an aortic valve prosthesis for calcific aortic stenosis: first human case description. Circulation. 2002;106:3006–8.

Dawkins S, Hobson AR, Kalra PR, et al. Permanent pacemaker implantation after isolated aortic valve replacement: incidence, indications, and predictors. Ann Thorac Surg. 2008;85:108–12.

Drews T, Pasic M, Buz S, et al. Transcranial Doppler sound detection of cerebral microembolism during transapical aortic valve implantation. Thorac Cardiovasc Surg. 2011;59:237–42.

Gurvitch R, Cheung A, Ye J, et al. Transcatheter valve-in-valve implantation for failed surgical bioprosthetic valves. J Am Coll Cardiol. 2011;58:2196–209.

Holmes Jr DR, Mack MJ. Transcatheter valve therapy: a professional society overview from the American College of Cardiology Foundation and the Society of Thoracic Surgeons. J Am Coll Cardiol. 2011;58: 445–55.

Khawaja MZ, Rajani R, Cook A, et al. Permanent pacemaker insertion after CoreValve transcatheter aortic valve implantation: incidence and contributing factors (the UK CoreValve Collaborative). Circulation. 2011;123:951–60.

Leon MB, Smith CV, Mack M. Transcatheter aortic-valve implantation for aortic stenosis in patients who cannot undergo surgery. N Engl J Med. 2010;363:1597–607.

Moat NE, Ludman P, de Belder MA, et al. Long-term outcomes after transcatheter aortic valve implantation in high-risk patients with severe aortic stenosis. J Am Coll Cardiol. 2011;58:2130–8.

O'Brien SM, Shahian DM, Filardo G. The society of thoracic surgeons 2008 cardiac risk models: part 2 – isolated valve surgery. Ann Thorac Surg. 2009;88: S23–42.

Pellikka PA, Sarano ME, Nishimura RA, et al. Outcome of 622 adults with asymptomatic, hemodynamically significant aortic stenosis during prolonged follow-up. Circulation. 2005;111:3290–5.

Reynolds MR, Magnuson EA, Lei Y. Cost effectiveness of transcatheter aortic valve replacement compared with surgical aortic valve replacement in patients with severe aortic stenosis: results from the PARTNER trial. J Am Coll Cardiol. 2011;58(Suppl B):xiii.

Smith CV, Leon MB, Mack MJ, et al. Transcatheter versus surgical aortic-valve replacement in high-risk patients. N Engl J Med. 2011;364:2187–98.

Taylor J. Clinical trials on transcatheter aortic valve implantation cannot be compared because of inconsistent endpoints. Eur Heart J. 2011;32:125–6.

Thuesen L, Andersen HR, Krusell R. Randomized comparison of apical transcatheter aortic valve implantation vs. surgical valve replacement for severe aortic stenosis in patients aged > 75 years. The STACCATO trial. J Am Coll Cardiol. 2011;58(supp B):xiii.

Tommaso CL, Bolman RM 3rd, Feldman T, et al. SCAI/AATS/ACCF/STS Multisociety expert consensus statement: operator & institutional requirements for transcatheter valve repair and replacement; part 1 TAVR. J Am Coll Cardiol. 2012.

Wenaweser P, Pilgrim T, Kadner A, et al. Clinical outcomes of patients with severe aortic stenosis at increased surgical risk according to treatment modality. J Am Coll Cardiol. 2011;58:2151–62.

Role of Statins in Valvular Heart Disease: Rheumatic Valve Disease and Bioprosthetic Valves

12

Francesco Antonini-Canterin, Luis Moura, and Nalini Marie Rajamannan

Statins and Rheumatic Valve Disease

Although rare nowadays in North America and Europe, rheumatic heart disease (RHD) continues to be an important healthcare problem in developing countries with an estimated prevalence of 15.6 million people worldwide and 470,000 newly diagnosed cases every year (Carapetis et al. 2005). Acute rheumatic fever leads to an abnormal immune response to the infection with rheumatogenic group A hemolytic streptococci leading to pancarditis with acute inflammation of the leaflets. Inflammation, fibrosis and calcification lead to alterations of the cusps and valvular apparatus, leading to mitral, aortic and/or tricuspid stenosis and/or regurgitation that will eventually become symptomatic. The mitral valve is commonly involved more often leading to mitral stenosis meanwhile isolated aortic or tricuspid involvement is rare (Marijon et al. 2007). Typical aspects of rheumatic involvement in valve disease are represented by adhesions and fusions of the commissures with cusp retraction and stiffening of the free borders of the cusps (Bonow et al. 2006).

The development and the time course of valvular heart disease differs in patients exposed to group A streptococcal infection since some subjects are genetically susceptible meanwhile others are not (Bryant et al. 2009). The progression from the initial rheumatic attack to calcification and clinically relevant valvular disease until recently was thought to be a consequence of chronic hemodinamic stress of a previously modified valve. Recent studies however have proven the presence of ongoing inflammation in chronic rheumatic valve disease, with the presence of inflammatory cytokines and T-lymphocytes infiltrate (Chiu-Braga et al. 2006). Elevated C-reactive protein (CRP) levels, circulating adhesion molecules, and other inflammatory cytokines as well as increased oxidative stress have been observed in these patients (Yetkin et al. 2001). Patients with multivalvular disease showed persistent and significantly higher plasma levels of CRP (Gölbasi et al. 2002). It has been also hypothesized that high sensitivity CRP levels could be related to rheumatic mitral stenosis progression (Alyan et al. 2009). The calcification process involved in both rheumatic and non-rheumatic valvular disease does resemble skeletal bone formation

F. Antonini-Canterin, M.D. (✉)
Department of Cardiology, Cardiologia, ARC, Azienda Ospedaliera S. Maria degli Angeli, Via Montereale, 24, 33170 Pordenone, Italy
e-mail: antonini.canterin@gmail.com

L. Moura, M.D.
Department of Cardiology, Hospital S. João/University of Porto Medical School, Porto, Portugal

N.M. Rajamannan, M.D.
Department of Molecular Biology and Biochemistry, Mayo Clinic, 200 First St SW, Rochester 55905, MN, USA

Department of Aerospace Engineering, University of Notre Dame, South Bend Indiana, Clay, IN, USA
e-mail: nrajamannan@gmail.com

N.M. Rajamannan (ed.), *Cardiac Valvular Medicine*,
DOI 10.1007/978-1-4471-4132-7_12, © Springer-Verlag London 2013

and is related to inflammation in a way similar to atherosclerosis and vascular calcifications. In explanted valves, calcifications have been shown to colocalize with vascular endothelial growth factor expression, a marker of neoangiogenesis, which is stimulated by an active inflammatory process (Figs. 12.1 and 12.2) (Rajamannan et al. 2005; Wylie-Sears et al. 2011). Altogether these data suggest that RHD is an active chronic inflammatory process. Thus, the factors that determine the rate of RHD progression could be related to a continuing rheumatic process with ongoing inflammation, continuing hemodinamic flow turbulence through a deformed valve orifice or both. Considering the aforementioned evidence inflammation became a potential therapeutic target in order to slow or even prevent valvular disease progression.

Although statins are used in clinical practice mainly for their cholesterol lowering effect, their non-low-density lipoprotein (LDL) lowering effects have also been studied. The non-cholesterol lowering properties, anti-inflammatory and anti-proliferative actions of statins have been generically termed as pleiotropic effects. The actions of statins result from their downstream effect of inhibiting 3-hydroxy-3-methylglutaryl coenzyme A, the enzyme responsible for cholesterol synthesis, but also by inhibiting mevalonic acid formation, a compound involved in intracellular signaling pathways related with cellular growth and differentiation (Mihos et al. 2010; Davidson 2005). This explains their anti-inflammatory properties and is the rationale for considering statin therapy for RHD. Apart from the anti-inflammatory properties of statins, their original role as anti-atherosclerotic drugs also might play an important role. An increasing body of evidence demonstrates features of atherosclerosis in the aortic valve, which are similar to the early stages of vascular atherosclerotic lesions and it is reasonable to hypothesize that pharmacological strategies effective in atherosclerosis might also be an effective therapy in aortic stenosis (Liebe et al. 2006). Also, recent studies describe similar pathophysiologic molecular markers in the development of rheumatic valve disease as in calcific aortic stenosis (Rajamannan et al. 2009).

On this basis several studies addressed the problem of statin therapy in valvular heart disease. Most of these studies addressed the more common issue of calcific aortic stenosis. However, the potential for statin therapy in slowing the progression of calcific aortic stenosis remains controversial as first non-randomized studies have shown benefits in this setting (Aronow et al. 2001; Bellamy et al. 2002; Rosenhek et al. 2004; Antonini-Canterin et al. 2008; Novaro et al. 2001; Moura et al. 2007) but the prospective randomized clinical trials to date have been negative (Cowell et al. 2005; Rossebø et al. 2008; Jassal et al. 2011).

There are however, differences in inflammation patterns described in degenerative lesions and those present in rheumatic valvular disease. Intense inflammatory infiltrate and vascular endothelial growth factor are found in areas of neoangiogenesis in the rheumatic valves compared with degenerative valves. The more intense inflammatory substrate associated with rheumatic lesions could make them a more suitable target for statin therapy. Statins have been shown to inhibit the inflammatory processes that induce the acute phase response and to reduce CRP levels (Jialal et al. 2001). Recently two retrospective studies in rheumatic valve disease patients showed positive results. Statin therapy in rheumatic aortic stenosis patients with a mean follow up of 8.5 ± 4.2 years (range 2–20 years) was associated with slower disease progression (annual change of peak aortic velocity: 0.05 ± 0.07 vs. 0.12 ± 0.11 m/s/year, $p = 0.001$) and a significantly reduced number of cases with fast progressive disease (Antonini-Canterin et al. 2009). In rheumatic mitral stenosis subjects also, statin treatment reduced the rate of decrease in mitral valve area (0.027 ± 0.056 versus 0.067 ± 0.082 cm^2/year; $p = 0.005$), the prevalence of fast progression mitral stenosis and less patients had an increase in systolic pulmonary artery pressure >10 mmHg over the mean follow-up period of 6.1 ± 4.0 years (Antonini-Canterin et al. 2010).

Once calcium and/or fibrosis are present in large amount in valvular and perivalvular tissue it is unlikely that any current drug could be of help. This underscores the tremendous importance of

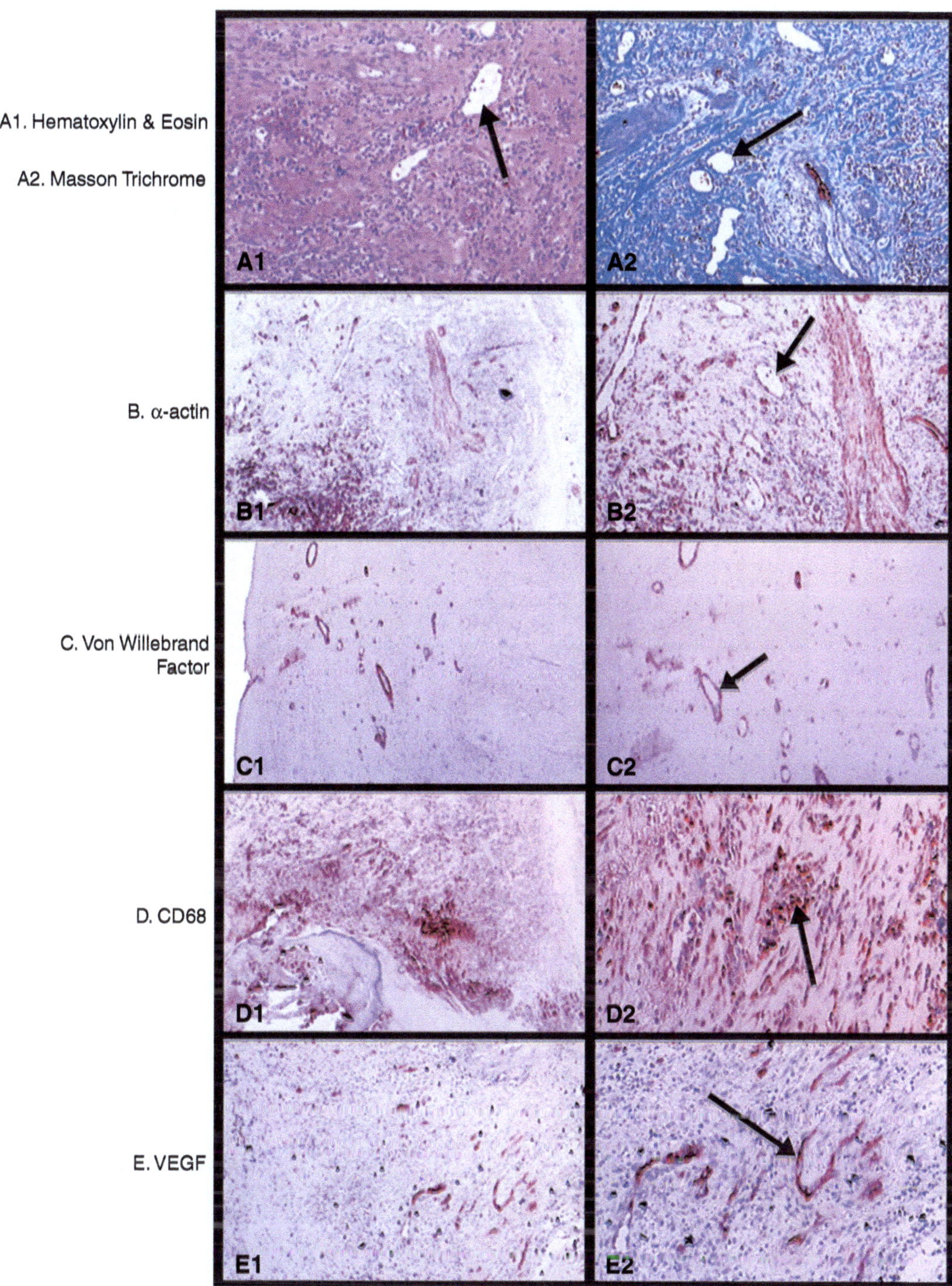

Fig. 12.1 Identification of neoangiogenesis markers in calcified rheumatic valves. (**a1**) Hematoxylin and eosin stain of calcified rheumatic valve. *Arrow* points to new vessels (magnification ×10). (**a2**) Masson trichrome stain. *Arrow* points to new vessels (magnification ×10). (**b1**) Actin immunostain (magnification ×10). (**b2**) Actin immunostain. *Arrow* points to neointima in neovasculature (magnification ×40). (**c1**) von Willebrand factor immunostain (magnification ×10). (**c2**) von Willebrand factor immunostain. *Arrow* points to endothelial layer staining positive for von Willebrand factor (magnification ×10). (**d1**) CD68 immunostain for human macrophages (magnification ×10). (**d2**) CD68 Immunostain for human macrophages. *Arrow* points to inflammatory staining cells (magnification ×40). (**e1**) VEGF immunostain (magnification ×10). (**e2**) VEGF immunostain. *Arrow* points to areas of VEGF stain in areas of inflammation (magnification ×40)

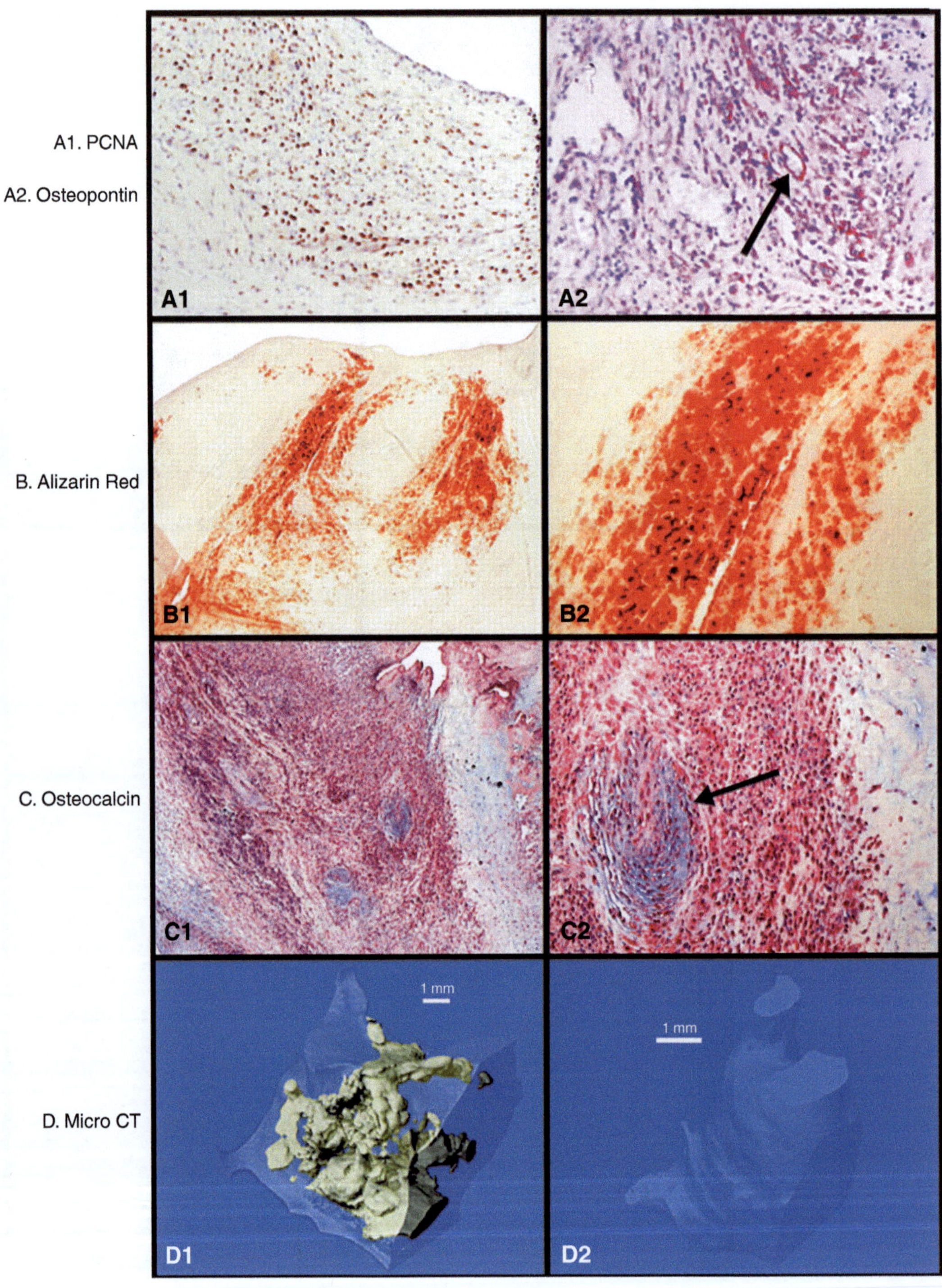

Fig. 12.2 Identification of bone matrix markers in calcified human rheumatic valves. (**a1**) PCNA immunostain (magnification ×10). (**a2**) Osteopontin immunostain. *Arrow* points to myofibroblast staining cells (magnification ×10). (**b1**) Alizarin red stain (magnification ×10). (**b2**) Alizarin red stain (magnification ×40). (**c1**) Osteocalcin immunostain (magnification ×10). (**c2**) Osteocalcin immunostain. *Arrow* points to myofibroblast staining cells (magnification ×40). (**d1**) MicroCT 3D reconstruction of calcified rheumatic valve. (**d2**) MicroCT 3D reconstruction of uncalcified degenerative mitral valve

interventions in an early stage of disease. Instead of addressing more than moderate valvular stenosis, in a timeframe when calcium is usually already present, it is presumable that the anti-inflammatory effects could exercise their maximum potential in an early stage of these. The retrospective studies that addressed the role of statins in rheumatic mitral and aortic stenosis actually included mild-to-moderate mitral and mild aortic stenosis, respectively. This aspect could account for their positive results. However, inherent limitations result from the retrospective nature of these studies and data from randomized trials is needed for further confirmation of the role of statins in RHD (Ben-Yehuda and DeMaria 2009). At this moment randomized trials addressing the potential use of statins in RHD are still missing.

Statins and Bioprosthetic Valves

A wide variety of prostheses, including mechanical, biological and human tissue prostheses are currently available for clinical use. There are major differences among the prosthetic valves types and the choice of prosthesis must fit the clinical context of the patient. Although mechanical valves have a greater long-term durability compared to their biological counterpart, their thrombogenic nature and the requirement of permanent anticoagulation are associated with a certain risk of hemorrhagic complications and also with patient discomfort (Hammermeister et al. 2000). Bioprosthetic valves instead have a low thrombogenicity and usually require only a brief period on anticoagulation therapy following implantation. However, bioprosthetic valves have the propensity to undergo structural degeneration limiting their durability and sometimes necessitating reoperation, at the cost of increased morbidity and mortality. This makes bioprostheses to be preferred in elderly patients and the proportion of tissue valves used for aortic valve replacement, currently the most common valvular surgery indication, is of about 70% in patients older than 70 years (Brown et al. 2009).

As population grows older and the incidence of aortic stenosis is increasing it is expected that the proportion of implanted bioprostheses will also increase in the near future. Therefore finding a way to slow down the progression of degenerative changes in bioprosthetic valves is likely to have an important clinical and socio-economic impact. In order to improve the lifespan of bioprostheses first we must understand the underlying physiopathology and the factors related to biological prosthetic valves degeneration. The factors responsible for calcification and degeneration of valvular bioprostheses are patient-related and valve-related. It has been demonstrated that the age of the patient at time of implant is closely correlated to structural valve deterioration. Younger patients are more likely to require reoperation and the relative risk of reoperation increases by 55% for each decade (Bloomfield et al. 1991). These aspects form the basis for the current recommendation of bioprostheses use preferably only in patients of 65 years or older (Vahanian et al. 2007). The current availability of percutaneous valvular procedures (i.e. transcatheter aortic valve implants [TAVI]) with the possibility of valve-in-valve implant could reduce further the age for preferring a biological valve as first choice (Webb et al. 2010). Hypercholesterolemia has been suggested as another patient-related risk factor for bioprosthetic valve degeneration and calcification even these result are controverted (Farivar and Cohn 2003; Nollert et al. 2003).

For a long time the mechanism of native valve degeneration was thought to be related only to passive calcium accumulation with age. Valve calcifications are currently believed to be an active atherosclerosis-like process (Rajamannan et al. 2011). Valvular endothelial cells actually resemble the endothelial cells found elsewhere in the circulatory tree. Just like the other endothelial cells they react in response to abnormal hemodynamic forces and shear stresses with tissue remodeling and inflammation, leading further to calcification and eventually clinically symptomatic valvular stenosis/failure (Balachandran et al. 2009). Lipids also play an important initiating role in the cell signaling of vascular and valvular calcification and this has also been proven by studies in patients with homozygous familial hypercholesterolemia. In a cholesterol-fed rabbit model, hypercholesterolemia induced atherosclerotic-like lesions in the aortic valve, and atorvastatin reduced the degree of structural changes in the aortic valve (Rajamannan et al. 2002). The same processes that lead to calcific deposits in natural diseased heart valves seem to be responsible also for degeneration of bioprostheses (Tomazic et al. 1995). Although commercially available bioprosthetic valves are pre-treated to remove lipids from the tissue, this could not prevent development of subsequent lipid deposits. Lipid insudation and inflammatory infiltrates occur in the cuspidal tissue of porcine bioprostheses similar to early atherosclerosis lesions and they can precipitate structural valve deterioration in the long-term, even in the absence of mineralization (Antonini-Canterin et al. 2006; Price et al. 2007).

Considering the common atherosclerosis-like process involved in degeneration of both native and prosthetic valves it is reasonable to assume that statins could be a therapeutic option to slow disease progression in both conditions (Lorusso et al. 2010). Although promising results emerged from the initial retrospective studies the evidence from prospective randomized trials does not support to date a strong role for statins in slowing progression of native aortic valve stenosis. Previous studies showed that human and porcine smooth muscle cells share a similar proliferation dependence on the mevalonate pathway, inhibited by statin treatment (Martínez-González and Badimon 1996; Antonini-Canterin et al. 2004). A positive effect of statin treatment on the vessel wall expression of a protein involved in the progression of atherosclerosis in a hypercholesterolemic porcine model has been demonstrated and this finding could partially explain a similar positive effect of statins in human and porcine valves (Martínez-González et al. 2001).

However as with RHD, there are some differences in the underlying physiopathological process that might explain the difference in the lifespan of bioprosthetic valves compared to their native counterparts. First, bioprosthesis remain "foreign bodies" so there are reasons to believe that the degree of inflammation present in a bioprosthesis is higher than in native valves. Second, the presence of a bioprosthesis is usually associated with higher transvalvular gradients compared to native valves. This can be due to the use of a stented valve, the surgical technique used or simply to the inherent imperfection of patient and prosthesis matching. All this aspects are associated with higher hemodinamic stress in biological prostheses compared with native valves. Actually native valve employs several decades of ages for developing significant degeneration and stenosis, while biological prostheses can degenerate in about 10 years. Thus, the bioprosthesis constitute a particular model of fast failure in which statins could be theoretically more effective.

Taken together more intense inflammation and higher shear stress of the biological valve compared to native valves might lead to a faster progression of degenerative lesions, prosthesis failure and need for replacement. This could also mean a better target for anti-inflammatory therapy. Current data show that pericardial valves are probably superior to porcine valves for aortic valve replacement (Rahimtoola 2003). Except for this difference, there is no hard evidence that, in patients with similar characteristics at baseline, outcome is better with newer than with older bioprosthetic aortic valves. A retrospective study analyzed 167 patients (97 men, mean age 71 ± 9 years) with both porcine and pericardial bioprostheses with a follow-up period of 46 ± 38 months (Antonini-Canterin et al. 2003). Statin treated patients had lower annual rate of increase in the peak trans prosthetic velocity (0.038 ± 0.074 vs. 0.140 ± 0.228 m/s/year, $p < 0.001$) and lower rate of decrease in the prosthetic indexed effective orifice area (0.019 ± 0.031 vs. 0.056 ± 0.086 cm^2/m^2/year, $p < 0.001$). A combined parameter of prosthetic degeneration progression, defined as the existence of either an annual rate of increase in peak velocity of 0.3 m/s/year or worsening of aortic regurgitation was more frequently found in

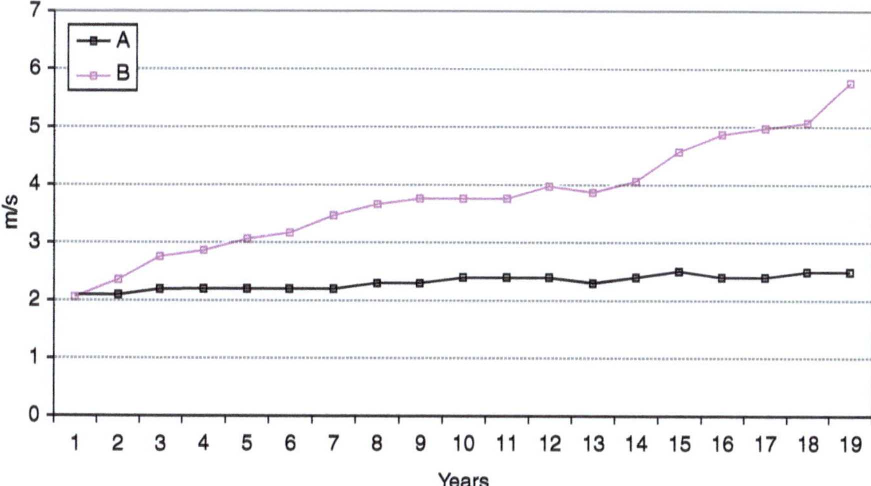

Fig. 12.3 Serial evaluation of peak aortic valve Doppler velocity in two patients with rheumatic heart disease during 20-year echocardiographic follow-up. Patient A (*black line*) was treated with simvastatin 40 mg/day and showed a slow progression of peak velocity (from 2.1 to 5.8 m/s in 20 years; rate of progression 0.185 m/s/year). Patient B (*pink line*) did not receive statins and showed a faster progression of peak velocity (from 2.1 to 5.8 m/s in 20 years; rate of progression (1.85 m/s/year)

the group without statins. Figure 12.3 shows the behaviour of peak aortic Doppler velocity in two emblematic patients with rheumatic aortic valve stenosis, the first one treated with statins and the second one not.

However, another recent observational study in 1,193 patients (mean age 71.7±8.7) who underwent aortic valve replacement with current generation bioprostheses (mean follow-up period of 4.5±3.1 years) did not demonstrated a benefit from early postoperative lipid-lowering therapy, including statins, and slowing of bioprosthesis deterioration (Kulik et al. 2010). The annualised linear rate of gradient progression following valve replacement was similar between the groups (peak gradient increase per year: 2.0±12.1 vs. 1.0±12.9 mmHg/year, lipid-lowering vs. no treatment, p=0.52). There were also no differences in respect of aortic regurgitation progression. The authors concluded that the structural durability of current bioprostheses could be the best explanation for their finding.

There are no prospective randomized trials to date addressing the issue of statin therapy for the prevention of bioprosthesis degeneration (Table 12.1) (Gilmanov et al. 2010). The potential impact can be tremendous considering not only the increasing incidence of older patients needing valve replacement surgery but also in light of the newer percutaneous procedures. The transcatheter aortic valve implants emerged as a solution for severe aortic stenosis patients ineligible for open heart surgery (Leon et al. 2010). The initial results are promising but data on the long-term durability of such valves is still missing and this is also one of the aspects preventing the expansion of current indications for this procedure to other aortic stenosis patients (Lazar 2010). In the future the indications for transcatheter aortic valve implants could be expanded and the possibility of having a medical therapy that prevents bioprosthesis degeneration could be of major interest.

Table 12.1 Published studies addressing the question of cholesterol levels and statin therapy in bioprosthetic valves degeneration

Year	Author	Study type	Results	Comments
2003	David and Ivanov (2003)	Retrospective cohort study	Hyperlipidemia was not a significant predictor of reoperation in any of the studied groups and the only significant independent predictor of reoperation was age	The probability of valve failure in patients with atherosclerosis risk factors was reduced because most of them were actually taking statins
2003	Farivar and Cohn (2003)	Retrospective cohort study with case–control analysis	The mean serum cholesterol level in the explanted valve group was significantly higher than that of those who did not need re-replacement	Hypercholesterolemia could be a risk factor for bioprosthetic valve failure and explantation. However, the study received criticism because first generation bioprosthesis are more susceptible for degeneration
2003	Nollert et al. (2003).	Retrospective cohort study	Cholesterol levels were a risk factor for reoperation. Also age younger than 57 years, female sex, diabetes mellitus and smoking were associated with reoperation	The studied patients received Hancock pericardial valves which are already out of market
2004	Antonini-Canterin et al. (2003)	Retrospective cohort study	Statin use was associated with a slower progression and a lower proportion of prosthesis degeneration	The retrospective nature of the study is the main limitation of the study
2006	Gring et al. (2006).	Prospective non-randomized trial	Preoperative cholesterol levels do not predict valvular degeneration in patients undergoing aortic valve replacement	Younger age, increased body weight, creatinine level and pericardial valve were related to bioprosthesis degeneration
2010	Kulik et al. (2010).	Retrospective observational study	The study demonstrated no association between early postoperative lipid lowering therapy and a slowing of bioprosthesis degeneration	The largest number of patients included and the use of contemporary prostheses are the main strengths of the study

References

Alyan O, Metin F, Kacmaz F, Ozdemir O, Maden O, Topaloglu S, Demir AD, Karahan Z, Karadede A, Ilkay E. High levels of high sensitivity C-reactive protein predict the progression of chronic rheumatic mitral stenosis. J Thromb Thrombolysis. 2009;28:63–9.

Antonini-Canterin F, Zuppiroli A, Popescu BA, Granata G, Cervesato E, Piazza R, Pavan D, Nicolosi GL. Effect of statins on the progression of bioprosthetic aortic valve degeneration. Am J Cardiol. 2003;92:1479–82.

Antonini-Canterin F, Popescu BA, Zuppiroli A, Nicolosi GL. Are statins effective in preventing bioprosthetic aortic valve failure? A need for a prospective, randomized trial. Ital Heart J. 2004;5:85–8.

Antonini-Canterin F, Zuppiroli A, Baldessin F, Popescu BA, Nicolosi GL. Is there a role of statins in the prevention of aortic biological prostheses degeneration? Cardiovasc Ultrasound. 2006;4:26.

Antonini-Canterin F, Hîrşu M, Popescu BA, Leiballi E, Piazza R, Pavan D, Ginghină C, Nicolosi GL. Stage-related effect of statin treatment on the progression of aortic valve sclerosis and stenosis. A long-term follow-up study in 1046 patients. Am J Cardiol. 2008;102:738–42.

Antonini-Canterin F, Leiballi E, Enache R, Popescu BA, Rosca M, Cervesato E, Piazza R, Ginghina C, Nicolosi GL. Hydroxymethylglutaryl coenzyme-A reductase inhibitors delay the progression of rheumatic aortic valve stenosis – a long-term echocardiographic study. J Am Coll Cardiol. 2009;53:1874–9.

Antonini-Canterin F, Moura L, Enache R, Leiballi E, Pavan D, Piazza R, Popescu BA, Ginghina C, Nicolosi GL, Rajamannan NM. Effect of hydroxymethylglutaryl coenzyme-A reductase inhibitors on the long-term progression of rheumatic mitral valve disease. Circulation. 2010;121:2130–6.

Aronow WS, Ahn C, Kronzon I, Goldman ME. Association of coronary risk factors and use of statins with progression of mild valvular aortic stenosis in older persons. Am J Cardiol. 2001;88:693–5.

Balachandran K, Sucosky P, Jo H, Yoganathan AP. Elevated cyclic stretch alters matrix remodeling in aortic valve cusps: implications for degenerative aortic valve disease. Am J Physiol. 2009;296:H756–64.

Bellamy MF, Pellikka PA, Klarich KW, Tajik AJ, Enriquez-Sarano M. Association of cholesterol levels, hydroxymethylglutaryl coenzyme-A reductase inhibitor treatment, and progression of aortic stenosis in the community. J Am Coll Cardiol. 2002;40:1723–30.

Ben-Yehuda O, DeMaria AN. Statins in rheumatic heart disease. Taking the bite out? J Am Coll Cardiol. 2009;53:1880–2.

Bloomfield P, Wheatley DJ, Prescott RJ, Miller HC. Twelve-year comparison of a Bjork-Shiley mechanical heart valve with porcine bioprosthesis. N Engl J Med. 1991;324:573–9.

Bonow RO, Carabello BA, Kanu C, de Leon AC, Jr FDP, Freed MD, Gaasch WH, Lytle BW, Nishimura RA, O'Gara PT, O'Rourke RA, Otto CM, Shah PM, Shanewise JS, Smith Jr SC, Jacobs AK, Adams CD, Anderson JL, Antman EM, Faxon DP, Fuster V, Halperin JL, Hiratzka LF, Hunt SA, Lytle BW, Nishimura R, Page RL, Riegel B. ACC/AHA 2006 guidelines for the management of patients with valvular heart disease: a report of the American College of Cardiology/American Heart Association Task Force on Practice Guidelines (Writing Committee to Revise the 1998 Guidelines for the Management of Patients With Valvular Heart Disease): developed in collaboration with the Society of Cardiovascular Anesthesiologists: endorsed by the Society for Cardiovascular Angiography and Interventions and the Society of Thoracic Surgeons. Circulation. 2006;114:e84–231.

Brown JM, O'Brien SM, Wu C, Sikora JA, Griffith BP, Gammie JS. Isolated aortic valve replacement in North America comprising 108,687 patients in 10 years: changes in risks, valve types, and outcomes in the Society of Thoracic Surgeons National Database. J Thorac Cardiovasc Surg. 2009;137:82–90.

Bryant PA, Robins-Browne R, Carapetis JR, Curtis N. Some of the people, some of the time: susceptibility to acute rheumatic fever. Circulation. 2009;119:742–53.

Carapetis JR, McDonald M, Wilson NJ. Acute rheumatic fever. Lancet. 2005;366:155–68.

Chiu-Braga YY, Hayashi SY, Schafranski M, Messias-Reason IJ. Further evidence of inflammation in chronic rheumatic valve disease (CRVD): high levels of advanced oxidation protein products (AOPP) and high sensitive C-reactive protein (hs-CRP). Int J Cardiol. 2006;109:275–6.

Cowell SJ, Newby DE, Prescott RJ, Bloomfield P, Reid J, Northridge DB, Boon NA, Scottish Aortic Stenosis and Lipid Lowering Trial, Impact on Regression (SALTIRE) Investigators. A randomized trial of intensive lipid-lowering therapy in calcific aortic stenosis. N Engl J Med. 2005;352:2389–97.

David TE, Ivanov J. Is degenerative calcification of the native aortic valve similar to calcification of bioprosthetic heart valves? J Thorac Cardiovasc Surg. 2003;126:939–41.

Davidson MH. Clinical significance of statin pleiotropic effects. Hypotheses versus evidence. Circulation. 2005;111:2280–1.

Farivar RS, Cohn LH. Hypercholesterolemia is a risk factor for bioprosthetic valve calcification and explantation. J Thorac Cardiovasc Surg. 2003;126:969–75.

Gilmanov D, Bevilacqua S, Mazzone A, Glauber M. Do statins slow the process of calcification of aortic tissue valves? Interact Cardiovasc Thorac Surg. 2010;11:297–301.

Gölbasi Z, Uçar O, Keles T, Sahin A, Cagli K, Camsari A, Diker E, Aydogdu S. Increased levels of high sensitive C-reactive protein in patients with chronic rheumatic valve disease: evidence of ongoing inflammation. Eur J Heart Fail. 2002;4:593–5.

Gring CN, Houghtaling P, Novaro GM, Roselli E, Smedira N, Banbury M, Blackstone E, Griffin BP. Preoperative cholesterol levels do not predict explant for structural valve deterioration in patients undergoing bioprosthetic aortic valve replacement. J Heart Valve Dis. 2006;15:261–8.

Hammermeister K, Sethi GK, Henderson WG, Grover FL, Oprian C, Rahimtoola S. Outcomes 15 years after valve replacement with a mechanical versus a bioprosthetic valve: final report of the Veterans Affairs Randomized Trial. J Am Coll Cardiol. 2000;36: 1152–8.

Jassal DS, Bhagirath KM, Karlstedt E, Zeglinski M, Dumesnil JG, Teo KK, Tam JW, Chan KL. Evaluating the effectiveness of rosuvastatin in preventing the progression of diastolic dysfunction in aortic stenosis: a substudy of the aortic stenosis progression observation measuring effects of rosuvastatin (ASTRONOMER) study. Cardiovasc Ultrasound. 2011;9:5.

Jialal I, Stein D, Balis D, Grundy SM, Adams-Huet B, Devaraj S. Effects of hydroxymethyl glutaryl coenzyme A reductase inhibitor therapy on high sensitive C-reactive protein levels. Circulation. 2001;103: 1933–5.

Kulik A, Masters RG, Bedard P, Hendry PJ, Lam BK, Rubens F, Mesana TG, Ruel M. Postoperative lipid-lowering therapy and bioprosthesis structural valve deterioration: justification for a randomised trial? Eur J Cardiothorac Surg. 2010;37:139–44.

Lazar H. Transcatheter aortic valves – where do we go from here? N Engl J Med. 2010;363:1667–8.

Leon MB, Smith CR, Mack M, Miller DC, Moses JW, Svensson LG, Tuzcu EM, Webb JG, Fontana GP, Makkar RR, Brown DL, Block PC, Guyton RA, Pichard AD, Bavaria JE, Herrmann HC, Douglas PS, Petersen JL, Akin JJ, Anderson WN, Wang D, Pocock S, PARTNER Trial Investigators. Transcatheter aortic-valve implantation for aortic stenosis in patients who cannot undergo surgery. N Engl J Med. 2010;363:1597–607.

Liebe V, Brueckmann M, Borggrefe M, Kaden JJ. Statin therapy of calcific aortic stenosis: hype or hope? Eur Heart J. 2006;27:773–8.

Lorusso R, Corradi D, Maestri R, Bosio S, Curulli A, Beghi C, Gerometta P, Russo C, Gelsomino S, Moreo A, De Cicco G, Rosano G, Volterrani M. Atorvastatin attenuates post-implant tissue degeneration of cardiac prosthetic valve bovine pericardial tissue in a subcutaneous animal model. Int J Cardiol. 2010;141:68–74.

Marijon E, Ou P, Celermajer DS, Ferriera B, Mocumbi AO, Jani D, Parquet C, Jacob S, Sidi D, Jouven X. Prevalence of rheumatic heart disease detected by echocardiographic screening. N Engl J Med. 2007;357: 470–6.

Martínez-González J, Badimon L. Human and porcine smooth muscle cells share similar proliferation dependence on the mevalonate pathway: implication for in vivo interventions in the porcine model. Eur J Clin Invest. 1996;26:1023–32.

Martínez-González J, Alfón J, Berrozpe M, Badimon L. HMG-CoA reductase inhibitors reduce vascular monocyte chemotactic protein-1 expression in early lesions from hypercholesterolemic swine independently of their effect on plasma cholesterol levels. Atherosclerosis. 2001;159:27–33.

Mihos CG, Salas MJ, Santana O. The pleiotropic effects of the hydroxy-methyl-glutaryl-CoA reductase inhibitors in cardiovascular disease: a comprehensive review. Cardiol Rev. 2010;18:298–304.

Moura LM, Ramos SF, Zamorano JL, Barros IM, Azevedo LF, Rocha-Gonçalves F, Rajamannan NM. Rosuvastatin affecting aortic valve endothelium to slow the progression of aortic stenosis. J Am Coll Cardiol. 2007;49:554–61.

Nollert G, Miksch J, Kreuzer E, Reichart B. Risk factors for atherosclerosis and the degeneration of pericardial valves after aortic valve replacement. J Thorac Cardiovasc Surg. 2003;126:965–8.

Novaro GM, Tiong IY, Pearce GL, Lauer MS, Sprecher DL, Griffin BP. Effect of hydroxymethylglutaryl coenzyme A reductase inhibitors on the progression of calcific aortic stenosis. Circulation. 2001;104:2205–9.

Price L, Sniderman A, Omerglu A, Lachapelle K. Bioprosthetic valve degeneration due to cholesterol deposition in a patient with a normal lipid profile. Can J Cardiol. 2007;23:233–4.

Rahimtoola SH. Choice of prosthetic heart valve for adult patients. J Am Coll Cardiol. 2003;41:893–904.

Rajamannan NM, Subramaniam M, Springett M, Sebo TC, Niekrasz M, McConnell JP, Singh RJ, Stone NJ, Bonow RO, Spelsberg TC. Atorvastatin inhibits hypercholesterolemia-induced cellular proliferation and bone matrix production in the rabbit aortic valve. Circulation. 2002;105:2660–5.

Rajamannan NM, Nealis TB, Subramaniam M, Pandya S, Stock SR, Ignatiev CI, Sebo TJ, Rosengart TK, Edwards WD, McCarthy PM, Bonow RO, Spelsberg TC. Calcified rheumatic valve neoangiogenesis is associated with vascular endothelial growth factor expression and osteoblast-like bone formation. Circulation. 2005;111:3296–301.

Rajamannan NM, Antonini-Canterin F, Moura L, Zamorano JL, Rosenhek RA, Best PJ, Lloyd MA, Rocha-Goncalves F, Chandra S, Alfieri O, Lancellotti P, Tornos P, Baliga RR, Wang A, Bashore T, Ramakrishnan S, Spargias K, Shuvy M, Beeri R, Lotan C, Suwaidi JA, Bahl V, Pierard LA, Maurer G, Nicolosi GL, Rahimtoola SH, Chopra K, Pandian NG. Medical therapy for rheumatic heart disease: is it time to be proactive rather than reactive? Indian Heart J. 2009;61:14–23.

Rajamannan NL, Evans F, Aikawa E, Grande-Allen K, Demer L, Heistad D, Simmons C, Masters K, Mathieu P, O'Brien K, Schoen F, Towler D, Yoganathan P, Otto CM. Calcific aortic valve disease: not simply a degenerative process. Circulation. 2011;124:1783–91.

Rosenhek R, Rader F, Loho N, Gabriel H, Heger M, Klaar U, Schemper M, Binder T, Maurer G, Baumgartner H. Statins but not angiotensin-converting enzyme inhibitors delay progression of aortic stenosis. Circulation. 2004;110:1291–5.

Rossebø AB, Pedersen TR, Boman K, Brudi P, Chambers JB, Egstrup K, Gerdts E, Gohlke-Bärwolf C, Holme I, Kesäniemi YA, Malbecq W, Nienaber CA, Ray S, Skjaerpe T, Wachtell K, Willenheimer R, SEAS Investigators. Intensive lipid lowering with simvastatin and ezetimibe in aortic stenosis. N Engl J Med. 2008;359:1–14.

Tomazic BB, Edwards WD, Schoen FJ. Physicochemical characterization of natural and bioprosthetic heart valve calcific deposits: implications for prevention. Ann Thorac Surg. 1995;60:S322–7.

Vahanian A, Baumgartner H, Bax J, Butchart E, Dion R, Filippatos G, Flachskampf F, Hall R, Iung B, Kasprzak J, Nataf P, Tornos P, Torracca L, Wenink A, Task Force on the Management of Valvular Hearth Disease of the European Society of Cardiology, ESC Committee for Practice Guidelines. Guidelines on the management of valvular heart disease. Eur Heart J. 2007;28:230–68.

Webb JG, Wood DA, Ye J, Gurvitch R, Masson JB, Rodés-Cabau J, Osten M, Horlick E, Wendler O, Dumont E, Carere RG, Wijesinghe N, Nietlispach F, Johnson M, Thompson CR, Moss R, Leipsic J, Munt B, Lichtenstein SV, Cheung A. Transcatheter valve-in-valve implantation for failed bioprosthetic heart valves. Circulation. 2010;121:1848–57.

Wylie-Sears J, Aikawa E, Levine RA, Yang JH, Bischoff J. Mitral valve endothelial cells with osteogenic differentiation potential. Arterioscler Thromb Vasc Biol. 2011;31:598–607.

Yetkin E, Erbay AR, Ileri M, Turhan H, Balci M, Cehreli S, Yetkin G, Demirkan D. Levels of circulating adhesion molecules in rheumatic mitral stenosis. Am J Cardiol. 2001;88:1209–11.

Slowing the Progression of Aortic Stenosis: The Emerging Role of Bisphosphonates

13

Sammy Elmariah

Introduction

Calcific aortic stenosis (AS) develops via an active process similar to atherosclerosis that frequently culminates in calcification and cortical bone formation (Fig. 13.1) (Elmariah and Mohler 2010; Goldbarg et al. 2007; Mohler et al. 2001). Significant evidence supports the notion that calcification within heart valves is a manifestation of generalized atherosclerosis (Allison et al. 2006; Yamamoto et al. 2003; Pohle et al. 2001) and that these lesions are associated with dramatically increased morbidity and mortality (Otto et al. 1999). HMG-CoA reductase inhibitors (statins) have been aggressively studied for the management of atherosclerosis and cardiovascular calcification (Mohler et al. 2007; Budoff and Raggi 2001; Callister et al. 1998; Shavelle et al. 2002; Aikawa et al. 2007a; Wu et al. 2005). In addition to lowering lipid levels by inhibiting the rate-limiting step in cholesterol biosynthesis, statin drugs may retard vascular and valvular calcification through various pleiotropic mechanisms (Wu et al. 2005; Luan et al. 2003; Osman et al. 2006; Liao 2002; Zhang and Casey 1996) The potent nitrogen-containing bisphosphonates (NCBPs) inhibit farnesyl-pyrophosphate synthase (FPPS), distal to HMG-CoA reductase in the mevalonate pathway (Fig. 13.2) (van Beek et al. 2003; Bergstrom et al. 2000), and have been found to possess many statin-like effects (Giraudo et al. 2004; Lai et al. 2007; Tamura et al. 2005; Adami et al. 2000; Montagnani et al. 2003; Ariyoshi et al. 2006; Nitta et al. 2004; Gozzetti et al. 2008). In addition, bisphosphonate inhibition of bone resorption may indirectly reduce calcification of cardiovascular tissues (Price et al. 2001). Interest is consequently growing in the use of NCBPs for calcific cardiovascular disease (Towler and Demer 2011). Here, we review the evidence suggesting a role for NCBPs in the management of aortic valve calcification (AVC) and the resultant valve obstruction.

Bisphosphonate Mechanisms of Action

Bisphosphonates are potent inhibitors of hydroxyapetite dissolution and osteoclast-mediated bone resorption (Fleisch et al. 1969) that are used in the treatment of numerous bone disorders in which osteoclasts play a pathologic role, such as osteoporosis, Paget's disease, hypercalcemia of malignancy, and metastatic osteolytic bone lesions. Bisphosphonates primarily adsorb to bone surfaces. There they are taken up by osteoclasts where they interfere with cellular functions (Russell and Rogers 1999; Benford et al. 1999). There are two classes of bisphosphonates, nitrogen-containing and non-nitrogen-containing bisphosphonates (non-NCBP). The potent NCBPs,

S. Elmariah, M.D., MPH
Interventional and Structural Heart Disease,
Division of Cardiology, Massachusetts General, Hospital,
Harvard Medical School, Boston, MA, USA
e-mail: selmariah@partners.org

N.M. Rajamannan (ed.), *Cardiac Valvular Medicine*,
DOI 10.1007/978-1-4471-4132-7_13, © Springer-Verlag London 2013

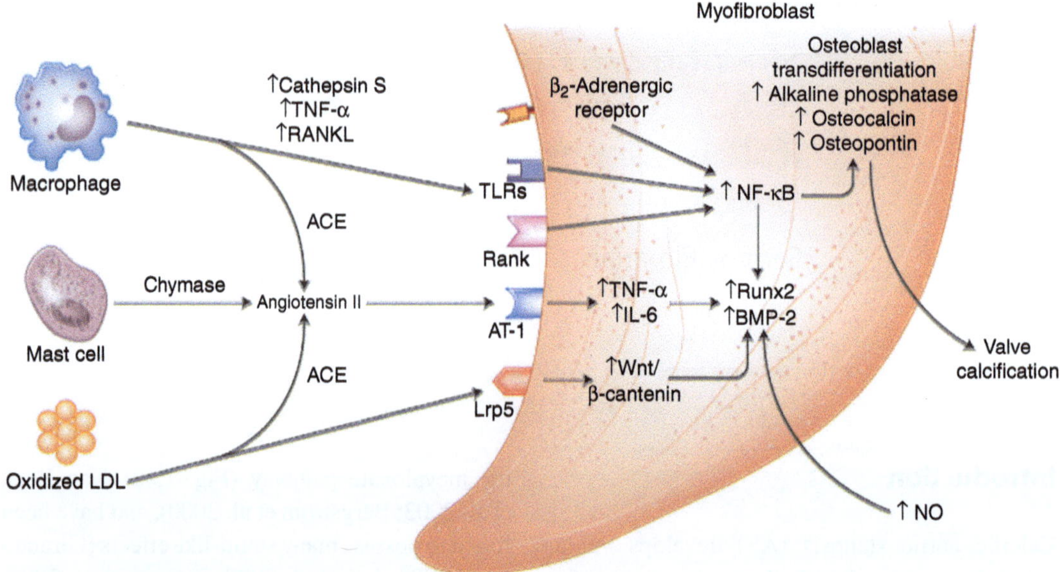

Fig. 13.1 Pathogenesis of calcific aortic stenosis. *ACE* angiotensin-converting enzyme, *AT-1* angiotensin II type 1 receptor, *BMP-2* bone morphogenic protein-2, *IL* interleukin, *LDL* low- density lipoprotein, *Lrp5* LDL receptor-related protein 5, *NF-κB* nuclear factor-κB, *NO* nitric oxide, *RANK* receptor activator of NF-κB, *RANKL* receptor activator of NF-κB ligand, *TLRs* toll-like receptors, *TNF-α* tumor necrosis factor-α (From Elmariah and Mohler (2010))

ibandronate, alendronate, risedronate, and zoledronate, inhibit farnesyl-PP synthase, distal to HMG-CoA reductase in the mevalonate pathway (Fig. 13.2) (van Beek et al. 2003; Bergstrom et al. 2000). Farnesyl-PP synthase is a key enzyme in the mevalonate pathway, affecting both protein prenylation and cholesterol biosynthesis. In osteoclasts, inhibition of protein prenylation disrupts cytoskeletal arrangements, membrane ruffling, trafficking of vesicles, and apoptosis (Russell and Rogers 1999). In a variety of other cell and tissue types, NCBP inhibition of the mevalonate pathway leads to effects similar to seen during statin therapy. The mechanism of action of the older non-NCBPs, such as etidronate and clodronate, appears to be due to the intracellular metabolism of these agents into a cytotoxic adenosine triphosphate (ATP) analogue (Benford et al. 1999; Frith et al. 1997; Rodan and Fleisch 1996). As opposed to NCBPs, non-NCBPs do not inhibit the mevalonate pathway or protein prenylation (Benford et al. 1999), although they have also been found to possess various vascular effects.

Experimental Evidence of Anti-atherosclerotic Bisphosphonate Effects

Non-nitrogen-containing Bisphosphonates

Non-NCBPs have been found to have several anti-atherosclerotic vascular effects. First and foremost, bisphosphonates demonstrate marked accumulate within vascular tissues (Ylitalo et al. 1996), and recent evidence suggests that such vascular accumulation is targeted to areas of osteogenesis and atherosclerotic calcification (Aikawa et al. 2007b). Clodronate, but not etidronate, significantly inhibits the secretion by macrophages of several inflammatory cytokines, including interleukin (IL)-1β, IL-6, and TNF (tumor necrosis factor)-α (Pennanen et al. 1995). Importantly, these effects were independent of cytotoxic effects on marcophages. Within segments of human internal mammary arteries, non-NCBPs reduce noradrenaline-induced arterial contractile force (Ylitalo et al. 1998).

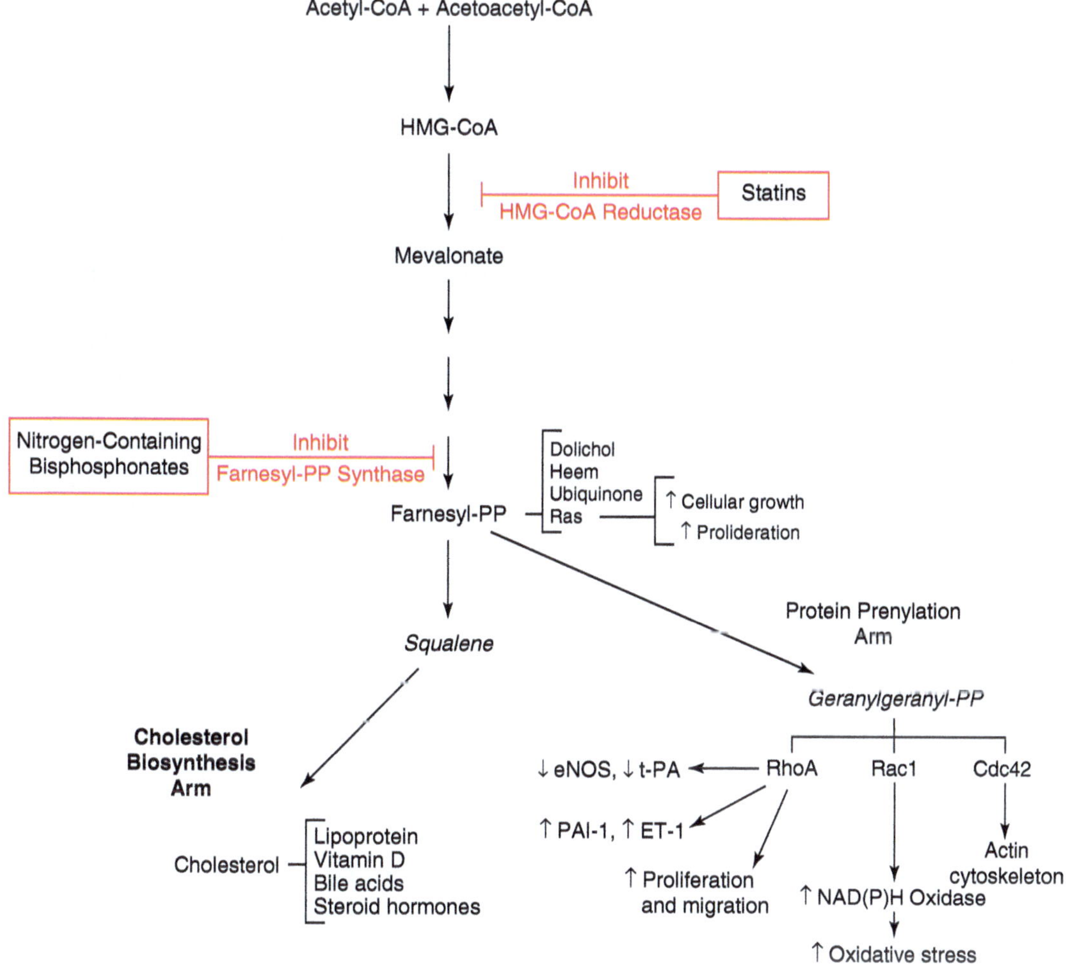

Fig. 13.2 Mevalonate pathway. NCBPs inhibit farnesyl pyrophosphate synthase (Adapted from Liao (2002)). *CoA* coenzyme A, *PP* pyrophosphate

In addition, injection of liposomal clodronate at the time of vascular injury inhibits neointimal hyperplasia presumably due to toxic effects on macrophages (Danenberg et al. 2002). Data support a role for non-NCBPs in specifically limiting vascular calcification as well. In partially nephrectomized rats, etidronate therapy significantly inhibited calcitriol-induced vascular calcification (Tamura et al. 2005). In summary, evidence suggests that non-NCBPs may help maintain vascular, and presumably valvular, health by inhibiting inflammation and neointimal hyperplasia, reducing vascular tone, and hindering calcification.

Nitrogen-Containing Bisphosphonates

Like statins and non-NCBPs, NCBPs exert multiple anti-inflammatory effects. In a macrophage-like cell line, pamidronate inhibits lipopolysaccharide-stimulated secretion of IL-1β, IL-6, and TNF-α (Pennanen et al. 1995). Alendronate similarly inhibits the production of these cytokines by activated monocytes in addition to inhibiting peripheral blood mononuclear cell proliferation (Sansoni et al. 1995). NCBPs also inhibit the secretion of MMP-2 and -9 in a variety of cell types, including infiltrating macrophages, and

Table 13.1 Anti-atherosclerotic bisphosphonate effects

Inflammation
↓ IL-1
↓ IL-6
↓ TNF-α
↓ MMP
↓ Angiogenesis
↓ Protein prenylation
↓ Bone resorption
↓ Ca/PO_4
↓ LDL
↑ HDL

Ca calcium, *HDL* high-density lipoprotein, *IL* interleukin, *LDL* low-density lipoprotein, *MMP* matrix metalloproteinase, *PO_4* phosphate, *TNF* tumor necrosis factor

have consequently been studied extensively as novel antiangiogenic agents for several cancers (Giraudo et al. 2004; Lai et al. 2007; Di Salvatore et al. 2011; Aft 2011). Whether NCBPs effectively inhibit neovascularization within the vascular or valvular tissues remains to be determined (Soini et al. 2003; Moreno et al. 2011). In hypercholesterolemic rabbits, injections of liposomal alendronate at the time of vascular injury reduced numbers of circulating monocytes and tissue macrophages and inhibited in-stent neointimal hyperplasia and arterial stenosis (Danenberg et al. 2003). Price and colleagues demonstrated that NCBPs dramatically inhibited vascular and valvular calcification in uremia- and warfarin-induced animal models of vascular calcification at doses comparable to those used for inhibiting bone resorption (Price et al. 2001, 2006). Together, these data support the hypothesis that NCBPs may slow the progression of calcific valve disease by inhibiting several pathologic components of the atherosclerotic process including inflammation, neovascularization, intimal hyperplasia, lipid accumulation, and calcification (Table 13.1).

The Calcification Paradox

Data from several observational studies have associated osteoporosis with cardiovascular calcification (Hyder et al. 2008; Pennisi et al. 2004; Parhami et al. 2000). The exact mechanisms responsible for the inverse relationship between cardiovascular calcification and bone mineral density (BMD) are unknown. One possibility is that bone resorption releases calcium-phosphate-fetuin-matrix-γ-carboxyglutamic acid protein complexes into the circulation, and that these calcific particles deposit in cardiovascular tissues and form a nidus for calcification (Price et al. 2001; Demer and Tintut 2011). If true, this hypothesis suggests that inhibitors of bone resorption may inhibit cardiovascular calcification indirectly simply by modulating bone metabolism (Fig. 13.3). While this mechanism may play a role, further observations suggest a paradoxical behavior of valve and bone cells to various factors. For example, in cell culture models, statins reduced calcification in aortic valve myofibroblasts and augmented calcification in a pre-osteoblast cell line (Wu et al. 2005). Similar paradoxical effects have been demonstrated in response to several inflammatory cytokines, the receptor activator of nuclear factor kappa-β (RANK)/RANK ligand/osteoprotegerin axis, and oxidized LDL in other models of vascular and bone calcification (Parhami et al. 1997, 2000; Demer and Tintut 2011; Kaden et al. 2004).

Clinical Evidence of Anti-atherosclerotic Bisphosphonate Effects

As with statins, NCBPs have a beneficial, albeit mild, effect on serum lipids, decreasing LDL by approximately 5–21% and raising HDL by 10–18% (Adami et al. 2000; Montagnani et al. 2003; Gozzetti et al. 2008). To our knowledge, these lipid effects have not been demonstrated with non-NCBPs. Regardless, non-NCBPs possess beneficial effects within the vasculature. In a study of Japanese diabetic patients with osteopenia, 1 year of etidronate therapy (200 mg/day for 2 weeks every 3 months) reduced carotid intima-media thickness (cIMT); whereas, cIMT increased in the control group (mean ± standard error: -0.038 ± 0.011 vs. 0.023 ± 0.015 mm, respectively; $p<0.005$) (Koshiyama et al. 2000). In a small study of patients on chronic hemodialysis therapy, those receiving etidronate (n = 8; 400 mg daily for 24 weeks) displayed a 64.1% reduction in mean thoracic aorta calcification scores quantified by

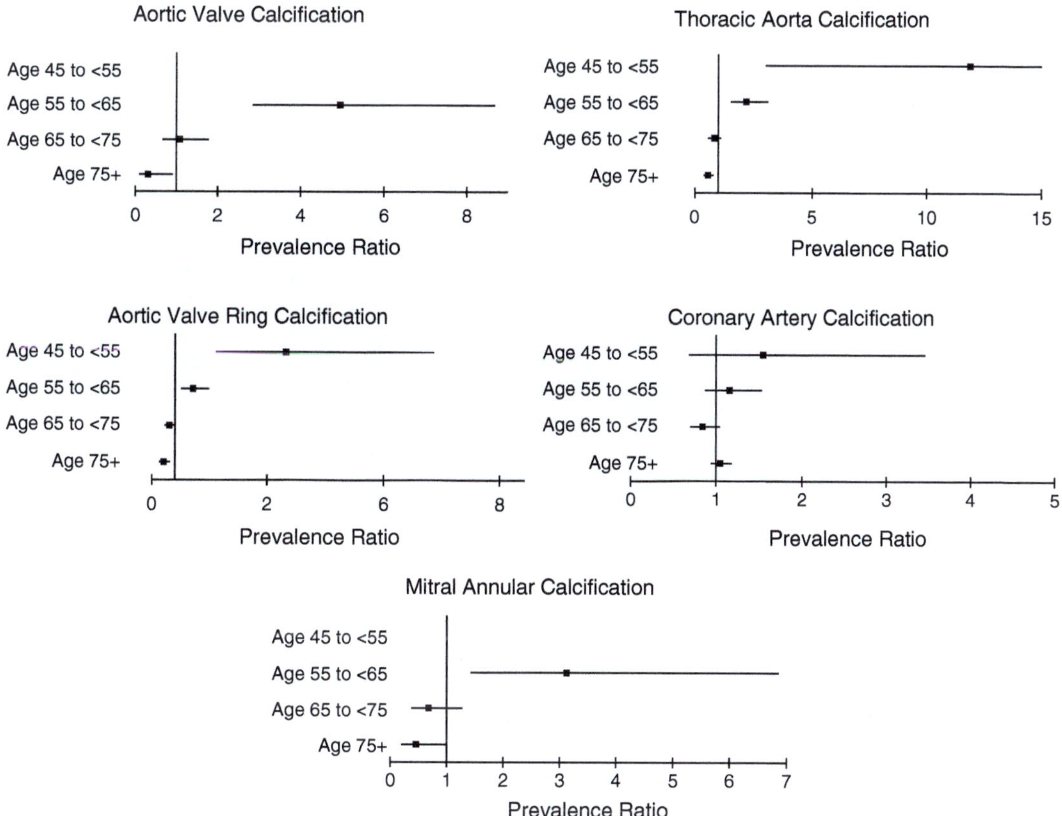

Fig. 13.3 Bisphosphonate-associated prevalence ratio of prevalent cardiovascular calcification stratified by age. The prevalence ratio of cardiovascular calcification associated with NCBP use is increased in young patients, but decreases with age and becomes significantly reduced in the elderly. Models adjust for age, body mass index, ethnicity, study site, education, income, health insurance, diabetes, hypertension, smoking, physical activity, blood pressure, serum cholesterol levels, and statin, hormone replacement, and renin-angiotensin inhibitor therapy (From Elmariah et al. (2010))

cardiac computed tomography at 1 year compared to a 130% increase in those not receiving a bisphosphonate (n=6) (Ariyoshi et al. 2006).

We recently evaluated the relationship between NCBP-use and cardiovascular calcification among female participants of the large and diverse Multi-Ethnic Study of Atherosclerosis (MESA) (Elmariah et al. 2010). We found a clear interaction of NCBP use with age such that there was reduced prevalence of vascular and valvular calcification in women ≥65 years of age and increased prevalence of cardiovascular calcification in younger women on treatment. Across all measures of cardiovascular calcification, aortic valve, aortic valve ring, mitral annulus, thoracic aorta, and coronary artery calcification (AVC, AVRC, MAC, TAC, and CAC, respectively) there was a consistent pattern of association across age strata (Fig. 13.4). In female subjects ≥65 years old, NCBP use was associated with less prevalent cardiovascular calcification (NCBP users vs. non-users: AVC 13% vs. 20%, $p=0.11$; AVRC 38% vs. 59%, $p<0.0001$; MAC 11% vs. 21%, $p<0.05$; TAC 38% vs. 54%, $p<0.001$; CAC 57% vs. 63%, $p=0.27$). In contrast, cardiovascular calcification was more prevalent in NCBP users younger than 65 years (AVC 18% vs. 4%, $p<0.0001$; AVRC 38% vs. 17%, $p=0.0001$; MAC 9% vs. 3%, $p<0.005$; TAC 31% vs. 11%, $p<0.0001$; CAC 36% vs. 25%, $p<0.05$). A similar relationship was observed in an analysis of severity of cardiovascular calcification. While the reason for this surprising relationship is elusive,

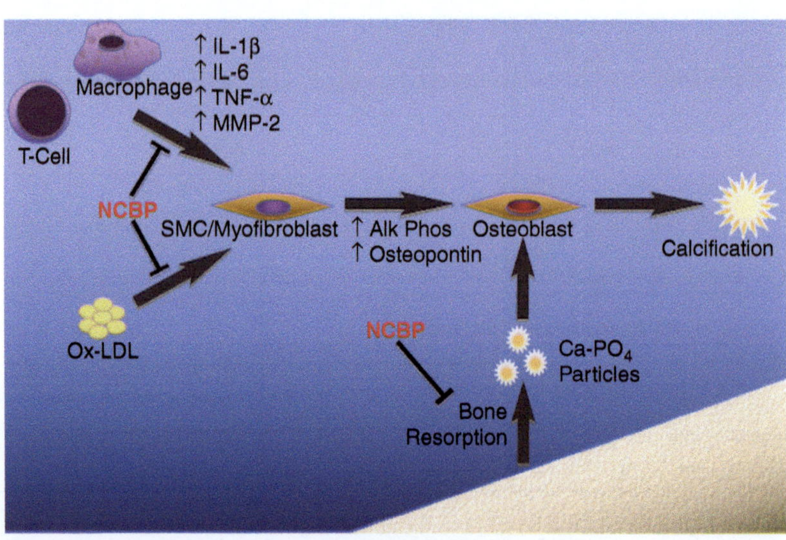

Fig. 13.4 Proposed mechanisms of action of nitrogen-containing bisphosphonates on cardiovascular calcification. *Alk Phos* alkaline phosphatase, *Ca* calcium, *IL* interleukin, *MMP* matrix metalloproteinase, *Ox-LDL* oxidized low-density lipoprotein, PO_4 phosphate, *SMC* smooth muscle cells, *TNF* tumor necrosis factor

several possible explanations exist. First, low BMD is associated with increased risk of cardiovascular calcification (Hyder et al. 2008; Pennisi et al. 2004; Parhami et al. 2000). Given that NCBP therapy is prescribed predominantly for patients with osteoporosis, NCBP therapy may initially serve as a marker for the increased risk of cardiovascular calcification associated with low BMD. With age, and presumably longer duration of NCBP use, the putative protective effect of these agents may overcome the BMD-associated cardiovascular risk thereby reversing the association. Alternatively, bisphosphonate use in younger women may be a marker for an aggressive osteoporotic process that may place them at higher risk of cardiovascular calcification. Lastly, a true age-dependent mechanism of NCBP action or of the relationship between osteoporosis and atherosclerosis remains. Unfortunately, the cross-sectional nature of the analysis, the mechanistic relationship between NCBP-use and cardiovascular calcification could not be elucidated.

Effects of Bisphosphonates on the Progression of Aortic Stenosis

Over the last 2 years, several small studies have evaluated the impact of bisphosphonate use on the progression of aortic stenosis. In the first, Skolnick et al. retrospectively evaluated data from 55 patients with mild or moderate AS who underwent a serial echocardiogram a mean 2.4 ± 1.0 years later (Skolnick et al. 2009). The authors identified 18 patients receiving osteoporosis therapy (OT), including bisphosphonates, calcitonin, or estrogen receptor modulators. Compared to those patients not receiving OT, patients receiving OT demonstrated slowed progression of AS (mean annual change in aortic valve area: -0.22 ± 0.22 vs. -0.10 ± 0.18 cm^2; $p = 0.025$). While this study evaluated several inhibitors of bone resorption, the majority of OT patients (67%) were on bisphosphonate therapy. A similar small study, aortic valve area decreased by 0.2 cm^2 in the reference group (n=68) and actually improved by 0.1 cm^2 with bisphosphonate use (n=8) over a mean follow-up of 23 months ($p < 0.001$) (Innasimuthu and Katz 2011).

In the largest study to date, Sterbakova and colleagues compared the progression of aortic stenosis in 28 bisphosphonate users to 75 non-users (Sterbakova et al. 2010). Importantly, the authors stratified their analysis by severity of aortic stenosis. In those with mild AS, bisphosphonates were associated with slowed AS progression. Specifically, over a mean follow-up of 29 ± 13 months, the annualized change in the mean aortic valve gradient was 0.1 ± 3.3 mmHg/year in bisphosphonate users compared to 2.8 ± 3.3 mmHg/year in non-users ($p = 0.002$; Table 13.2). Bisphosphonate use had no impact

Table 13.2 Comparison of echocardiographic characteristics between the bisphosphonate-treated and untreated patients in the whole study sample and within the subgroups of mild and moderate-to-severe AS

	All patients (n = 103)			Mild AS (n = 57)			Moderate-to-severe AS (n = 46)		
	Bisphosphonate-treated (n = 28)	Untreated (n = 75)	P	Bisphosphonate-treated (n = 22)	Untreated (n = 35)	P	Bisphosphonate-treated (n = 6)	Untreated (n = 40)	P
Baseline									
LVEF, %	61 ± 9	60 ± 9	0.446	61 ± 9	57 ± 10	0.096	62 ± 6	68 ± 8	0.561
LVd, mm	49 ± 7	49 ± 7	0.755	49 ± 7	51 ± 6	0.252	51 ± 8	48 ± 7	0.396
Maximal gradient, mmHg	35 ± 28	52 ± 26	<0.001	22 ± 8	30 ± 11	0.003	82 ± 25	70 ± 20	0.219
Mean gradient, mmHg	23 ± 20	33 ± 19	<0.001	14 ± 4.9	17 ± 6.1	0.010	56 ± 18	46 ± 15	0.202
Final									
LVEF, %	56 ± 13	57 ± 13	0.535	57 ± 12	55 ± 15	0.694	52 ± 17	59 ± 11	0.228
LVd, mm	49 ± 9	49 ± 8	0.707	49 ± 8	51 ± 7	0.252	50 ± 9	48 ± 9	0.452
Maximal gradient, mmHg	39 ± 33	62 ± 29	<0.001	27 ± 16	41 ± 16	<0.001	86 ± 37	81 ± 24	0.566
Mean gradient, mmHg	23 ± 20	38 ± 19	<0.001	15 ± 9	24 ± 10	0.001	53 ± 21	51 ± 16	0.632
Annualized maximal gradient change mmHg/Year	1.5 ± 6.7	4.7 ± 7.2	0.008	1.2 ± 5.2	4.3 ± 5.7	0.013	2.3 ± 11	5.1 ± 8	0.300
Annualized mean gradient change mmHg/Year	−0.3 ± 4.8	2.0 ± 5.7	0.007	0.1 ± 3.3	2.8 ± 3.3	0.002	−1.7 ± 9	1.3 ± 7	0.264

From Sterbakova et al. (2010)
Values are shown as means as standard deviations
LVEF left ventricular ejection fraction, *LVd* left ventricular diastolic dimension

on the progression of AS in those with moderate-to-severe AS. Despite stratifying by AS severity, however, the baseline mean aortic valve gradient was significantly greater in the untreated group than in the bisphosphonate group (24 ± 10 vs. 15 ± 9 mmHg, respectively; $p = 0.001$). The higher baseline gradient may explain the more rapid AS progression in bisphosphonate non-users, but a multivariable analysis adjusting for baseline mean gradient and several clinical confounders identified bisphosphonates as the only independent predictor of slower AS progression. These studies, while small, support the hypothesis that bisphosphonate use may slow the progression of aortic stenosis and lay the foundation for future work in this field.

Summary

Calcific aortic valve disease occurs via an active process similar to artherosclerosis. As such, therapies effective in limiting atherosclerosis, such as statins, may slow the progression of AVC and AS. To date, experimental data are inconclusive regarding the effects of statins on AS; however, inhibition of the mevalonate pathway has shown promise. NCBPs inhibit the mevalonate pathway and share several pleiotropic effects with statins. NCBPs exhibit anti-inflammatory effects, reduce serum LDL-cholesterol, raise HDL-cholesterol, limit vascular calcification, and inhibit AVC in animal models. Several small, retrospective studies have demonstrated that bisphosphonate therapy is associated with slowed progression of AS. Additionally, analyses from MESA suggest that NCBPs may exert a beneficial effect on valve and vascular calcification. With such growing evidence, prospective clinical trials testing the hypothesis that NCBPs inhibit the progression of calcific aortic valve disease are clearly needed. It will be important to focus such trials on early stages of disease as it is unlikely that pharmacologic therapy will affect heavily calcified and stenotic valves. Additionally, further efforts are needed to identify mechanistic pathways modulated by NCBPs within the aortic valve.

References

Adami S, Braga V, Guidi G, et al. Chronic intravenous aminobisphosphonate therapy increases high-density lipoprotein cholesterol and decreases low-density lipoprotein cholesterol. J Bone Miner Res. 2000;15(3):599–604.

Aft R. Bisphosphonates in breast cancer: clinical activity and implications of preclinical data. Clin Adv Hematol Oncol. 2011;9(3):194–205.

Aikawa E, Nahrendorf M, Figueiredo JL, et al. Osteogenesis associates with inflammation in early-stage atherosclerosis evaluated by molecular imaging in vivo. Circulation. 2007a;116(24):2841–50.

Aikawa E, Nahrendorf M, Sosnovik D, et al. Multimodality molecular imaging identifies proteolytic and osteogenic activities in early aortic valve disease. Circulation. 2007b;115(3):377–86.

Allison MA, Cheung P, Criqui MH, et al. Mitral and aortic annular calcification are highly associated with systemic calcified atherosclerosis. Circulation. 2006; 113(6):861–6.

Ariyoshi T, Eishi K, Sakamoto I, et al. Effect of etidronic acid on arterial calcification in dialysis patients. Clin Drug Investig. 2006;26(4):215–22.

Benford HL, Frith JC, Auriola S, et al. Farnesol and geranylgeraniol prevent activation of caspases by aminobisphosphonates: biochemical evidence for two distinct pharmacological classes of bisphosphonate drugs. Mol Pharmacol. 1999;56(1):131–40.

Bergstrom JD, Bostedor RG, Masarachia PJ, et al. Alendronate is a specific, nanomolar inhibitor of farnesyl diphosphate synthase. Arch Biochem Biophys. 2000;373(1):231–41.

Budoff MJ, Raggi P. Coronary artery disease progression assessed by electron-beam computed tomography. Am J Cardiol. 2001;88(2A):46E–50.

Callister TQ, Raggi P, Cooil B, et al. Effect of HMG-CoA reductase inhibitors on coronary artery disease as assessed by electron-beam computed tomography. N Engl J Med. 1998;339(27):1972–8.

Danenberg HD, Fishbein I, Gao J, et al. Macrophage depletion by clodronate-containing liposomes reduces neointimal formation after balloon injury in rats and rabbits. Circulation. 2002;106(5):599–605.

Danenberg HD, Golomb G, Groothuis A, et al. Liposomal alendronate inhibits systemic innate immunity and reduces in-stent neointimal hyperplasia in rabbits. Circulation. 2003;108(22):2798–804.

Demer L, Tintut Y. The roles of lipid oxidation products and receptor activator of nuclear factor-kappaB signaling in atherosclerotic calcification. Circ Res. 2011;108(12):1482–93.

Di Salvatore M, Orlandi A, Bagala C, et al. Anti-tumour and anti-angiogenetic effects of zoledronic acid on human non-small-cell lung cancer cell line. Cell Prolif. 2011;44(2):139–46.

Elmariah S, Mohler 3rd ER. The pathogenesis and treatment of the valvulopathy of aortic stenosis: beyond the SEAS. Curr Cardiol Rep. 2010;12(2):125–32.

Elmariah S, Delaney JA, O'Brien KD, et al. Bisphosphonate use and prevalence of valvular and vascular calcification in women MESA (the multi-ethnic study of atherosclerosis). J Am Coll Cardiol. 2010;56(21):1752–9.

Fleisch H, Russell RG, Francis MD. Diphosphonates inhibit hydroxyapatite dissolution in vitro and bone resorption in tissue culture and in vivo. Science (New York, NY). 1969;165(899):1262–4.

Frith JC, Monkkonen J, Blackburn GM, et al. Clodronate and liposome-encapsulated clodronate are metabolized to a toxic ATP analog, adenosine 5′-(beta, gamma-dichloromethylene) triphosphate, by mammalian cells in vitro. J Bone Miner Res. 1997;12(9):1358–67.

Giraudo E, Inoue M, Hanahan D. An amino-bisphosphonate targets MMP-9-expressing macrophages and angiogenesis to impair cervical carcinogenesis. J Clin Invest. 2004;114(5):623–33.

Goldbarg SH, Elmariah S, Miller MA, et al. Insights into degenerative aortic valve disease. J Am Coll Cardiol. 2007;50(13):1205–13.

Gozzetti A, Gennari L, Merlotti D, et al. The effects of zoledronic acid on serum lipids in multiple myeloma patients. Calcif Tissue Int. 2008;82(4):258–62.

Hyder JA, Allison MA, Wong N, et al. Association of coronary artery and aortic calcium with lumbar bone density: the MESA Abdominal Aortic Calcium Study. Am J Epidemiol. 2008;169(2):186–94.

Innasimuthu AL, Katz WE. Effect of bisphosphonates on the progression of degenerative aortic stenosis. Echocardiography. 2011;28(1):1–7.

Kaden JJ, Bickelhaupt S, Grobholz R, et al. Receptor activator of nuclear factor kappaB ligand and osteoprotegerin regulate aortic valve calcification. J Mol Cell Cardiol. 2004;36(1):57–66.

Koshiyama H, Nakamura Y, Tanaka S, et al. Decrease in carotid intima-media thickness after 1-year therapy with etidronate for osteopenia associated with type 2 diabetes. J Clin Endocrinol Metabol. 2000;85(8):2793–6.

Lai TJ, Hsu SF, Li TM, et al. Alendronate inhibits cell invasion and MMP-2 secretion in human chondrosarcoma cell line. Acta Pharmacol Sin. 2007;28(8): 1231–5.

Liao JK. Isoprenoids as mediators of the biological effects of statins. J Clin Invest. 2002;110(3):285–8.

Luan Z, Chase AJ, Newby AC. Statins inhibit secretion of metalloproteinases 1, 2, 3, and -9 from vascular smooth muscle cells and macrophages. Arterioscler Thromb Vasc Biol. 2003;23(5):769–75.

Mohler 3rd ER, Gannon F, Reynolds C, et al. Bone formation and inflammation in cardiac valves. Circulation. 2001;103(11):1522–8.

Mohler 3rd ER, Wang H, Medenilla E, et al. Effect of statin treatment on aortic valve and coronary artery calcification. J Heart Valve Dis. 2007;16(4):378–86.

Montagnani A, Gonnelli S, Cepollaro C, et al. Changes in serum HDL and LDL cholesterol in patients with Paget's bone disease treated with pamidronate. Bone. 2003;32(1):15–9.

Moreno PR, Astudillo L, Elmariah S, et al. Increased macrophage infiltration and neovascularization in congenital bicuspid aortic valve stenosis. J Thorac Cardiovasc Surg. 2011;142(4):895–901.

Nitta K, Akiba T, Suzuki K, et al. Effects of cyclic intermittent etidronate therapy on coronary artery calcification in patients receiving long-term hemodialysis. Am J Kidney Dis. 2004;44(4):680–8.

Osman L, Yacoub MH, Latif N, et al. Role of human valve interstitial cells in valve calcification and their response to atorvastatin. Circulation. 2006;114 (1 Suppl):I547–52.

Otto CM, Lind BK, Kitzman DW, et al. Association of aortic-valve sclerosis with cardiovascular mortality and morbidity in the elderly. N Engl J Med. 1999;341(3):142–7.

Parhami F, Morrow AD, Balucan J, et al. Lipid oxidation products have opposite effects on calcifying vascular cell and bone cell differentiation. A possible explanation for the paradox of arterial calcification in osteoporotic patients. Arterioscler Thromb Vasc Biol. 1997; 17(4):680–7.

Parhami F, Garfinkel A, Demer LL. Role of lipids in osteoporosis. Arterioscler Thromb Vasc Biol. 2000; 20(11):2346–8.

Pennanen N, Lapinjoki S, Urtti A, et al. Effect of liposomal and free bisphosphonates on the IL-1 beta, IL-6 and TNF alpha secretion from RAW 264 cells in vitro. Pharm Res. 1995;12(6):916–22.

Pennisi P, Signorelli SS, Riccobene S, et al. Low bone density and abnormal bone turnover in patients with atherosclerosis of peripheral vessels. Osteoporos Int. 2004;15(5):389–95.

Pohle K, Maffert R, Ropers D, et al. Progression of aortic valve calcification: association with coronary atherosclerosis and cardiovascular risk factors. Circulation. 2001;104(16):1927–32.

Price PA, Faus SA, Williamson MK. Bisphosphonates alendronate and ibandronate inhibit artery calcification at doses comparable to those that inhibit bone resorption. Arterioscler Thromb Vasc Biol. 2001;21(5):817–24.

Price PA, Roublick AM, Williamson MK. Artery calcification in uremic rats is increased by a low protein diet and prevented by treatment with ibandronate. Kidney Int. 2006;70(9):1577–83.

Rodan GA, Fleisch HA. Bisphosphonates: mechanisms of action. J Clin Invest. 1996;97(12):2692–6.

Russell RG, Rogers MJ. Bisphosphonates: from the laboratory to the clinic and back again. Bone. 1999;25(1): 97–106.

Sansoni P, Passeri G, Fagnoni F, et al. Inhibition of antigen-presenting cell function by alendronate in vitro. J Bone Miner Res. 1995;10(11):1719–25.

Shavelle DM, Takasu J, Budoff MJ, et al. HMG CoA reductase inhibitor (statin) and aortic valve calcium. Lancet. 2002;359(9312):1125–6.

Skolnick AH, Osranek M, Formica P, et al. Osteoporosis treatment and progression of aortic stenosis. Am J Cardiol. 2009;104(1):122–4.

Soini Y, Salo T, Satta J. Angiogenesis is involved in the pathogenesis of nonrheumatic aortic valve stenosis. Hum Pathol. 2003;34(8):756–63.

Sterbakova G, Vyskocil V, Linhartova K. Bisphosphonates in calcific aortic stenosis: association with slower progression in mild disease – a pilot retrospective study. Cardiology. 2010;117(3):184–9.

Tamura K, Suzuki Y, Hashiba H, et al. Effect of etidronate on aortic calcification and bone metabolism in calcitriol-treated rats with subtotal nephrectomy. J Pharmacol Sci. 2005;99(1):89–94.

Towler DA, Demer LL. Thematic series on the pathobiology of vascular calcification: an introduction. Circ Res. 2011;108(11):1378–80.

van Beek ER, Cohen LH, Leroy IM, et al. Differentiating the mechanisms of antiresorptive action of nitrogen containing bisphosphonates. Bone. 2003;33(5):805–11.

Wu B, Elmariah S, Kaplan FS, et al. Paradoxical effects of statins on aortic valve myofibroblasts and osteoblasts: implications for end-stage valvular heart disease. Arterioscler Thromb Vasc Biol. 2005;25(3):592–7.

Yamamoto H, Shavelle D, Takasu J, et al. Valvular and thoracic aortic calcium as a marker of the extent and severity of angiographic coronary artery disease. Am Heart J. 2003;146(1):153–9.

Ylitalo R, Monkkonen J, Urtti A, et al. Accumulation of bisphosphonates in the aorta and some other tissues of healthy and atherosclerotic rabbits. J Lab Clin Med. 1996;127(2):200–6.

Ylitalo R, Kalliovalkama J, Wu X, et al. Accumulation of bisphosphonates in human artery and their effects on human and rat arterial function in vitro. Pharmacol Toxicol. 1998;83(3):125–31.

Zhang FL, Casey PJ. Protein prenylation: molecular mechanisms and functional consequences. Annu Rev Biochem. 1996;65:241–69.

LDL-Density-Theory: Clinical Trial Design for Aortic Valve Disease

14

Nalini Marie Rajamannan

Introduction

The cellular mechanisms are evolving rapidly in the field of calcific aortic valve biology. The experimental studies will have future translational implications for the treatment of this disease process. This chapter provides the premise for the role of lipids to activate atherosclerosis within the heart to initiate the development of bone formation. Lessons from the experimental studies have evolved into a series of clinical parameters, which provide the foundation for an algorithm to treat aortic valve disease: the LDL-Density-Radius and the LDL-Density-Pressure Theories. The LDL Density Theories provides a premise for the translational role of the Lrp 5/6 receptor biology in the treatment of calcific aortic valve disease.

The LDL-Density-Radius Theory assumes the initiating event in aortic valve disease is atherosclerosis, then, the possibility for medical therapy for aortic valve disease resides in two fundamental differences in vascular versus valvular biology: first is calculating the magnitude of LDL lowering necessary to treat the process, and second is the difference in the radius between the aortic valve and that of the vessel. The LDL-Density-Pressure theory accounts for the hemodynamic pressure differential which regulates the Lrp5/6 receptors. The combination of these theories provide a biological and a hemodynamic approach towards understanding the development of valvular heart disease and the implications in the field of bone molecular biology. This chapter will review the theories, provide a basis for the development of valve disease and indicate future therapeutic approaches for this disease process in the future.

Lrp5 Receptor Biology

The low-density lipoprotein-related receptor 5 and 6 (Lrp5 and Lrp6) genes were cloned in 1998 based on their homology with the low-density lipoprotein receptor (LDLR) (Dong et al. 1998; Brown et al. 1998; Hey et al. 1998; Kim et al. 1998). Mutations in either LRP5 or LRP6, proteins have caused a number of disease processed in the field of bone (Gong et al. 2001; Little et al. 2002), and have been associated with cardiovascular disease (Kim et al. 1998; Fujino et al. 2003a; Rajamannan et al. 2005a; Caira et al. 2006). The most recent perspectives in the field of Lrp5/6 (Williams and Insogna 2009) in signaling in the bone and Lrp5 in the regulation of bone mass (Johnson and Summerfield 2005)demonstrate the most comprehensive reviews in this field and provide the background for the structure and function of these co-receptors.

N.M. Rajamannan, M.D.
Department of Molecular Biology and Biochemistry, Mayo Clinic, 200 First St SW, Rochester, MN 55905, USA

Department of Aerospace Engineering, University of Notre Dame, South Bend, IN, USA
e-mail: nrajamannan@gmail.com

N.M. Rajamannan (ed.), *Cardiac Valvular Medicine*,
DOI 10.1007/978-1-4471-4132-7_14, © Springer-Verlag London 2013

The low density lipoprotein co-receptor Lrp5/6 is a member of the family of structurally closely related cell surface low density lipoprotein receptors that have diverse biological functions in different organs, tissues and cell types which are important in development and disease mechanisms. The most prominent role in this evolutionary ancient family is cholesterol homeostasis. In humans, cholesterol in the blood is captured by low-density lipoprotein (LDL) and metabolized by the liver via endocytosis of the LDL receptor. There is recent evidence that members of the LDL receptor gene family are active in the cell signaling pathways between specialized cells in many multicellular organisms.

The LRP5 pathway regulates bone formation in different diseases of bone (Gong et al. 2001; Boyden et al. 2002). The discovery of the LRP5 receptor in the gain of function (Boyden et al. 2002) and loss of function (Gong et al. 2001) mutations in the development of bone diseases, resulted in a number of studies which have shown that activation of the canonical Wnt pathway is important in osteoblastogenesis (Fujino et al. 2003b; Babij et al. 2003; Westendorf et al. 2004; Holmen et al. 2004). Three studies to date have confirmed the regulation of the LRP5/Wnt pathway for cardiovascular calcification *in vivo* and *ex vivo* (Rajamannan et al. 2005a; Caira et al. 2006; Shao et al. 2005). The LRP5 receptor signaling in

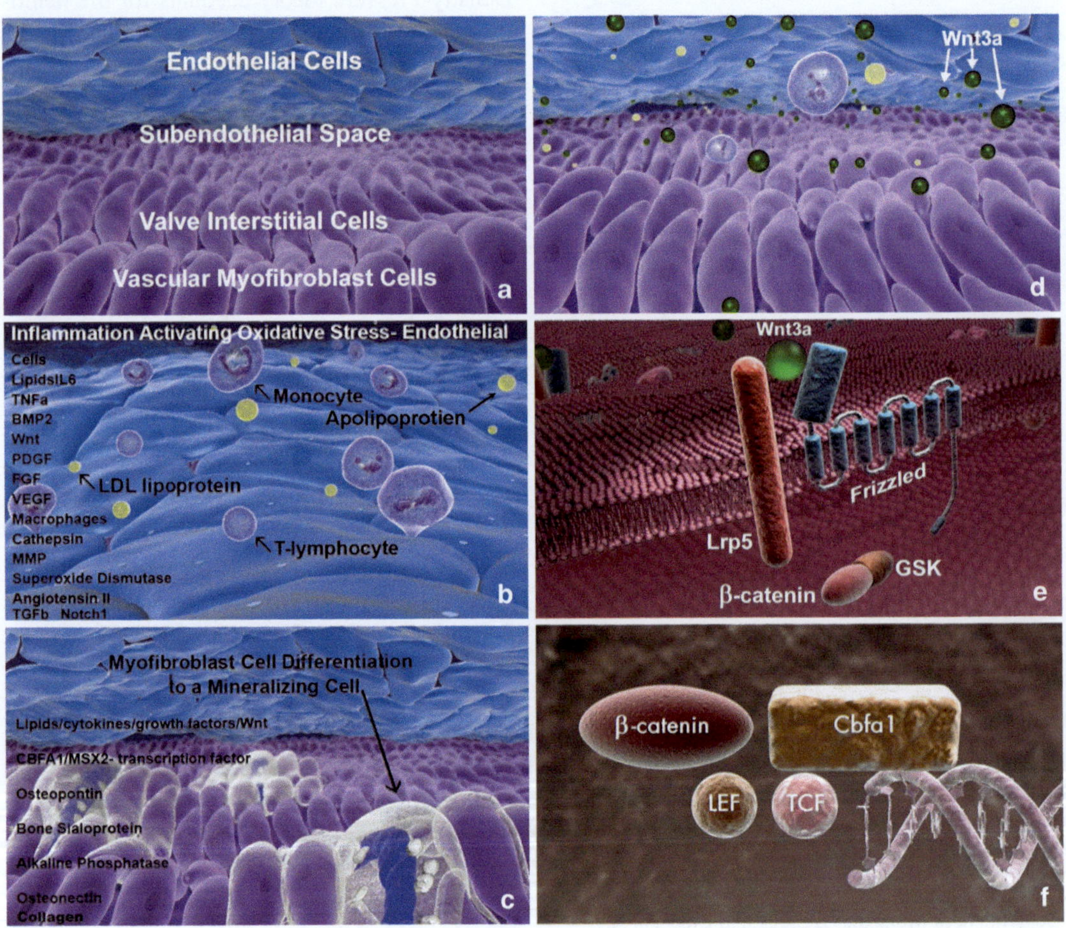

Fig. 14.1 Cell signaling events involved in the development of calcific aortic stenosis *Panel* **a**: Cell layers along the Aortic Valve Fibrosa surface where calcified nodules develop. *Panel* **b**: Endothelial layer of the aortic valve: Effects of Oxidative Stress. *Panel* **c**: Signaling pathways important in the development of myofibroblast calcification. *Panel* **d**: Secretion of Wnt3a in the activation of the Lrp5 receptor pathway. *Panel* **e**: Formation of the Lrp5/Wnt3a/Frizzled receptor complex along the surface of the myofibroblast extracellular membrane. *Panel* **f**: Transcriptional activation of the Cbfa1 osteoblast differentiation pathway in the myofibroblast cell

bone is mediated via the canonical Wnt pathway as shown in Fig. 14.1. In this pathway, Wnt proteins bind to receptors composed of a frizzled protein and either of the low-density lipoprotein receptor-related proteins LRP5 or LRP6. Signaling via Disheveled and/or Axin then results in inactivation of a multiprotein complex including Axin, adenomatous polyposis coli (APC), and glycogen synthase kinase-3β that normally renders β-catenin unstable. By inhibiting this complex, Wnt signals lead to accumulation of β-catenin in the cytosol and its entry into the nucleus. Once in the nucleus, β-catenin binds to proteins of the T-cell factor/lymphoid enhancer factor-1 family and modulates the expression of several target genes which include Cyclin D, Msx2, Cbfa1, and Sox9. Bone and cartilage are major tissues in the vertebrate skeletal system, which is primarily composed of three cell types: osteoblasts, chrondrocytes, and osteoclasts. In the developing embryo, osteoblast and chrondrocytes, both differentiate from common mesenchymal progenitors in situ, where as osteoclasts are of hematopoietic origin and brought in later by invading blood vessels. Osteoblast differentiation and maturation lead to bone formation controlled by two distinct mechanisms: intramembranous and endochondral ossification, both starting from mesenchymal condensations.

Studies have demonstrated that osteoblastogenesis and chrondrogenesis is critical in the development of valvular heart disease. The presence of calcification in the aortic valve is responsible for valve stenosis. Severe aortic stenosis can result in symptomatic chest pain, as well as syncope and congestive heart failure in patients with severe aortic valve stenosis. For years, aortic valve stenosis was thought to be a degenerative process. However, the pathologic lesion of calcified aortic valves demonstrate indicate the presence of complex calcification in these tissues. Furthermore, there are a growing number of descriptive studies delineating the presence of bone formation in the aortic valve (O'Brien et al. 1995a; Mohler et al. 1997, 2001).

Until recently the etiology of valvular heart disease has been thought to be a degenerative process related to the passive accumulation of calcium binding to the surface of the valve leaflet. Recent descriptive studies have demonstrated the critical features of aortic valve calcification, including osteoblast expression, cell proliferation and atherosclerosis (Mohler et al. 2001; O'Brien et al. 1995b; Rajamannan et al. 2002, 2003a) and mitral valve degeneration, glycosaminglycan accumulation, proteoglycan expression, and abnormal collagen expression (Whittaker et al. 1987; Wooley et al. 1991; Grande-Allen et al. 2004, 2005). These studies define the biochemical and histological characterization of these valve lesions. Studies have also shown that specific bone cell phenotypes are present in calcifying valve specimens in human specimens (Caira et al. 2006; Jian et al. 2001). These data provide the evidence that the aortic valve calcification follows the spectrum of bone formation in calcifying tissues. Genes which code for the bone extracellular matrix proteins in osteoblast cells include alkaline phosphatase (AP), osteopontin (OP), osteocalcin (OC), and bone sialoprotein (BSP). This data supports a potential regulatory mechanism that these matrix proteins play a role in the development of biomineralization. To date, many of these markers have been shown to be critical in the extracellular mineralization and bone formation that develops in normal osteoblast differentiation. Figure 14.1 demonstrates the dual role of Lrp5/6 in the activation of Wnt signaling: (1) lipid binding and (2) mechanostat effect in the activation of the Wnt Signaling pathway.

Figure 14.1 demonstrates the secretion of Wnt (Hawse et al. 2008) from the endothelial cells into the subendothelial space to bind and form the Lrp5/Wnt/Frizzled complex on the myofibroblast extracellular membrane (Rajamannan et al. 2005a). a. Formation of this trimeric complex activates the Cbfa1/Msx2/Sox9 (Rajamannan et al. 2005a; Caira et al. 2006; Shao et al. 2005) transcription factors important in the gene expression of osteogenic bone formation as shown in Fig. 14.1. Over time activation of the bone matrix proteins mineralize and calcify to induce stenosis. In summary, three important aspects in the cellular biology of calcific AV disease include atherosclerotic risk factors, genetics and signaling pathways specific to bone differentiation. Clinically, the presence of a moderately-to-severely calcified aortic valve is a significant predictor of poor outcome (Rosenhek et al. 2000), as compared to patients with mild-to-moderate aortic stenosis (Rosenhek et al. 2004), and has also subsequently been studied using quantitative electron beam computed tomography to measure calcium in the valve. Calcification, AS severity and progression are all important prognostic parameters. Furthermore these factors are interrelated since calcification predicts disease progression, which is in turn directly relates to AS severity.

Phenotypic Expression of Calcification in the Heart: The Bernoulli Equation

Fluid hemodynamics in the heart is dependent on multiple factors as derived by the Bernoulli's equation for fluid flow (Bernoulli 1738). Bernoulli described flow through a column is directly proportional to the change in pressure across the column and indirectly proportional to the resistance. The formula for flow through the heart, is similar to Ohm's law for electricity as shown in Eq. 14.1.

$$Q = \frac{\Delta P}{R} \quad (14.1)$$

The entire formula for resistance for steady state flow through a circular tube, is shown in Eq. 14.2, where η = viscosity, r = radius of the tube.

$$R = \frac{8n\,L}{\pi r^4} \quad (14.2)$$

Equations 14.1 and 14.2 can be combined to give the flow rate through a circular tube in terms of a pressure drop which is described as Poiseuille's law:

$$Q = \frac{\pi r^4}{8nL}\Delta P \quad (14.3)$$

The differences in the rate of fluid flow are dependent on the radius of the anatomic structure, which is inversely proportional to the resistance. In addition, it is important to note the inverse r^4 dependence of the resistance to fluid flow. If the radius of the tube is halved, the pressure drop for a given flow rate and viscosity is increased by a factor of 16. Since the flow rate is then proportional to the fourth power of the radius. The size of the radius becomes important as blood flows through the heart.

For example, the average diameter of a left main coronary artery is 4.5 ± 0.5 mm (Dodge et al. 1992), and the average diameter of for the left ventricular outflow tract is 2.0 ± 0.2 cm (Oh et al. 2007). From a circulatory perspective, these differences in the radii lengths become relevant as the effect of the calcification is correlated with the hemodynamic flow properties. These differences in radii will have different effects on resistance. This concept becomes important as the rates of occlusion for vascular occlusion vs. valvular stenosis are considered in the treatment of these two disease processes. Vascular occlusion occurs secondary to an increase in vascular atheroma which in many cases is a calcified artery, similar to valvular atherosclerosis and eventual calcification, however, both have different rates of progression depending on risk factors, genetics and signaling events. Treatment of these two diseases will have different rates of improvement because of multiple factors including: risk factors, genetics and the anatomic location of the disease which affects the physiology of flow. If both disease processes are treated at the same time, vascular occlusion will respond faster than the valve stenosis because of the size of the radius. Therefore, the fundamental difference in treating these two different diseases will be dependent not only on the targeting biologic signaling events important in calcification, but also understanding that the differences in rate of improvement depends on the size of the radius for the different disease processes. Theoretical understanding of the effect of fluid hemodynamics on the calcification phenotype, and the signaling mechanisms involved in the development of calcification, provides the foundation for why randomized vascular trials demonstrate positive results more rapidly than randomized valvular trials, if the trials are designed the same.

Clinical Studies in Aortic Valve Disease

The pioneers in valve clinical trials designed studies prior to the publication of many of the experimental models. The trials were designed with the traditional trial design for lipid lowering using vascular and valvular end points. The first randomized prospective study testing the effects of statins in aortic valve disease was published in 2005 (Cowell et al. 2005). In this double-blind, placebo-controlled trial, patients with calcific aortic stenosis were randomly assigned to receive either 80 mg of atorvastatin daily or a matched placebo. Aortic-valve stenosis and calcification were assessed with the use of Doppler echocardiography and helical computed tomography, respectively. The primary end points were change in aortic-jet velocity and aortic-valve calcium score, secondary end points were traditional vascular end-points. The SALTIRE investigators demonstrated a trend in slowing of the progression of the aortic valve stenosis but not a statistically significant study for primary end-points. The vascular end-points demonstrated statistically significant improvement. The SALTIRE investigators concluded that intensive lipid-lowering therapy does not halt the progression of calcific aortic stenosis or induce its regression (Cowell et al. 2005) and the reason for this negative trial is the timing of therapy (Newby et al. 2006).

In the RAAVE trial, Moura et al. (Moura et al. 2007), performed a prospective trial of AS with Rosuvastatin targeting serum LDL slowed progression of echo hemodynamic measurements, and improved inflammatory biomarkers providing the first clinical evidence for targeted therapy in patients with asymptomatic AS. The study's aim was to assess Rosuvastatin on the hemodynamic progression and the inflammatory markers of AS by treating LDL in patients with aortic stenosis according to the NCEP-ATPIII guidelines for 1.5 year. Prospective treatment of moderate aortic stenosis with Rosuvastatin targeting serum LDL did slow progression of echocardiographic parameters of aortic stenosis, improved inflammatory biomarkers and improved vascular end-points showing the first clinical evidence for targeted therapy in asymptomatic moderate to severe aortic stenosis (Moura et al. 2007).

The largest randomized clinical trial SEAS, Intensive Lipid Lowering with Simvastatin and Ezetimibe in Aortic Stenosis (Rossebo et al. 2008) This trial is a randomized, double-blind trial involving 1,873 patients with mild-to-moderate, asymptomatic aortic stenosis. Again, similar to SALTIRE, there were fewer patients with ischemic cardiovascular events in the Simvastatin–Ezetimibe group (148 patients) than in the placebo group (187 patients); the authors noted that this is mainly because of the smaller number of patients who underwent coronary-artery bypass grafting. Cancer occurred more frequently in the Simvastatin–Ezetimibe group (105 vs. 70, P=0.01). The investigators concluded that the medication did not reduce the composite outcome of combined aortic-valve events in patient with aortic stenosis including echo progression and vascular end-points. These three clinical trials have different results. However, the design of the clinical trials for SALTIRE and SEAS was the traditional vascular trial studies. RAAVE was designed by clinical echocardiographers and a valve biologist with the perspective of many years of testing the effects of statins in *in vivo* animal models. Therefore, the results are positive with the design of the trial to include the cellular and hemodynamic mechanisms of aortic valve disease.

Translating Experimental Studies into the Treatment of Valvular Heart Disease: The LDL-Density-Radius Theory

Lessons from the experimental studies have evolved into a series of clinical parameters, which provide the foundation for an algorithm to treat aortic valve disease. the LDL-Density-Radius Theory. From a valve biologist perspective, the possibility for medical therapy for aortic valve disease resides in two fundamental differences in vascular versus valvular biology: first is calculating the magnitude of LDL lowering necessary to treat the process, and second is the difference in the radius between the aortic valve and that of the vessel. These differences are important to understand for the final analysis of these trials, and for the future trial design for aortic valve disease.

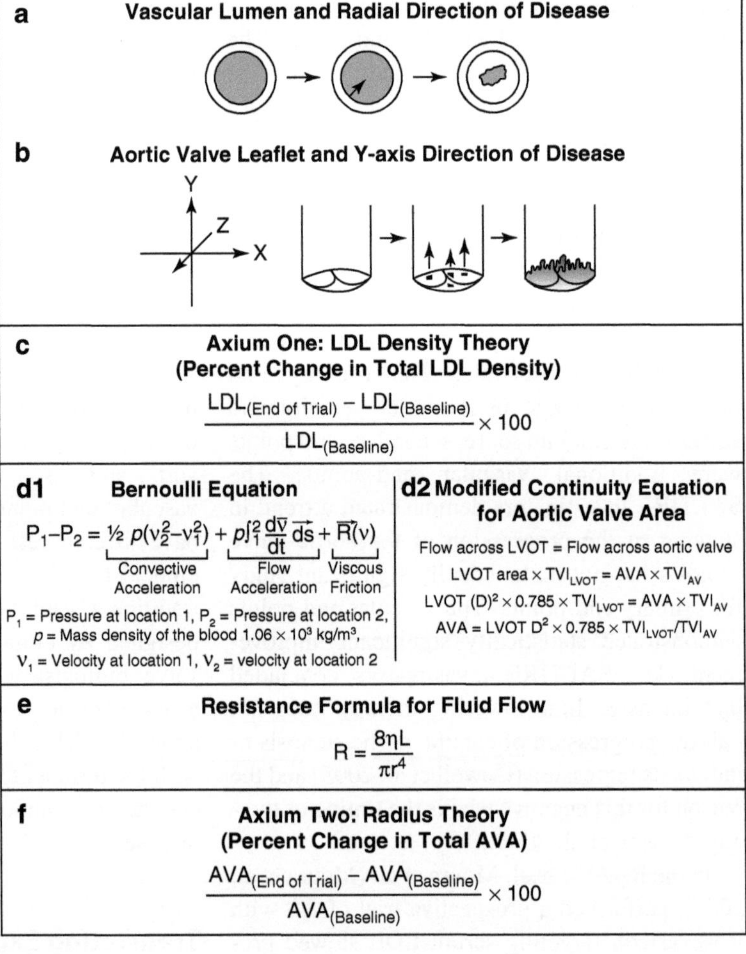

Fig. 14.2 The LDL-Density-Radius theory *Panel* **a**: Vascular lumen and radial direction of disease. *Panel* **b**: Aortic valve leaflet and Y-axis direction of disease. *Panel* **c**: Axiom one: LDL-Density theory. *Panel* **d1**: Bernoulli equation. *Panel* **d2**: Modified continuity equation for aortic valve area. *Panel* **e**: Resistance for fluid flow. *Panel* **f**: Axiom two: radius theory

The hypothesis to measure the effects of lipid lowering in slowing the progression of calcific aortic stenosis is dependent on two axioms, biology and hemodynamics. The experimental data demonstrates that lipids activate the bone differentiation within the valve myofibroblast (Rajamannan et al. 2005a) and atheroma in the vessel. The first axiom is the LDL density theory. The first axiom accounts for the effect of Low-density lipoprotein (LDL) biology in atherosclerosis. If the risk factors of elevated cholesterol and LDL are important in this disease then measuring lipid lowering using standard established assays for LDL in the treatment of valve disease becomes necessary. This approach does not take into account the effect of other inflammatory contributors to this disease including sharp (Hsu et al. 2006), HDL (Yilmaz et al. 2004), homocysteine (Agmon et al. 2001; Gunduz et al. 2005), CD40 (Moura et al. 2007, 2008; Novaro et al. 2007; Galante et al. 2001), and small particle LDL (Busseuil et al. 2008; Mohty et al. 2008) which also contribute to the pathogenesis of valvular heart disease but are not routinely measured in everyday clinical practice.

The direction of the LDL affects the vascular lumen in an inward direction causing occlusion overtime, as shown in Fig. 14.2, Panel a. The direction of this LDL affects the valve is an upward direction along the y axis along the aortic surface of the valvular fibrosa (O'Brien et al. 1996). Overtime, the leaflets stiffen and can fuse in some valves (Kumar et al. 2007) the overall effect on the radius is a reduction in the aortic valve opening and obstruction which leads to progressive stenosis (Drolet et al. 2003) of the outflow tract Fig. 14.2,

Panel b. Figure 14.2, Panel c, demonstrates a formula to calculate the percent reduction of the LDL density before and after therapy similar to the calculation derived in the Reversal trial measuring reductions in atheroma volume in coronary artery disease (Nissen et al. 2004). Calculation of the percent lowering of LDL density in a valve trial allows for the potential to calculate the improvement on the biologic effect of LDL on this disease.

The second axiom for the theory is the radius theory. This hemodynamic radius principle is based on the biologic direction of this disease. The second axiom calculates the biologic effect of the changes in the radius for specific the anatomic location in the heart. Figure 14.2, Panel d1, the formula for Bernoulli flow through a pipe, as modified (Hatle et al. 1980) for echocardiography. Figure 14.2, Panel d2, is the formula to calculate aortic valve areas by echocardiography using the doppler technique (Smith et al. 1986). The derivation of the Bernoulli Principal for this equation includes the drop of the calculation for the flow acceleration and the viscous friction because the velocity profile in the center of the lumen is usually so low that the effect of viscous friction becomes insignificant and not necessary to calculate. Clinically, the viscous friction factor has been ignored as part of the continuity equation in aortic valve disease as defined by the echocardiography physiologists (Hatle et al. 1978).

However, the concept of viscous friction becomes important when comparing vascular trials to valvular trials. The size of the radius plays a very important role in the time to see treatment effects which are defined by vascular clinical end-points such as ischemia and acute myocardial infarction. To date SEAS and SALTIRE were designed using the vascular trial approach which includes randomizing patients to therapy versus no therapy and measuring echo and vascular end-points. However, because the flow in the lumen of the vasculature is not flat due to a smaller radius (Bernoulli 1738), the viscous friction factor must be taken into account in evaluating the treatment effects within the vasculature as derived by Bernoulli's original equation (Bernoulli 1738). Therefore, the treatment effect of LDL lowering will have a more rapid effect on the vasculature as compared to the heart valve.

The importance of the smaller radius is shown in Fig. 14.2, Panel e, which is the calculation of resistance of fluid through a pipe. If the size of the radius(r) is significant in the calculation of flow, then the inverse r^4 dependence of the resistance becomes important in the treatment a smaller radius versus a larger radius in the aortic valve area as viscosity increases by a factor of 16. Therefore, comparing the rates of improvement in a vascular trial versus a valvular trial will be different due the differences in the size of the radius and the derivation of the modified Bernoulli equation for the echocardiographic formula for valve areas. The Continuity Equation drops the calculation of viscous friction due to the large size of the radius of the outflow tract of the left ventricle.

To measure the treatment effect for aortic valve disease: Fig. 14.2, Panel f, is the calculation for the percent improvement for the aortic valve area. Mathematically and biologically, clinical trials for aortic valve disease may consider the following two axioms for targeting the disease biology in terms of the radial direction of disease and the magnitude of the LDL density to activate the atherosclerotic process according to Bernoulli's original formula and the effect on resistance and fluid flow. The effect will require a longer period of time to see slowing of progression in the Aortic valve area for the reasons described in the LDL-Density-Radius Theory. Furthermore, the effect may be masked in the results of the published trials as the patients were randomized to treatment and the two axioms described in this theory are not accounted for in the randomization protocol.

LDL-Density-Pressure Theory: Hypothesis for the Role of Lrp5/6 Signaling in Valvular Heart Disease

This hypothesis evaluates the effect of pressure in the development of calcification is dependent on two axioms, biology and hemodynamics. The experimental data demonstrates that lipids activate the bone differentiation

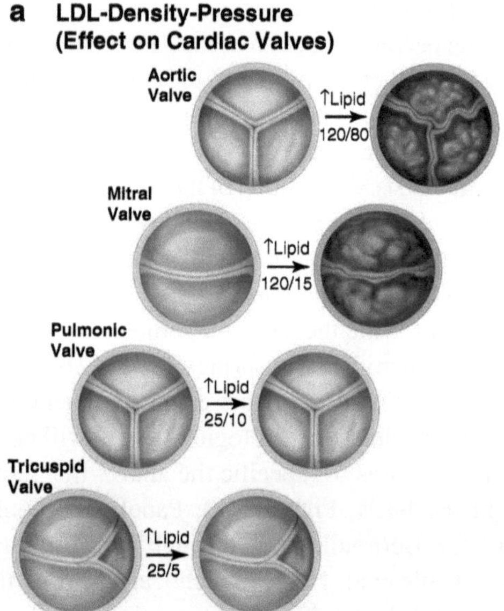

b Axiom One: LDL-Density-Pressure (Percent Change in Total LDL Density)

$$\frac{LDL_{(end\ of\ trail)} - LDL_{(Baseline)}}{LDL_{(Baseline)}} \times 100$$

c1 Bernoulli Equation

$$P_1 - P_2 = \underbrace{\tfrac{1}{2}\rho(V_2^2 - V_1^2)}_{\text{Convective Acceleration}} + \underbrace{\rho\int_1^2 \frac{d\vec{V}}{dt}\,d\vec{s}}_{\text{Flow Acceleration}} + \underbrace{R(\vec{V})}_{\text{Viscous Friction}}$$

P_1 = Pressure at location 1, P_2 = Pressure at location 2, ρ = Mass density of the blood $1.06 \times 10^3\ kg/m^3$, V_1 = Velocity at location 1, V_2 = velocity at location 2

c2 Modified Continuty Equation for Aortic Valve Area

Flow across LVOT = Flow across aortic valve

$$\text{LVOT area} \times TVI_{LVOT} = AVA \times TVI_{AV}$$

$$\text{LVOT } (D)^2 \times 0.785 \times TVI_{LVOT} = AVA \times TVI_{AV}$$

$$AVA = \text{LVOT } D^2 \times 0.785 \times TVI_{LVOT}/TVI_{AV}$$

d Pressure Formula for Fluid Flow

$$\Delta P = Q\frac{8\mu L}{\pi r^4}$$

e Axiom Two: Pressure Theory (Percent Change in Total Blood Pressure)

$$\frac{BP_{(end\ of\ trail)} - BP_{(Baseline)}}{BP_{(Baseline)}} \times 100$$

Fig. 14.3 The LDL-Density-Pressure theory (effect on cardiac valves). The serum lipid levels affect all four heart valves as the lipids circulate throughout the heart. However, the pressure is different depending on the chamber and location in the heart. *Panel* **a**: The effect of lipids and the different pressures in the heart. *Panel* **b**: Axiom one: LDL-Density-Pressure- percent change in the LDL density. *Panel* **c1**: Bernoulli equation. *Panel* **c2**: Modified continuity equation for aortic valve area. *Panel* **d**: Pressure formula for fluid flow. *Panel* **e**: Axiom two: pressure theory (percent change in total blood pressure)

(Rajamannan et al. 2005a) in the valve. The first axiom is the effect of Low-density lipoprotein (LDL) in atherosclerotic biology. LDL affects the left sided heart valves, as shown in Fig. 14.3, Panel a. In the presence of experimental hypercholesterolemic the LDL only manifests disease in the left sided valves where the pressure in the heart is higher Overtime, the leaflets fuse which to occlude the aortic valve Fig. 14.3, Panel b. Calculation of the percent lowering of LDL density will target specifically the biologic effect of LDL on this disease. Figure 14.3, Panel c, demonstrates a formula to calculate the percent reduction of the LDL density before and after therapy.

The second axiom is the effect of the radius on fluid flow. The Bernoulli equation (Bernoulli 1738) Fig. 14.3, Panel c1, the formula for flow through a pipe, was modified (Hatle et al. 1980) Fig. 14.3, Panel c2, to calculate aortic valve areas by echocardiography using the doppler technique. The modification of this equation for aortic valve areas includes the drop of the calculation for the flow acceleration and the viscous friction because the velocity profile in the center of the lumen is usually flat, therefore, the viscous friction factor can be ignored in the clinical setting of aortic valve disease. However, the flow in the lumen of a vessel is not flat due to smaller radius, therefore, the viscous friction factor must be taken into account. The importance of the smaller radius is shown in Fig. 14.3, Panel d, which is the calculation of resistance of fluid through a pipe. This size of the radius becomes important in the calculation of flow as the inverse r^4 dependence of the resistance to fluid flow will increase viscosity by a factor of 16 requiring the effect of viscous friction to become important with smaller radii. Reductions of the LDL density will therefore, have a quicker effect in the reduction of the vascular lesion as it affects the lumen circumference directly as shown in Fig. 14.3, Panel a. To measure the treatment effect for blood pressure on aortic valve disease: Fig. 14.3, Panel f, is the calculation for the percent improvement in the blood pressure as an effect on the hemodynamic progression of the valve disease. This hypothesis provides a mathematical foundation for treating this disease in the heart.

Hemodynamic Phenotype of Cardiac Valve Disease: Role of Lrp5/6 in Cardiac Valve Disease

The development of heart valve disease occurs in the left side of the heart the aortic valve and the mitral valve, which manifests as calcific aortic valve disease and myxomatous mitral valve disease. The LDL-Density-Pressure theory provides a scientific explanation for the manifestation of this phenotype. In experimental hypercholesterolemia the left-sided heart valves aortic (Rajamannan et al. 2001, 2002, 2003b, 2005a, b) and the mitral valve (Makkena et al. 2005) develop the atherosclerotic lesion and not the right sided heart valves: pulmonic and tricuspid valves. Figure 14.4, demonstrates the differences of the pressures in the heart and the expression of the phenotype of the heart valve. The lipids bind to the Lrp5/6 receptors to activate the Canonical Wnt pathway and the bone formation. Since the Lrp5 plays a role in the mechanostat theory (Johnson and Summerfield 2005)- this mechanism provides the foundation for the Pressure theory on mechanical effects on Lrp5 in the heart. Normal pressures in the heart increase from the right atrium, to the right ventricle, to the left atrium and finally to the left ventricle for normal cardiac physiology as shown in the Fig. 14.4. However, this theory hypothesizes that in the presence of hyperlipidemia the phenotypic expression of the valve changes in response to the different pressures in the heart. Human phenotypic studies of cardiac valve disease have demonstrated that the aortic valve expresses an osteoblast phenotype (Caira et al. 2006; Rajamannan et al. 2003b) and the mitral valve expresses a chondrogenic phenotype (Caira et al. 2006). It is known that the mitral valve has a lower pressure present in the left atrium as compared to the aorta. Therefore the pressure on the mitral valve is enough to produce cartilage and the pressure on the aortic valve is higher to drive the Lrp5 mechanostat mechanism to form bone. The mitral annulus which has slightly higher pressures than the valve leaflet can form bone if the pressures are high enough causing mitral annular calcification (Boon et al. 1997; Aronow et al. 2001). The results of these studies further confirm the mechanostat theory for the role of Lrp5 in the presence of the different pressures in the heart. The highest pressure aortic valve differentiates to form bone and the mitral valve which has lower pressures only develops calcification at the mitral annulus and in the leaflets develops a cartilage phenotype. Even though the lipids are present throughout the systemic circulation, the right sided valves with the lowest pressures in the hearts do not calcify or form cartilage as shown in Fig. 14.4. The human study (Caira et al. 2006) further confirms the hemodynamic pressures correlating with the expression of Lrp5/6 in the human diseased valves by immunohistochemistry staining with the Lrp5/6 antibody. This paradox between bone and the heart is demonstrated in Fig. 14.5.

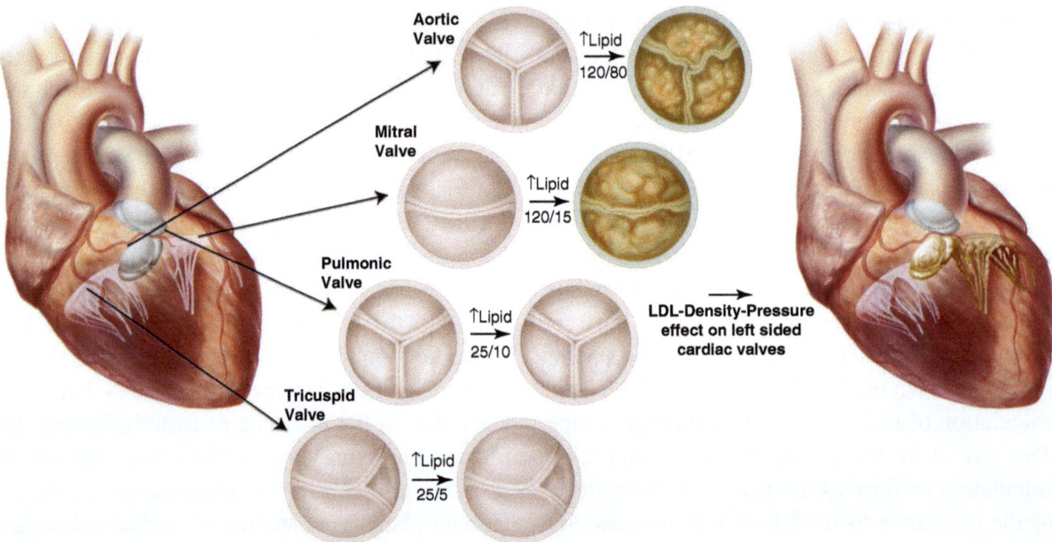

Fig. 14.4 Schematic for the role of hemodynamic pressures in the heart in the lipid-pressure activation of Lrp5/6 in the valves

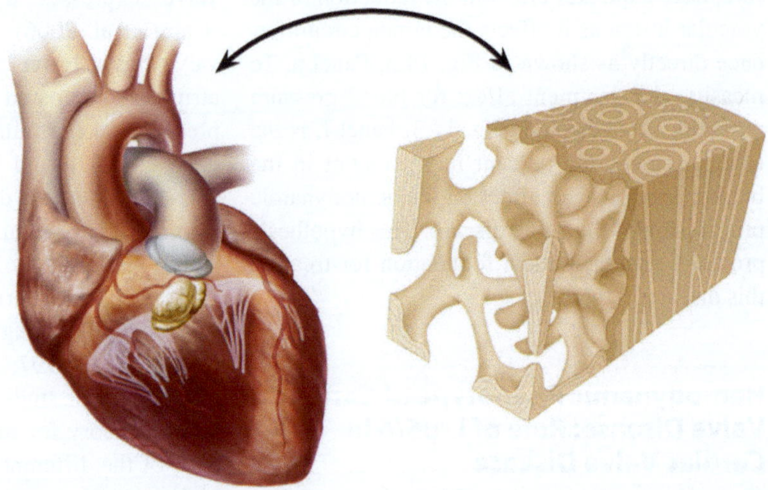

Fig. 14.5 The cardiovascular-bone paradox: atherosclerotic calcification and atherosclerotic osteoporosis

Summary

Mathematically and biologically, medical therapy for aortic valve disease can consider the following two axioms for targeting the disease biology in terms of the magnitude of the LDL density to activate the atherosclerotic process and the change in blood pressure in aortic valve disease. This theory provides a biologic-hemodynamic foundation for the mechanism of Lrp5/6 activation in the heart. This chapter provides a novel foundation for the role of lipids and blood pressure in the development of bone formation in the heart. Future clinical studies in the field of valvular heart disease may include these theories in determining if medical therapy indeed can slow progression of this disease.

Acknowledgements This work was completed with the support of an American Heart Association Grant-in-Aid (0555714Z) and a grant from the National Institute of Health (5K08HL073927-04, 1R01HL085591-01A1). Nalini M. Rajamannan is an inventor on a patent for the use of statins in degeneration of aortic valve disease. This patent is owned by the Mayo Clinic and Dr. Rajamannan does not receive any royalties from this patent.

References

Agmon Y, Khandheria BK, Meissner I, Sicks JR, O'Fallon WM, Wiebers DO, Whisnant JP, Seward JB, Tajik AJ. Aortic valve sclerosis and aortic atherosclerosis: different manifestations of the same disease? Insights from a population-based study. J Am Coll Cardiol. 2001;38(3):827–34.

Aronow WS, Ahn C, Kronzon I. Association of mitral annular calcium with symptomatic peripheral arterial disease in older persons. Am J Cardiol. 2001;88(3):333–4.

Babij P, Zhao W, Small C, Kharode Y, Yaworsky PJ, Bouxsein ML, Reddy PS, Bodine PV, Robinson JA, Bhat B, Marzolf J, Moran RA, Bex F. High bone mass in mice expressing a mutant LRP5 gene. J Bone Miner Res. 2003;18(6):960–74.

Bernoulli D. Hydrodynamica sive de viribus et motibus fluidorum commentarrii. Strasbourg: Argentoratum; 1738. p. St.31.

Boon A, Cheriex E, Lodder J, Kessels F. Cardiac valve calcification: characteristics of patients with calcification of the mitral annulus or aortic valve. Heart (British Cardiac Society). 1997;78(5):472–4.

Boyden LM, Mao J, Belsky J, Mitzner L, Farhi A, Mitnick MA, Wu D, Insogna K, Lifton RP. High bone density due to a mutation in LDL-receptor-related protein 5. N Engl J Med. 2002;346(20):1513–21.

Brown SD, Twells RC, Hey PJ, Cox RD, Levy ER, Soderman AR, Metzker ML, Caskey CT, Todd JA, Hess JF. Isolation and characterization of LRP6, a novel member of the low density lipoprotein receptor gene family. Biochem Biophys Res Commun. 1998;248(3):879–88.

Busseuil D, Shi Y, Mecteau M, Brand G, Kernaleguen AE, Thorin E, Latour JG, Rheaume E, Tardif JC. Regression of aortic valve stenosis by ApoA-I mimetic peptide infusions in rabbits. Br J Pharmacol. 2008;154(4): 765–73.

Caira FC, Stock SR, Gleason TG, McGee EC, Huang J, Bonow RO, Spelsberg TC, McCarthy PM, Rahimtoola SH, Rajamannan NM. Human degenerative valve disease is associated with up-regulation of low-density lipoprotein receptor-related protein 5 receptor-mediated bone formation. J Am Coll Cardiol. 2006;47(8):1707–12.

Cowell SJ, Newby DE, Prescott RJ, Bloomfield P, Reid J, Northridge DB, Boon NA. A randomized trial of intensive lipid lowering therapy in calcific aortic stenosis. N Engl J Med. 2005;352(23):2389–97.

Dodge Jr JT, Brown BG, Bolson EL, Dodge HT. Lumen diameter of normal human coronary arteries. Influence of age, sex, anatomic variation, and left ventricular hypertrophy or dilation. Circulation. 1992; 86(1):232–46.

Dong Y, Lathrop W, Weaver D, Qiu Q, Cini J, Bertolini D, Chen D. Molecular cloning and characterization of LR3, a novel LDL receptor family protein with mitogenic activity. Biochem Biophys Res Commun. 1998;251(3):784–90.

Drolet MC, Arsenault M, Couet J. Experimental aortic valve stenosis in rabbits. J Am Coll Cardiol. 2003; 41(7):1211–7.

Fujino T, Asaba H, Kang MJ, Ikeda Y, Sone H, Takada S, Kim DH, Ioka RX, Ono M, Tomoyori H, Okubo M, Murase T, Kamataki A, Yamamoto J, Magoori K, Takahashi S, Miyamoto Y, Oishi H, Nose M, Okazaki M, Usui S, Imaizumi K, Yanagisawa M, Sakai J, Yamamoto TT. Low-density lipoprotein receptor-related protein 5 (LRP5) is essential for normal cholesterol metabolism and glucose-induced insulin secretion. Proc Natl Acad Sci U S A. 2003;100(1):229–34.

Galante A, Pietroiusti A, Vellini M, Piccolo P, Possati G, De Bonis M, Grillo RL, Fontana C, Favalli C. C-reactive protein is increased in patients with degenerative aortic valvular stenosis. J Am Coll Cardiol. 2001;38(4):1078–82.

Gong Y, Slee RB, Fukai N, Rawadi G, Roman-Roman S, Reginato AM, Wang H, Cundy T, Glorieux FH, Lev D, Zacharin M, Oexle K, Marcelino J, Suwairi W, Heeger S, Sabatakos G, Apte S, Adkins WN, Allgrove J, Arslan-Kirchner M, Batch JA, Beighton P, Black GC, Boles RG, Boon LM, Borrone C, Brunner HG, Carle GF, Dallapiccola B, De Paepe A, Floege B, Halfhide ML, Hall B, Hennekam RC, Hirose T, Jans A, Juppner H, Kim CA, Keppler-Noreuil K, Kohlschuetter A, LaCombe D, Lambert M, Lemyre E, Letteboer T, Peltonen L, Ramesar RS, Romanengo M, Somer H, Steichen-Gersdorf E, Steinmann B, Sullivan B, Superti-Furga A, Swoboda W, van den Boogaard MJ, Van Hul W, Vikkula M, Votruba M, Zabel B, Garcia T, Baron R, Olsen BR, Warman ML, Osteoporosis-Pseudoglioma Syndrome Collaborative G. LDL receptor-related protein 5 (LRP5) affects bone accrual and eye development. Cell. 2001;107(4):513–23.

Grande-Allen KJ, Calabro A, Gupta V, Wight TN, Hascall VC, Vesely I. Glycosaminoglycans and proteoglycans in normal mitral valve leaflets and chordae: association with regions of tensile and compressive loading. Glycobiology. 2004;14:621–33.

Grande-Allen KJ, Borowski AG, Troughton RW, Houghtaling PL, Dipaola NR, Moravec CS, Vesely I, Griffin BP. Apparently normal mitral valves in patients with heart failure demonstrate biochemical and structural derangements: an extracellular matrix and echocardiographic study [see comment]. J Am Coll Cardiol. 2005;45:54–61.

Gunduz H, Arinc H, Tamer A, Akdemir R, Ozhan H, Binak E, Uyan C. The relation between homocysteine and calcific aortic valve stenosis. Cardiology. 2005; 103(4):207–11.

Hatle L, Brubakk A, Tromsdal A, Angelsen B. Noninvasive assessment of pressure drop in mitral stenosis by Doppler ultrasound. Br Heart J. 1978;40(2):131–40.

Hatle L, Angelsen BA, Tromsdal A. Non-invasive assessment of aortic stenosis by Doppler ultrasound. Br Heart J. 1980;43(3):284–92.

Hawse JR, Iwaniec UT, Bensamoun SF, Monroe DG, Peters KD, Ilharreborde B, Rajamannan NM, Oursler MJ, Turner RT, Spelsberg TC, Subramaniam M. TIEG-null mice display an osteopenic gender-specific phenotype. Bone. 2008;42(6):1025–31.

Hey PJ, Twells RC, Phillips MS, Yusuke N, Brown SD, Kawaguchi Y, Cox R, Guochun X, Dugan V, Hammond

H, Metzker ML, Todd JA, Hess JF. Cloning of a novel member of the low-density lipoprotein receptor family. Gene. 1998;216(1):103–11.

Holmen SL, Giambernardi TA, Zylstra CR, Buckner-Berghuis BD, Resau JH, Hess JF, Glatt V, Bouxsein ML, Ai M, Warman ML, Williams BO. Decreased BMD and limb deformities in mice carrying mutations in both Lrp5 and Lrp6. J Bone Miner Res. 2004; 19(12):2033–40.

Hsu SY, Hung KC, Chang SH, Wen MS, Hsieh IC. C-reactive protein in predicting coronary artery disease in subjects with aortic valve sclerosis before diagnostic coronary angiography. Am J Med Sci. 2006;331(5):264–9.

Jian B, Jones PL, Li Q, Mohler 3rd ER, Schoen FJ, Levy RJ. Matrix metalloproteinase-2 is associated with tenascin-C in calcific aortic stenosis. Am J Pathol. 2001;159(1):321–7.

Johnson ML, Summerfield DT. Parameters of LRP5 from a structural and molecular perspective. Crit Rev Eukaryot Gene Expr. 2005;15(3):229–42.

Kim DH, Inagaki Y, Suzuki T, Ioka RX, Yoshioka SZ, Magoori K, Kang MJ, Cho Y, Nakano AZ, Liu Q, Fujino T, Suzuki H, Sasano H, Yamamoto TT. A new low density lipoprotein receptor related protein, LRP5, is expressed in hepatocytes and adrenal cortex, and recognizes apolipoprotein E. J Biochem. 1998;124(6): 1072–6.

Kumar V, Abbas A, Fausto N, Richard N. Robbins basic pathology. 8th ed. Philadelphia: Saunders; 2007. p. 402.

Little RD, Carulli JP, Del Mastro RG, Dupuis J, Osborne M, Folz C, Manning SP, Swain PM, Zhao SC, Eustace B, Lappe MM, Spitzer L, Zweier S, Braunschweiger K, Benchekroun Y, Hu X, Adair R, Chee L, FitzGerald MG, Tulig C, Caruso A, Tzellas N, Bawa A, Franklin B, McGuire S, Nogues X, Gong G, Allen KM, Anisowicz A, Morales AJ, Lomedico PT, Recker SM, Van Eerdewegh P, Recker RR, Johnson ML. A mutation in the LDL receptor-related protein 5 gene results in the autosomal dominant high-bone-mass trait. Am J Hum Genet. 2002;70(1):11–9.

Makkena B, Salti H, Subramaniam M, Thennapan S, Bonow RH, Caira F, Bonow RO, Spelsberg TC, Rajamannan NM. Atorvastatin decreases cellular proliferation and bone matrix expression in the hypercholesterolemic mitral valve. J Am Coll Cardiol. 2005;45(4):631–3.

Mohler 3rd ER, Adam LP, McClelland P, Graham L, Hathaway DR. Detection of osteopontin in calcified human aortic valves. Arterioscler Thromb Vasc Biol. 1997;17(3):547–52.

Mohler 3rd ER, Gannon F, Reynolds C, Zimmerman R, Keane MG, Kaplan FS. Bone formation and inflammation in cardiac valves. Circulation. 2001; 103(11):1522–8.

Mohty D, Pibarot P, Despres JP, Cote C, Arsenault B, Cartier A, Cosnay P, Couture C, Mathieu P. Association between plasma LDL particle size, valvular accumulation of oxidized LDL, and inflammation in patients with aortic stenosis. Arterioscler Thromb Vasc Biol. 2008;28(1):187–93.

Moura LM, Ramos SF, Zamorano JL, Barros IM, Azevedo LF, Rocha-Goncalves F, Rajamannan NM. Rosuvastatin affecting aortic valve endothelium to slow the progression of aortic stenosis. J Am Coll Cardiol. 2007;49(5):554–61.

Moura LM, Rocha-Goncalves F, Zamorano JL, Barros I, Bettencourt P, Rajamannan N. New cardiovascular biomarkers: clinical implications in patients with valvular heart disease. Expert Rev Cardiovasc Ther. 2008;6(7):945–54.

Newby DE, Cowell SJ, Boon NA. Emerging medical treatments for aortic stenosis: statins, angiotensin converting enzyme inhibitors, or both? Heart (British Cardiac Society). 2006;92(6):729–34.

Nissen SE, Tuzcu EM, Schoenhagen P, Brown BG, Ganz P, Vogel RA, Crowe T, Howard G, Cooper CJ, Brodie B, Grines CL, DeMaria AN. Effect of intensive compared with moderate lipid-lowering therapy on progression of coronary atherosclerosis: a randomized controlled trial. JAMA. 2004;291(9):1071–80.

Novaro GM, Katz R, Aviles RJ, Gottdiener JS, Cushman M, Psaty BM, Otto CM, Griffin BP. Clinical factors, but not C-reactive protein, predict progression of calcific aortic-valve disease: the cardiovascular health study. J Am Coll Cardiol. 2007;50(20):1992–8.

O'Brien KD, Kuusisto J, Reichenbach DD, Ferguson M, Giachelli C, Alpers CE, Otto CM. Osteopontin is expressed in human aortic valvular lesions. Circulation. 1995;92(8):2163–8.

O'Brien KD, Reichenbach DD, Marcovina SM, Kuusisto J, Alpers CE, Otto CM. Apolipoproteins B, (a), and E accumulate in the morphologically early lesion of 'degenerative' valvular aortic stenosis. Arterioscler Thromb Vasc Biol. 1996;16(4):523–32.

Oh J, Seward J, Tajik A. The Echo Manual. Wolters Kluwer. 2006; 59–70, 189–201.

Rajamannan NM, Sangiorgi G, Springett M, Arnold K, Mohacsi T, Spagnoli LG, Edwards WD, Tajik AJ, Schwartz RS. Experimental hypercholesterolemia induces apoptosis in the aortic valve. J Heart Valve Dis. 2001;10(3):371–4.

Rajamannan NM, Subramaniam M, Springett M, Sebo TC, Niekrasz M, McConnell JP, Singh RJ, Stone NJ, Bonow RO, Spelsberg TC. Atorvastatin inhibits hypercholesterolemia-induced cellular proliferation and bone matrix production in the rabbit aortic valve. Circulation. 2002;105(22):2260–5.

Rajamannan NM, Subramaniam M, Rickard D, Stock SR, Donovan J, Springett M, Orszulak T, Fullerton DA, Tajik AJ, Bonow RO, Spelsberg T. Human aortic valve calcification is associated with an osteoblast phenotype. Circulation. 2003a;107(17):2181–4.

Rajamannan NM, Edwards WD, Spelsberg TC. Hypercholesterolemic aortic-valve disease. N Engl J Med. 2003b;349(7):717–8.

Rajamannan NM, Subramaniam M, Caira F, Stock SR, Spelsberg TC. Atorvastatin inhibits hypercholesterolemia-induced calcification in the aortic valves via the Lrp5 receptor pathway. Circulation. 2005a;112(9 Suppl):I229–34.

Rajamannan NM, Subramaniam M, Stock SR, Stone NJ, Springett M, Ignatiev KI, McConnell JP, Singh RJ, Bonow RO, Spelsberg TC. Atorvastatin inhibits calcification and enhances nitric oxide synthase production in the hypercholesterolaemic aortic valve. Heart (British Cardiac Society). 2005b;91(6):806–10.

Rosenhek R, Binder T, Porenta G, et al. Predictors of outcome in severe asymptomatic aortic stenosis. NEJM. 2000;343:611–7.

Rosenhek R, Klaar U, Schemper M, Scholten C, Heger M, Gabriel H, Binder T, Maurer G, Baumgartner H. Mild and moderate aortic stenosis. Natural history and risk stratification by echocardiography. Eur Heart J. 2004;25(3):199–205.

Rossebo AB, Pedersen TR, Boman K, Brudi P, Chambers JB, Egstrup K, Gerdts E, Gohlke-Barwolf C, Holme I, Kesaniemi YA, Malbecq W, Nienaber CA, Ray S, Skjaerpe T, Wachtell K, Willenheimer R. Intensive lipid lowering with simvastatin and ezetimibe in aortic stenosis. N Engl J Med. 2008;359:1343–56.

Shao JS, Cheng SL, Pingsterhaus JM, Charlton-Kachigian N, Loewy AP, Towler DA. Msx2 promotes cardiovascular calcification by activating paracrine Wnt signals. J Clin Invest. 2005;115(5):1210–20.

Smith MD, Kwan OL, DeMaria AN. Value and limitations of continuous-wave Doppler echocardiography in estimating severity of valvular stenosis. JAMA. 1986;255(22):3145–51.

Westendorf JJ, Kahler RA, Schroeder TM. Wnt signaling in osteoblasts and bone diseases. Gene. 2004;341:19–39.

Whittaker P, Boughner DR, Perkins DG, Canham PB. Quantitative structural analysis of collagen in chordae tendineae and its relation to floppy mitral valves and proteoglycan infiltration. Br Heart J. 1987;57(3):264–9.

Williams BO, Insogna KL. Where Wnts went: the exploding field of Lrp5 and Lrp6 signaling in bone. J Bone Miner Res. 2009;24(2):171–8.

Wooley CF, Baker PB, Kolibash AJ, Kilman JW, Sparks EA, Boudoulas H. The floppy, myxomatous mitral valve, mitral valve prolapse, and mitral regurgitation. Prog Cardiovasc Dis. 1991;33(6):397–433.

Yilmaz MB, Guray U, Guray Y, Cihan G, Caldir V, Cay S, Kisacik HL, Korkmaz S. Lipid profile of patients with aortic stenosis might be predictive of rate of progression. Am Heart J. 2004;147(5):915–8.

15 Infective Endocarditis: New Recommendations and Perspectives

Franck Thuny and Gilbert Habib

Introduction

Infective endocarditis (IE) is a serious disease with an incidence ranging from 30 to 100 episodes/million patient-years (van der Meer et al. 1992a; Hogevik et al. 1995; Hoen et al. 2005). Mortality is high since more than one-third of patients will die within the first year of diagnosis (Cabell et al. 2002; Thuny et al. 2005). Prevention strategies have not lowered the incidence of this life-threatening disease (van der Meer et al. 1992a; Hogevik et al. 1995; Hoen et al. 2002; Berlin et al. 1995). Despite improvements in the diagnostic and therapeutic strategies, the fatality rate due to IE has not significantly decreased since the end of the 1970s. Important changes in the epidemiological profile of this disease that have occurred over the past few decades can explain a part of this situation. In fact, the age of patients and the incidence of health care-associated IE have increased as a consequence of the medical progress (Fowler et al. 2005; Benito et al. 2009; Sy and Kritharides 2010). Thus, the most frequent causative agents now tend to be aggressive pathogens such as staphylococci, resistant-enterococci, or fungi. Although significant geographical variations exist, a significant increase in the rate of staphylococcal IE has been reported in industrialized countries (Fig. 15.1) (Cabell et al. 2002; Fowler et al. 2005). Therefore, efforts should be made to develop new strategies at each step of IE management to reduce the residual causes of IE-related deaths. Challenges in IE management include (i) cost-effective measures of prevention, (ii) improvement of diagnostic strategies to reduce the delays for the initiation of the appropriate treatment, (iii) and better identification patients who require close monitoring and urgent surgery (Thuny et al. 2012).

Recently, many national and international guidelines have been published (Baddour et al. 2005; Westling et al. 2007; Daly et al. 2008; Richey et al. 2008; Habib et al. 2009). They provide new recommendations on several points such as IE prevention, diagnosis and surgical indications, in order to assist medical professionals in clinical decision-making. This chapter, review the main modifications provided by the recent guidelines of the European Society of Cardiology (ESC) (Habib et al. 2009, 2010). Perspectives and future directions in the management of IE are also discussed.

New Recommendations 1: Prevention of IE

Prevention of IE has been subject to important changes during the past decade; the importance of nonspecific hygiene is now placed above the prophylactic antibiotic therapy, the use of which is restricted (Habib et al. 2009). Almost all current national or international guidelines, including those from the USA (Wilson et al. 2007), Europe

F. Thuny, M.D. (✉) • G. Habib, M.D.
Department of Cardiology,
La Timone Hospital, Marseille, France
e-mail: gilbert.habib@free.fr

N.M. Rajamannan (ed.), *Cardiac Valvular Medicine*,
DOI 10.1007/978-1-4471-4132-7_15,

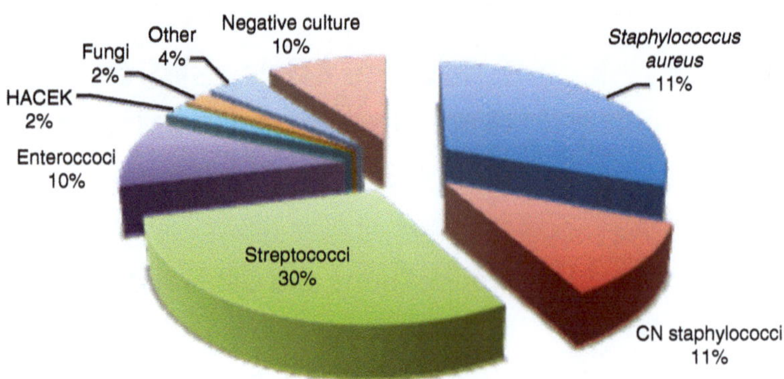

Fig. 15.1 Causative pathogens of IE. *CN* coagulase negative (Data summarized from Murdoch et al. 2009)

(Habib et al. 2009), and Australia (Daly et al. 2008) have narrowed these recommendations radically, but still recommend prophylaxis for certain dental procedures in high-risk cardiac patients. The British guidelines from the National Institute for Health and Clinical Excellence (Richey et al. 2008) are alone in recommending no antibiotic prophylaxis for any cardiac patients.

Restriction of the Antibiotic Prophylaxis

The previous recommendations for prophylaxis were based in part on the results of animal studies showing that antibiotics could prevent the development of experimental IE after inoculation of bacteria. Several reasons justify the revision of previous recommendations. The reported incidence of transient bacteremia after dental procedures is highly variable (Lockhart 2000) and is even less well established after other types of medical procedures. In contrast, transient bacteremia is reported to occur frequently in the context of daily routine activities such as tooth brushing, flossing, or chewing (Forner et al. 2006). It therefore appears plausible that a large proportion of IE-causing bacteremia may derive from these daily routine activities. These findings emphasize the importance of good oral hygiene and regular dental review rather than antibiotic prophylaxis to prevent IE (Duval and Leport 2008). Moreover, studies reporting on the efficacy of antibiotic prophylaxis to prevent or alter bacteremia in humans after dental procedures are contradictory, (Hall et al. 1993; Lockhart et al. 2008) and so far there are no data demonstrating that reduced duration or frequency of bacteremia after any medical procedure leads to a reduced procedure-related risk of IE. Similarly, no sufficient evidence exists from case–control studies (Van der Meer et al. 1992b; Lacassin et al. 1995; Strom et al. 1998) to support the necessity of IE prophylaxis. In addition, the concept of antibiotic prophylaxis efficacy itself has never been investigated in a prospective randomized controlled trial. Finally, antibiotic administration carries a small risk of anaphylaxis. Thus, the ESC and ACC/AHA Task Forces decided to maintain the principle of antibiotic prophylaxis when performing procedures at risk of IE in patients with predisposing cardiac conditions, but to limit its indication to patients with the highest risk of IE (Table 15.1) undergoing the highest risk procedures (Table 15.2) (Habib et al. 2009; Wilson et al. 2007). The antibiotics recommended are summarized in Table 15.3.

Importance of the Other Preventive Measures

The importance of nonspecific hygiene is now placed above the prophylactic antibiotic therapy. Education of patients at risk of IE is paramount. Good oral hygiene and regular dental review are of particular importance for the prevention of IE. Piercing and tattooing should be discouraged. Procedures causing health care-associated IE represent up to 30% of all cases of IE and are characterized by an increasing incidence and a severe prognosis, thus representing an important health problem (Fernandez-Hidalgo et al. 2010). Although routine antimicrobial prophylaxis administered before most invasive procedures is

Table 15.1 Cardiac conditions at highest risk of IE for which antibiotic prophylaxis is recommended when high risk procedure is performed

Recommendations: prophylaxis	Class	Level
Antibotic prophylaxis should only be considered for patients at highest risk of IE	IIa	C
1. Patients with prosthetic valve or a material used for cardiac valve repair		
2. Patients with previous IE		
3. Patients with congenital heart disease (CHD)		
(a) cyanotic CHD, without surgical repair, or with residual defects, palliative shunts or conduits		
(b) CHD with complete repair with prosthetic material whether placed by surgery or by percutaneous technique, up to 6 months after the procedure		
(c) When a residual defect persists at the site of implantation of a prosthetic material or device by cardiac surgery or percuatneous technique		
Antibiotic prophylaxis is no longer recommended in other forms of valvular or congenital heart disease	III	C

Adapted from Habib et al. (2009), with permission

Although AHA guidelines recommend prophylaxis in cardiac transplant recipients who develop cardiac valvulopathy, this is not supported by strong evidence. In addition, although the risk of adverse outcome is high when IE occurs in transplant patients, the probability of IE from dental origin is extremely low in these patients. The ESC Task Force does not recommend prophylaxis in such situations

Table 15.2 Recommendations for antibiotic prophylaxis in highest risk patients according to the type of procedure at risk

Recommendations: prophylaxis	Class	Level
A. Dental procedures:		
Antibiotic prophylaxis should only be considered for dental procedures requiring manipulation of the gingival or periapical region of the teeth or perforation of the oral mucosa	IIa	C
Antibiotic prophylaxis is not recommended for local anesthetic injections in non-infected tissue, removal of sutures, dental X-rays, placement or adjustment of removal prosthodontic or othodontic appliances or braces. Prophylaxis is also not recommended following the shedding of deciduous teeth or trauma to the lips and oral mucosa	III	C
B. Respiratory tract procedures:		
Antibiotic prophylaxis is not recommended for respiratory tract procedures, including bronchoscopy or laryngoscopy, transnasal or endotracheal intubation	III	C
C. Gastro-intestinal or urogenital procedures:		
Antibiotic prophylaxis is not recommended for gastroscopy, colonoscopy, cystoscopy or transoesophageal echocardiography	III	C
D. Skin and soft tissue:		
Antibiotic prophylaxis is not recommended for any procedure	III	C

Adapted from Habib et al. (2009), with permission

Table 15.3 Recommended prophylaxis for dental procedures at risk

		Single dose 30–60 min before procedure	
Situation	Antibiotic	Adults	Children
No allergy to penicillin or ampicillin	Amoxicillin or ampicilin[a]	2 g p.o. or i.v.	50 mg/kg p.o. or i.v.
Allergy to penicillin or ampicillin	Clindamycine	600 mg p.o. or i.v.	20 mg/kg p.o. or i.v.

Adapted from Habib et al. (2009), with permission

Cephalosporins should not be used in patients with anaphylaxis, angio-oedema or urticaria after intake of penicillin and ampicillin

[a]Alternatively cephalexin 2 g i.v. or 50 mg/kg i.v. for children, ceftriaxone 1 g i.v. for adults or 50 mg/kg i.v. for children

not recommended, aseptic measures during the insertion and manipulation of venous catheters and during any invasive procedures are mandatory to reduce the rate of this infection.

New Recommendations 2: Diagnosis of IE

Clinical Presentation

In cases with a high suspicion of IE, the appropriate antibiotics must be used as soon as possible because a delay in antibiotic therapy has negative effects on clinical outcomes in acute bacterial infectious diseases (Lodise et al. 2003). Thus, efforts should be made to rapidly identify patients with a definite or highly probable diagnosis and the causative pathogen to ensure that the appropriate antibiotic therapy will begin promptly. Infective endocarditis diagnosis usually relies on the association of an infectious syndrome and a recent endocardial involvement (Table 15.4). However, clinical presentations are highly variable. Therefore, a high index of suspicion and a low threshold for investigation are essential. Using this strategy, blood cultures and echocardiography remain the cornerstone for diagnosis, but their results can be negative or doubtful and then require more advanced investigations.

Table 15.4 Clinical presentation of IE

IE must be suspected in the following situations

1. New regurgitant heart murmur
2. Embolic events of unknown origin
3. Sepsis of unknown origin (especialy if associated with IE causative organism)
4. Fever: the most frequent sign of IE

   IE should be suspected if fever is associated with:

   (a) Intracardiac prosthetic material (e.g. prosthetic valve, pacemaker, implantable defibrillator, surgical baffle/conduit)
   (b) Previous history of IE
   (c) Previous valvular or congenital heart disease
   (d) Other predisposition for IE (e.g. immunocompromised state, IVDA)
   (e) Predisposition and recent intervention with associated bacteraemia
   (f) Evidence of congestive heart failure
   (g) New conduction disturbance
   (h) Positive blood cultures with typical IE causative organism or positive serology for chronic Q fever
   (i) Vascular or immunologic phenomena: embolic event, Roth spots, splinter haemorrhages, Janway lesions, Osler's nodes
   (j) Focal or non-specific neurological symptoms and signs
   (k) Evidence of pulmonary embolism/infiltration (right-sided IE)
   (l) Peripheral abscesses (renal, splenic, cerebral vertebral) of unknown cause

Adapted from Habib et al. (2009), with permission

Echocardiography

Echocardiography remains an accurate tool to detect endocardial involvement during IE and must be performed rapidly and repeated once a week as soon as IE is suspected. Transthoracic echocardiography (TTE) is the initial technique of choice for investigating IE. A normal scan in low-risk patients provides a rapid, non-invasive confirmation that the diagnosis is unlikely (Evangelista and Gonzalez-Alujas 2004). Moreover, TTE is superior to trans-oesophageal echocardiography (TEE) for the detection of anterior cardiac abscesses and in the haemodynamic assessment of valvular dysfunction. ESC and EAE guidelines provided clear new recommendations regarding the use of TTE and TEE that are summarized in Fig. 15.2 (Habib et al. 2009, 2010). The identification of vegetation, abscess, valvular perforation or new prosthetic-valve dehiscence will allow the confirmation of diagnosis in the majority of cases (Fig. 15.3); however, sometimes neither technique is sufficient to confirm IE. Diagnosis of IE may be particularly challenging in some situations, including intracardiac devices, valvular prosthesis, presence of pre-existing severe lesions, very small vegetations, and when no vegetation or abscess is present.

Microbiological Diagnosis

The challenge is to obtain a rapid recognition of the causative pathogen and identify the rare cases of non-infective IE. Positive blood cultures remain the cornerstones of diagnosis and provide

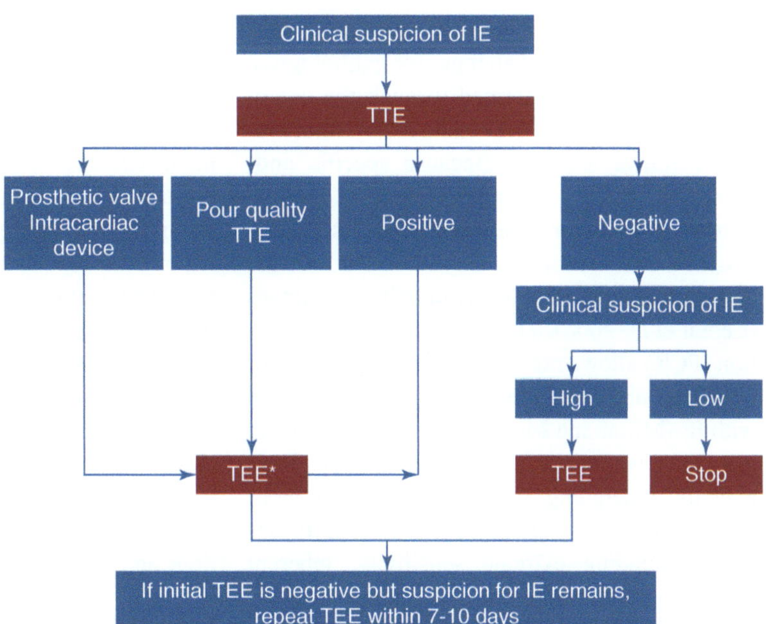

Fig. 15.2 Indications for echocardiography in suspected infective endocarditis. *IE* infective endocarditis, *TEE* transesophageal echocardiography, *TTE* transthoracic echocardiography. *TEE is not mandatory in isolated right-sided native valve IE with good quality TTE examination and unequivocal echocardiographic findings (Adapted from Habib et al. 2009, with permission)

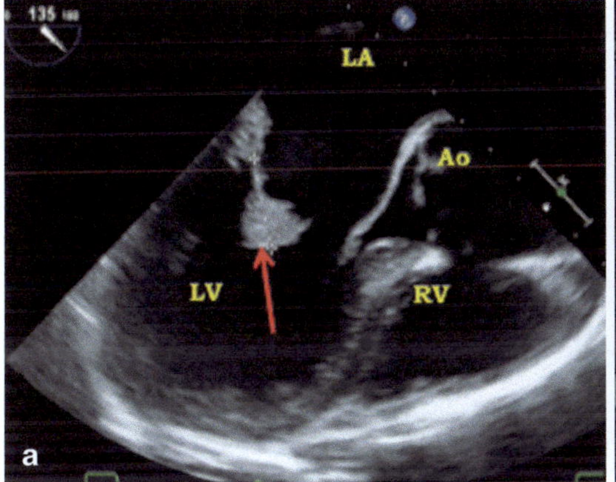

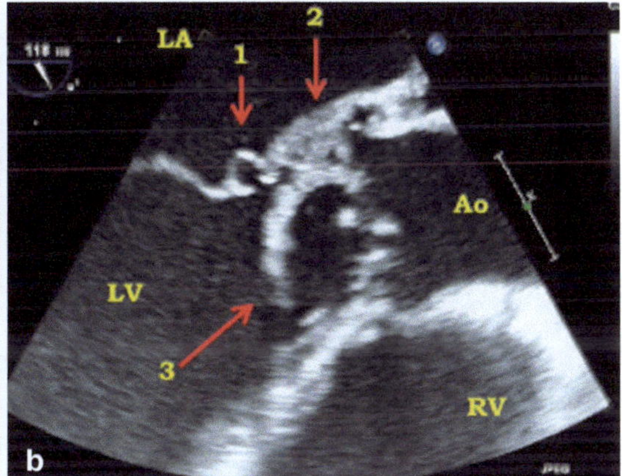

Fig. 15.3 examples of typical echographic findings in IE. (**a**) large vegetation on the anterior mitral valve (*arrow*). (**b**) complex lesions in an acute aortic IE: (*arrows*): *1* aneurysm of the anterior mitral valve, *2* abscess of the mitral aortic intervalvular fibrosa. *3* huge vegetation on the aortic valve. *LV* left ventricle, *LA* left atrium, *RV* right ventricle, *Ao* aorta

live bacteria for susceptibility testing. However, blood cultures are negative in 25–31% of cases (Lamas and Eykyn 2003; Houpikian and Raoult 2005; Raoult et al. 2005). Although blood culture-negative endocarditis (BCNE) are often related to a previous antibiotic therapy, a significant incidence of culture-negative IE results from infection with obligate intracellular bacteria, fungi, and fastidious pathogens (Raoult et al. 2005; Fournier et al. 2010). Isolation of these organisms requires culturing them on specialized media, and their growth is relatively slow on artificial culture media. Moreover, systematic serological testing must be performed in case of BCNE including specific antibodies directed against *Coxiella burnetii*, *Bartonella* spp., *Brucella* spp., *Chlamydia* spp., *Mycoplasma pneumoniae*, *Legionella pneumophila*, and *Aspergillus* spp. Other microbiological testing can be used according to the clinical presentation and the samples (blood and/or valvular tissue) provided. Culturing valvular tissue can also identify causative pathogens. However, pathogen detection often poses a challenge for pathologists. Detection can be performed through the use of nonspecific histochemical stains or by immunohistochemical analyses. Because specific antibodies are often not available, another method termed autoimmunohistochemistry, using the patient's own serum, has been described for the detection of microorganisms in valve specimens (Lepidi et al. 2006). The polymerase chain reaction (PCR) allows rapid and reliable detection of fastidious and non-culturable agents in patients with IE (Millar and Moore 2004). The technique has been validated using valve tissue from patients undergoing surgery for IE (Breitkopf et al. 2005). Although there are several advantages, including extreme sensitivity, inherent limitations include the lack of reliable application to whole blood samples, risk of contamination, false negatives due to the presence of PCR inhibitors in clinical samples, inability to provide information concerning bacterial sensitivity to antimicrobial agents, and persistent positivity despite clinical remission. The PCR results still require careful specialist interpretation. PCR of excised valve tissue or embolic material should be systematically performed in patients with negative blood cultures who undergo valve surgery.

Modified Duke Criteria

The modified Duke criteria are based upon clinical, echocardiographic, and microbiological findings (Li et al. 2000). They provide a sensitivity and specificity of around 80% for both. Clear deficiencies remain and clinical judgment remains essential, especially in settings where sensitivity of the modified criteria is diminished, e.g. BCNE, in prosthetic valve or pacemaker lead IE, and when IE affects the right heart (particularly in IVDAs).

New Recommendations 3: IE Prognostic Assessment

Owing to the severity of the disease, the quick identification of patients at highest risk of death may offer the opportunity to change the course of the disease and improve prognosis. It will also allow identification of patients with the worst immediate outcome who will benefit from closer follow-up and a more aggressive treatment strategy. Using simple clinical, microbiological and echocardiographic parameters, this risk stratification will help the clinician to choose the best therapeutic option. For optimal risk stratification, several factors must be taken into account, including the presence of predictors of poor outcome related to the disease, the presence of predictors of poor outcome related to the patient (comorbidities), and the operative risk (Table 15.5). In each case, the overall benefit of surgery should be weighed against the operative risk that is related to the previous IE complications and the patients' comorbidities.

Table 15.5 predictors of poor outcome in infective endocarditis

Predictors related to the patients characteristics
Older age
Diabetes mellitus
Other comorbidities
Prosthetic valve
Predictors related to the disease
Heart failure
Stroke, abnormal mental status
Septic shock
Persisting fever >7–10 days
Large or enlarging vegetation
Perivalvular complications (abscess, pseudo-aneurysm, fistula)
New heart block
Severe left-sided regurgitation, severe prosthetic dysfunction
Low left ventricular ejection fraction
Signs of elevated left cavities filling pressures
Pulmonary hypertension
Microorganism other than viridans streptococci, especially *S. aureus*, Fungi, and Gram-negative bacilli
Acute renal failure
Predictors of high operative risk
Pre-operative shock
Heart failure
Pre-operative stroke
Renal insufficiency
Low left ventricular ejection fraction
Prosthetic valve
Perivalvular complications
High logistic Euroscore

Table 15.6 Indications and timing of surgery in native and prosthetic valve infective endocarditis

Indication for surgery	Timing	Class	Level of evidence
Heart failure			
Aortic or mitral IE or PVE with severe acute regurgitation, obstruction or fistula causing refractory pulmonary oedema or cardiogenic shock	Emergency	I	B
Aortic or mitral IE with severe acute regurgitation or obstruction and persisting heart failure or echocardiographic signs of poor hemodynamic tolerance (early mitral closure or pulmonary hypertension)	Urgent	I	B
Aortic or mitral IE or PVE with severe regurgitation and no HF	Elective	IIa	B
Right HF secondary to severe tricuspid regurgitation with poor response to diuretic therapy	Urgent/elective	IIa	C
Uncontrolled infection			
Locally uncontrolled infection (abscess, false aneurysm, fistula, enlarging vegetation)	Urgent	I	B
Persisting fever and positive blood cultures >7–10 days	Urgent	I	B
Infection caused by fungi or multiresistant organisms	Urgent/elective	I	B
PVE caused by staphylococci or gram negative bacteria	Urgent/elective	IIa	C
Prevention of embolism			
Aortic or mitral IE or PVE with large vegetations (>10 mm) following one or more embolic episodes despite appropriate antibiotic therapy	Urgent	I	B
Aortic or mitral IE or PVE with large vegetations (>10 mm) and other predictors of complicated course (heart failure, persistent infection, abscess)	Urgent	I	C
Aortic or mitral IE or PVE with isolated very large vegetations (>15 mm)[a]	Urgent	IIb	C
Persistent tricuspid valve vegetations >20 mm after recurrent pulmonary emboli	Urgent/elective	IIa	C

Adapted from Habib et al. (2009), with permission

IE infective endocarditis, *PVE* prosthetic valve endocarditis

[a]Surgery may be preferred if procedure preserving the native valve is feasible

New Recommendations 4: Indications and Timing of Surgery

The treatment of IE relies on the combination of prolonged antimicrobial therapy and - in about half patients – surgical eradication of the infected tissues. The new ESC guidelines (16) give clear and simple indications for surgery in infective endocarditis, based on the presence or risk of heart failure, infection, and/or embolism. (Table 15.6). In addition, recommendations are given on the optimal timing of surgery, separating patients needing surgery on an emergency (within 24 h), urgent (within 1 week), or elective (after 1 or 2 weeks antibiotic therapy) basis.

However, the decision whether a patient with IE must be operated on or not is always difficult. It must be discussed using a multidisciplinary approach in the individual patient and must take into account both the comorbities and the operative risk.

New Recommendations 5: Conclusion and Perspectives

Despite the improvements in the management of patients with infective endocarditis, the mortality of this disease is still high, justifying improvements in our diagnostic and therapeutic strategies.

- Improvements must begin with a better (or different) prevention of the disease, taking into account the fact that IE is a changing disease, with a clear reduction of the number of cases related to a dental procedure, but 30% patients suffering from a nosocomial portal of entry. Reducing the rate of nosocomial IE is a new challenge for the future.
- Improvements in diagnosis of IE are also desirable. Diagnosis of IE is still difficult and frequently delayed. Diagnostic strategies allowing an earlier diagnosis are needed, including the use of optimal imaging tools

(3D echo, CT-scan, MRI, 18F-FDG PET-CT) and biomarkers, and improvements in microbiological testing, including the Polymerase Chain Reaction (PCR).

- Finally, improvements in therapeutic management should be obtained with the standardization of therapeutic protocols, the use of a systematic multidisciplinary approach, and the use of earlier surgery associated with more valve repair.

These objective will be ideally reached in reference centers with high degree of expertise and high specialisation in the field of IE, allowing an earlier diagnosis, a prompt antibiotic treatment and prognostic assessment, an immediate surgery if needed, and a close short-term and long-term follow-up of the patient.

References

Baddour LM, Wilson WR, Bayer AS, et al. Infective endocarditis: diagnosis, antimicrobial therapy, and management of complications: a statement for healthcare professionals from the Committee on Rheumatic Fever, Endocarditis, and Kawasaki Disease, Council on Cardiovascular Disease in the Young, and the Councils on Clinical Cardiology, Stroke, and Cardiovascular Surgery and Anesthesia, American heart Association: endorsed by the Infectious Diseases Society of America. Circulation. 2005;111:e394–434.

Benito N, Miro JM, de Lazzari E, et al. Health care-associated native valve endocarditis: importance of non-nosocomial acquisition. Ann Intern Med. 2009;150:586–94.

Berlin JA, Abrutyn E, Strom BL, et al. Incidence of infective endocarditis in the Delaware Valley, 1988–1990. Am J Cardiol. 1995;76:933–6.

Breitkopf C, Hammel D, Scheld HH, Peters G, Becker K. Impact of a molecular approach to improve the microbiological diagnosis of infective heart valve endocarditis. Circulation. 2005;111:1415–21.

Cabell CH, Jollis JG, Peterson GE, et al. Changing patient characteristics and the effect on mortality in endocarditis. Arch Intern Med. 2002;162:90–4.

Daly CG, Currie BJ, Jeyasingham MS, et al. A change of heart: the new infective endocarditis prophylaxis guidelines. Aust Dent J. 2008;53:196–200; quiz 97.

Duval X, Leport C. Prophylaxis of infective endocarditis: current tendencies, continuing controversies. Lancet Infect Dis. 2008;8:225–32.

Evangelista A, Gonzalez-Alujas MT. Echocardiography in infective endocarditis. Heart. 2004;90:614–7.

Fernandez-Hidalgo N, Almirante B, Tornos P, et al. Prognosis of left-sided infective endocarditis in patients transferred to a tertiary-care hospital-prospective analysis of referral bias and influence of inadequate antimicrobial treatment. Clin Microbiol Infect. 2010;17:769–75.

Forner L, Larsen T, Kilian M, Holmstrup P. Incidence of bacteremia after chewing, tooth brushing and scaling in individuals with periodontal inflammation. J Clin Periodontol. 2006;33:401–7.

Fournier PE, Thuny F, Richet H, et al. Comprehensive diagnostic strategy for blood culture-negative endocarditis: a prospective study of 819 new cases. Clin Infect Dis. 2010;51:131–40.

Fowler Jr VG, Miro JM, Hoen B, et al. Staphylococcus aureus endocarditis: a consequence of medical progress. JAMA. 2005;293:3012–21.

Habib G, Hoen B, Tornos P, et al. Guidelines on the prevention, diagnosis, and treatment of infective endocarditis (new version 2009): the Task Force on the Prevention, Diagnosis, and Treatment of Infective Endocarditis of the European Society of Cardiology (ESC). Eur Heart J. 2009;30:2369–413.

Habib G, Badano L, Tribouilloy C, et al. Recommendations for the practice of echocardiography in infective endocarditis. Eur J Echocardiogr. 2010;11:202–19.

Hall G, Hedstrom SA, Heimdahl A, Nord CE. Prophylactic administration of penicillins for endocarditis does not reduce the incidence of postextraction bacteremia. Clin Infect Dis. 1993;17:188–94.

Hoen B, Alla F, Selton-Suty C, et al. Changing profile of infective endocarditis: results of a 1-year survey in France. JAMA. 2002;288:75–81.

Hoen B, Chirouze C, Cabell CH, et al. Emergence of endocarditis due to group D streptococci: findings derived from the merged database of the International Collaboration on Endocarditis. Eur J Clin Microbiol Infect Dis. 2005;24:12–6.

Hogevik H, Olaison L, Andersson R, Lindberg J, Alestig K. Epidemiologic aspects of infective endocarditis in an urban population. A 5-year prospective study. Medicine (Baltimore). 1995;74:324–39.

Houpikian P, Raoult D. Blood culture-negative endocarditis in a reference center: etiologic diagnosis of 348 cases. Medicine (Baltimore). 2005;84:162–73.

Lacassin F, Hoen B, Leport C, et al. Procedures associated with infective endocarditis in adults. A case control study. Eur Heart J. 1995;16:1968–74.

Lamas CC, Eykyn SJ. Blood culture negative endocarditis: analysis of 63 cases presenting over 25 years. Heart. 2003;89:258–62.

Lepidi H, Coulibaly B, Casalta JP, Raoult D. Autoimmunohistochemistry: a new method for the histologic diagnosis of infective endocarditis. J Infect Dis. 2006;193:1711–7.

Li JS, Sexton DJ, Mick N, et al. Proposed modifications to the Duke criteria for the diagnosis of infective endocarditis. Clin Infect Dis. 2000;30:633–8.

Lockhart PB. The risk for endocarditis in dental practice. Periodontol 2000. 2000;23:127–35.

Lockhart PB, Brennan MT, Sasser HC, Fox PC, Paster BJ, Bahrani-Mougeot FK. Bacteremia associated with toothbrushing and dental extraction. Circulation. 2008;117:3118–25.

Lodise TP, McKinnon PS, Swiderski L, Rybak MJ. Outcomes analysis of delayed antibiotic treatment for hospital-acquired Staphylococcus aureus bacteremia. Clin Infect Dis. 2003;36:1418–23.

Millar BC, Moore JE. Current trends in the molecular diagnosis of infective endocarditis. Eur J Clin Microbiol Infect Dis. 2004;23:353–65.

Murdoch DR, Corey GR, Hoen B, et al. Clinical presentation, etiology, and outcome of infective endocarditis in the 21st century: the International Collaboration on Endocarditis-Prospective Cohort Study. Arch Intern Med. 2009;169:463–73.

Raoult D, Casalta JP, Richet H, et al. Contribution of systematic serological testing in diagnosis of infective endocarditis. J Clin Microbiol. 2005;43:5238–42.

Richey R, Wray D, Stokes T. Prophylaxis against infective endocarditis: summary of NICE guidance. BMJ. 2008;336:770–1.

Strom BL, Abrutyn E, Berlin JA, et al. Dental and cardiac risk factors for infective endocarditis. A population-based, case-control study. Ann Intern Med. 1998;129: 761–9.

Sy RW, Kritharides L. Health care exposure and age in infective endocarditis: results of a contemporary population-based profile of 1536 patients in Australia. Eur Heart J. 2010;31:1890–7.

Thuny F, Di Salvo G, Belliard O, et al. Risk of embolism and death in infective endocarditis: prognostic value of echocardiography: a prospective multicenter study. Circulation. 2005;112:69–75.

Thuny F, Grisoli D, Collart F, Habib G, Raoult D. Management of infective endocarditis: challenges and perspectives. Lancet. 2012;379:965–75.

van der Meer JT, Thompson J, Valkenburg HA, Michel MF. Epidemiology of bacterial endocarditis in the Netherlands. I. Patient characteristics. Arch Intern Med. 1992a;152:1863–8.

Van der Meer JT, Van Wijk W, Thompson J, Vandenbroucke JP, Valkenburg HA, Michel MF. Efficacy of antibiotic prophylaxis for prevention of native-valve endocarditis. Lancet. 1992b;339:135–9.

Westling K, Aufwerber E, Ekdahl C, et al. Swedish guidelines for diagnosis and treatment of infective endocarditis. Scand J Infect Dis. 2007;39:929–46.

Wilson W, Taubert KA, Gewitz M, et al. Prevention of infective endocarditis: guidelines from the American Heart Association: a guideline from the American Heart Association Rheumatic Fever, Endocarditis, and Kawasaki Disease Committee, Council on Cardiovascular Disease in the Young, and the Council on Clinical Cardiology, Council on Cardiovascular Surgery and Anesthesia, and the Quality of Care and Outcomes Research Interdisciplinary Working Group. Circulation. 2007;116:1736–54.

Assessment and Timing to Intervention of Mitral Regurgitation

16

José Juan Gómez de Diego
and Nalini Marie Rajamannan

Introduction

There is no doubt about the fact that mitral regurgitation (MR) is one of the most frequent and challenging diagnosis in daily work in any echocardiography lab. Chronic organic MR, due to increasing prevalence of myxomatous disease and the increasing mean age of population, is presenting as often as aortic stenosis: moderate or severe MR is found in 1.7% of the general population and in up to 9.3% of those over 75 years (Iung and Vahanian 2011). Echocardiography is the main tool for MR evaluation. In the modern times of mitral valve (MV) repair surgery, echocardiography has become even more important because the study has to cover not only the MR diagnosis, but the evaluation of the valvular lesions and the mechanisms of disease to guide the election between the different therapeutic options. This combination of aspects related to the complexity of mitral regurgitation is the primary driving force to develop an all encompassing assessment of MR to allow the clinician and surgeon to achieve the superior clinical outcomes.

Brief Overview of Mitral Valve Anatomy for the Echo

The mitral valve has a complex and elegant functional structure. It is composed by different elements that have to work together as a single unit to get the final goal of a complete valve closure in systole (Castillo et al. 2011) (Fig. 16.1).

- **Annulus**. MV annulus is a D-shaped structure. The anterior zone is in close contact to the aortic valve annulus and is in fact part of the fibrous skeleton of the heart. Therefore, this anterior zone has a strong mechanical support. The posterior zone of the mitral annulus has no rigid structure and is more vulnerable to stress forces transmitted from the left ventricle.
- **Leaflets.** MV is composed by two leaflets, anterior and posterior. Both leaflets are not symmetrical, because the anterior leaflet is shorter and wider and has the insertion only in the anterior 1/3 of the annulus whereas the posterior leaflet is larger and takes up the remainder posterior 2/3 of the ring. Each leaflet is subdivided in three components or scallops, division that is more apparent in the posterior leaflet. In both leaflets scallops are

J.J.G. de Diego, M.D. (✉)
Cardiac Imaging Laboratory, Hospital Clinico San Carlos, Madrid, Spain
e-mail: josejgd@gmail.com

N.M. Rajamannan, M.D.
Department of Molecular Biology and Biochemistry, Mayo Clinic, 200 First St SW, Rochester, MN 55905, USA

Department of Aerospace Engineering, University of Notre Dame, South Bend, IN, USA
e-mail: nrajamannan@gmail.com

N.M. Rajamannan (ed.), *Cardiac Valvular Medicine*,
DOI 10.1007/978-1-4471-4132-7_16, © Springer-Verlag London 2013

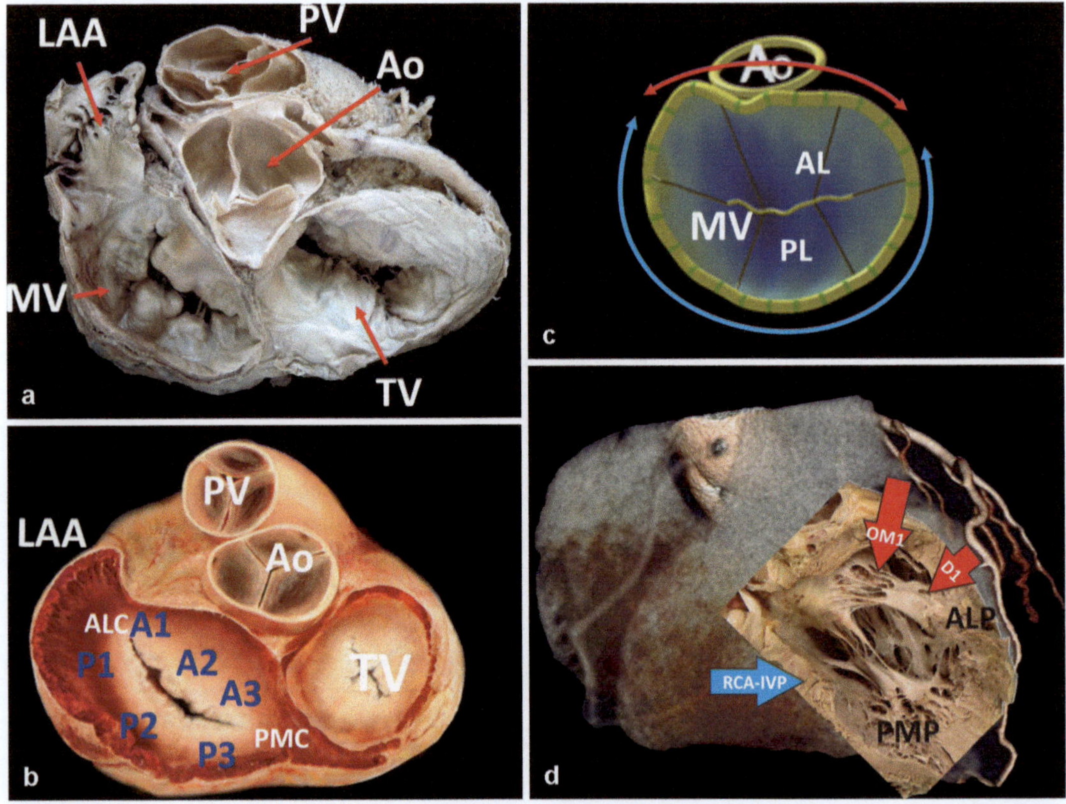

Fig. 16.1 Mitral valve anatomy. (**a**) Mitral valve view from atrial face in an anatomical specimen. (**b**) Mitral valve ring diagram. Anterior zone (*red line*) is shorter and near to aortic valve ring. (**c**) Mitral valve diagram. The figure parallels the anatomical image to show and label leaflets, commissures and scallops. (**d**) Mitral papillary muscles and chords in a anatomical specimen showed inside a Cardiac CT image to show relations with the coronary arteries. *MV* Mitral valve, *LAA* left atrial appendage, *PV* pulmonary valve, *Ao* aortic valve, *TV* tricuspid valve, *AL* anterior leaflet, *A1 A2 A3* anterior leaflet scallops, *PL* posterior leaflet, *P1 P2 P3* posterior scallops, *ALC* anterolateral commissure, *PMC* posteromedial commissure, *ALP* anterolateral papillary muscle, *PMP* posteromedial papillary muscle, *IVP* interventricular posterior coronary artery, *OM1* first obtuse marginal branch, *D1* first diagonal branch

labeled from 1 in the superior part of the leaflet to 3 in the inferior zone. Both leaflets are separated by the commissures and contact in systole along a C shaped closure line in a security area that includes the 3–4 distal millimeters of both free edges.

- **Chordae tendineae**. Chords are fibrous filaments that join the papillary muscles and leaflets. There are approximately 20–25 chordae that begin in the papillary muscles and progressively subdivide like tree branches to insert in the leaflets. There are marginal chords that support the free border of the leaflet, intermediate chords for the leaflet body and, in the case of the posterior leaflet, basal chords that give support to leaflet basal zone and ring.
- **Papillary Muscles**. There are two main groups of papillary muscles. The anterolateral papillary muscle (ALP) is bigger had has an only body whereas posteromedial (PMP) uses to be smaller and split in two different bodies. Is important to have in mind that PMP has coronary flow only from posterior interventricular coronary artery while AMP has redundant sources from marginal

branches of the circumflex coronary artery and from diagonal branches of the descending anterior coronary artery. This is the reason why PMP is more vulnerable to ischemic damage.

- **Left ventricle**: Not really a MV structure, but it gives support to the MV annulus and both papillary muscles and therefore left ventricle diseases have a direct translation on the valve function.

Location of Disease

2D TEE Evaluation of Mitral Valve

Transthoracic echocardiography (TTE) is the basic tool for MV evaluation. Although TTE can give a general overview of the MV anatomy, a careful study needs in most of cases the use of the transesophageal (TEE) approach (Lancellotti et al. 2011). Most of the cardiac imaging laboratories use the conventional 2D TEE for MV evaluation. In 2D studies, the ultrasound beam shows different structures of the MV depending on the relative spatial orientation of the ultrasound beam and the valve. 2D technique for MV study can be sometimes a hard work because it is needed to get multiple views and to mix them up in a mental reconstruction to have a clear view of the overall the structure of the valve. However, a careful protocol of study can give excellent results. Other problem related to 2D TEE evaluation of MV is there are many schemas in the literature showing the relationships between TEE planes and structures that are not congruent because are based on different relative positions for the observer and the valve. This methodological inconsistency gives some additional complexity to the teaching of the technique.

The evaluation of MV disease should give a final result that can be easily understood for the clinician and the surgeon who is to repair the valve. This is the reason why we strongly suggest using the surgeon's view to make the study and to explain the results. Surely this will be the easiest way to assure consistency for all the medical team. In the surgeon's view, the observer is facing the mitral valve from the atrial side and the left atrial appendage and the aortic valve are in anterior (or upper) position (at 11:00 in the clock sphere for the left atrial appendage and at 13:00 for the aortic valve). In this orientation tricuspid valve is on the right side of MV and the left ventricle can be seen below the MV plane. In TEE studies, the probe is placed behind the left atrium, in a viewpoint very similar to surgeon's eyes looking to MV from the same atrial side. With this orientation in mind, the 0° view has a horizontal orientation passing over left and the right ventricle and to move the degree ultrasound beam orientation control equals to turn clockwise the ultrasound plane (Fig. 16.2).

The main views in 2D TEE for MV evaluation are the 0° view and the 60° view because it parallels the valve closure line. The 0° view

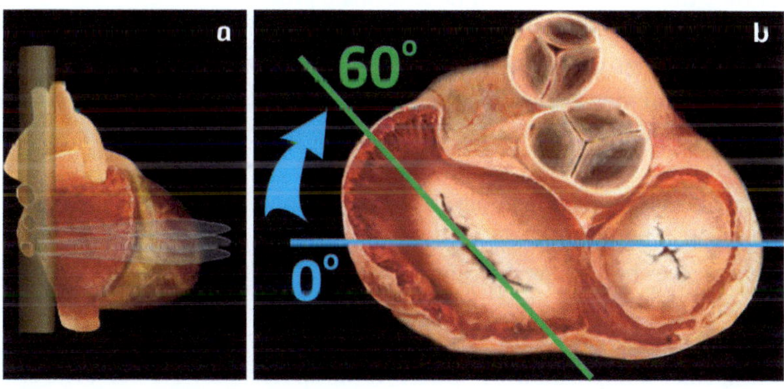

Fig. 16.2 Spatial orientation of 2D TEE in mitral valve evaluation. (**a**) Relative position of TEE probe and the heart. (**b**) Relative position of mitral valve and 2D TEE planes (explanation in the text)

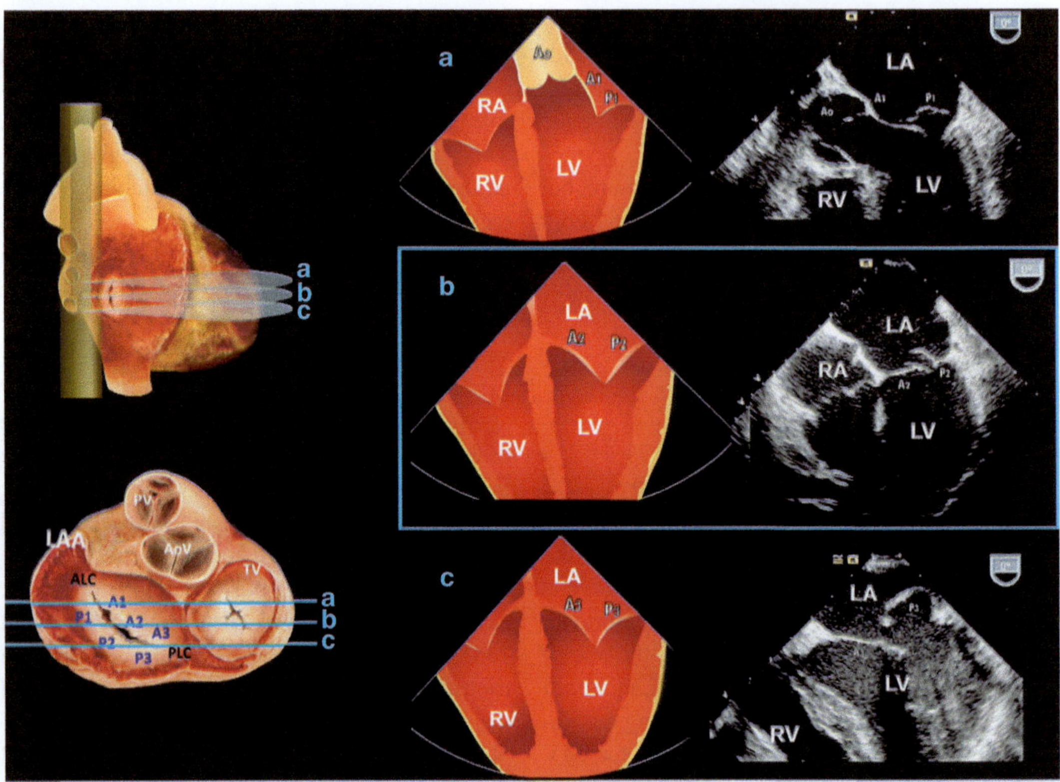

Fig. 16.3 2D TEE planes at 0° orientation. *Left figures* shows the spatial position of TEE probe and planes in *upper* (**a**), medium (**b**, *blue box*) and distal (**c**) probe positions. *LA* left atrium, *RA* right atrium, *LV* left ventricle, *RV* right ventricle, *A1 A2 A3* anterior leaflet scallops, *P1 P2 P3* posterior scallops

shows the MV in a four chamber long axis image of the heart. With this angle for the ultrasound beam, to move the probe to an upper position in the esophagus allow to see the most superior parts of the valve and to move the probe distally gives images of the inferior zone (Fig. 16.3). The 60° view gives a nicely exploration of the MV closure line. In this beam angle, to turn the probe to the left or the right sides gives clear images of the anterior and the posterior leaflets (Fig. 16.4). Other useful views (Fig. 16.5) are the 135° orientation, which shows the central zones of both leaflets and the transgastric view that gives a short axis view including both scallops and commissures. The transgastric view in 90° orientation is the best view to study the papillary muscles.

In 2D TEE there are two useful rules to make the mental composition of structures in space. The first rule is to have in mind that all the structures near the Aortic valve are Always in an Anterior position (this is the A rule). The second rule is to remember that like in sport classifications, number 1 structures (for scallops) are always up in the podium (or in the valve).

3D TEE Evaluation of Mitral Valve

3D TEE has been a clear improvement in the evaluation of MV diseases. 3D TEE gives in only one acquisition a highly detailed image of the entire valve (Fig. 16.6) that can be used to study at the same time the different structures and their relative space positions. 3D TEE is not only more accurate for diagnosis, but also a useful tool to show the study results in an understandable way for the non echo specialist.

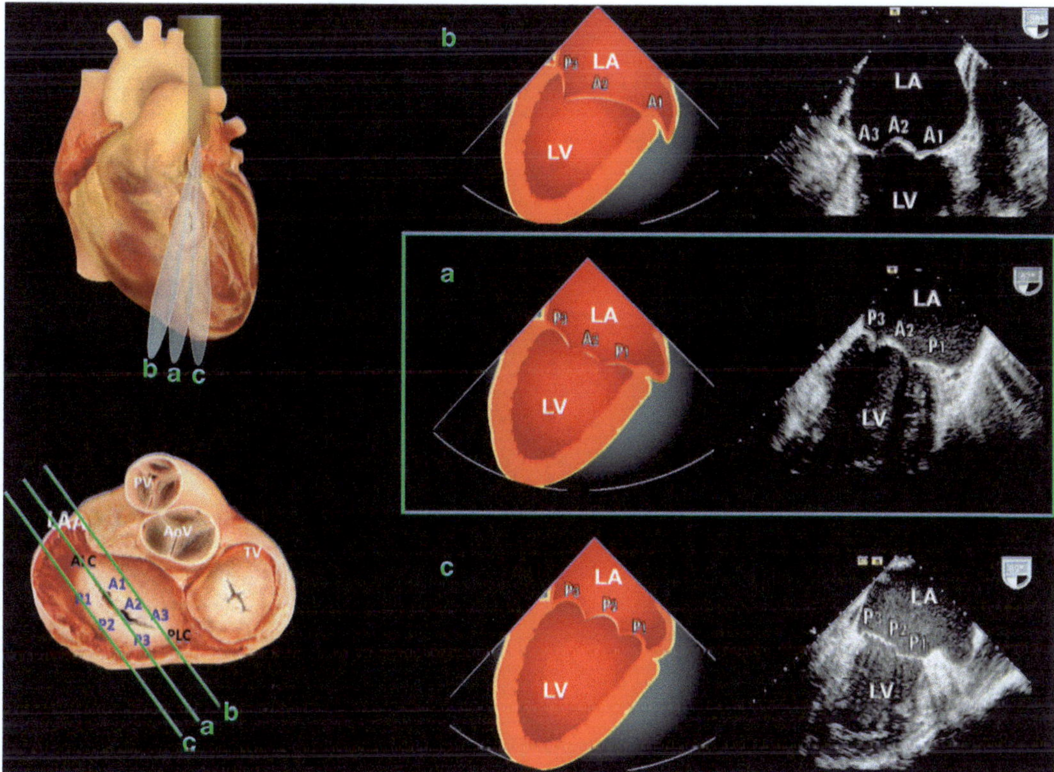

Fig. 16.4 2D TEE planes at 60° orientation. *Left figures* shows the spatial position of TEE probe and planes in neutral (**a**, *green box*), left (**b**) and right (**c**) probe positions. *LA* left atrium, *RA* right atrium, *LV* left ventricle, *RV* right ventricle, *A1 A2 A3* anterior leaflet scallops, *P1 P2 P3* posterior scallops

Mechanisms of Disease

The final pathophysiologic mechanism involved in MR is the existence of flow between the left ventricle and the left atrium in systole that causes left ventricle volume overload, dilatation and progressive left ventricular dysfunction and heart failure. There are many possible valve lesions that can cause first a reduction of the leaflets coaptation surface area and after a defect of leaflet coaptation and MR. In a general approach, we can made a broad distinction between organic valve diseases, in which the MR cause are anatomical lesions in valvular structures and functional valve alterations where the valve is anatomically normal but becomes regurgitant due to alterations in their support structures.

The systematic study of the location, severity and extension of all the valve lesions is basic to assess the chances for valve repair. In his pioneer work, Carpentier nicely showed the need to distinguish between the valve disease that is the cause of the lesions and the mechanisms that are involved to become the valve regurgitant. The Carpentier classification (Carpentier et al. 2010) of MV mechanisms of disease (Fig. 16.7) is a conceptual framework widely used to understand MV diseases and to have a common language for the echocardiographer and cardiac surgeon.

The Type I of MV dysfunction is the MR in spite of normal valve leaflets movement. There are two main broad valve alterations included in this pattern. Type Ia is the MR caused by annulus dilatation due to left ventricular dilatation. The most frequent causes are ischemic heart disease and dilated cardiomyopathy. The ventricle dilatation stretches the posterior zone of the

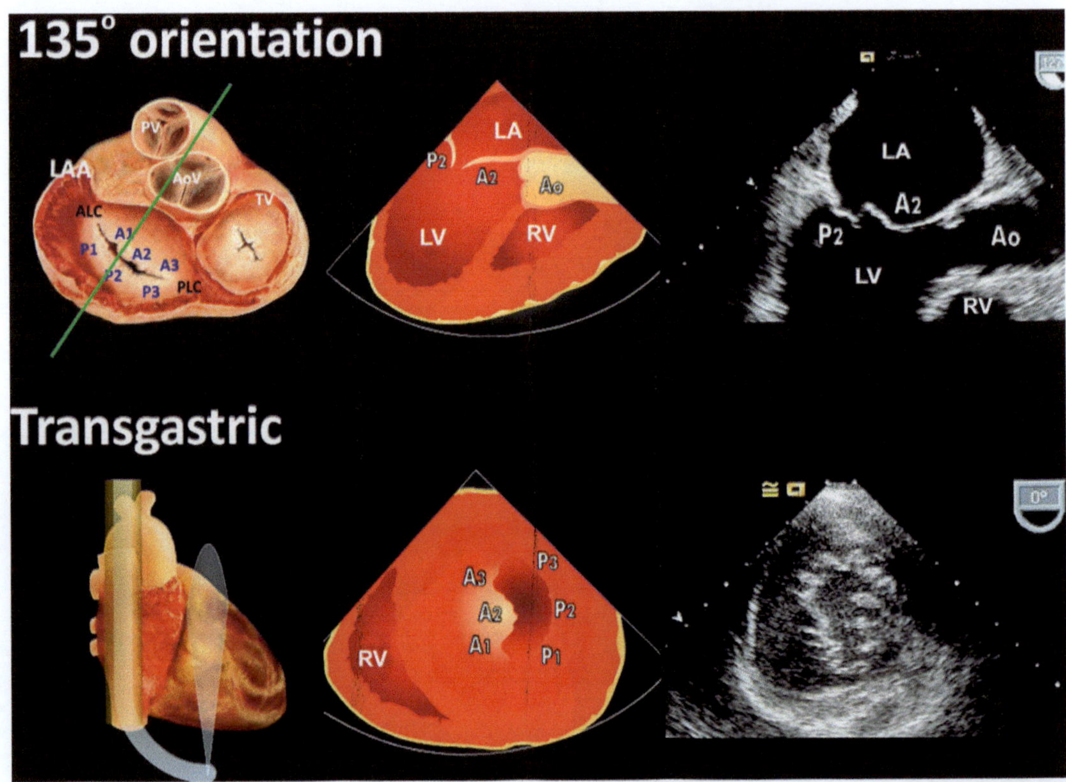

Fig. 16.5 Other 2D TEE useful planes. *Upper figures* for the 135° orientation view. *Lower figures* shows transgastric views. *LA* left atrium, *RA* right atrium, *LV* left ventricle, *RV* right ventricle, *A1 A2 A3* anterior leaflet scallops, *P1 P2 P3* posterior scallops

mitral ring and move apart both leaflets causing a functional coaptation defect along all the closure line and a MR jet that is typically central oriented. The second group of diseases or Ib Type are the MR cases due to defects of the leaflets. Typical examples are the leaflet perforation caused for endocarditis or congenital clefts. In this case, the MR has an organic cause and both the origin and the orientation of the MV jet are very variable.

Type II MV dysfunction is the caused by an excess of movement of one or both leaflets. Involved lesions include pathological elongation or rupture of chordae tendineae or papillary muscles. The most frequent cause is degenerative mitral valve disease (in the different clinical presentations from fibroelastic deficiency to Barlow disease) but it can be seen also due to trauma, endocarditis, ischemic heart disease or the Ehler-Danlos disease. In all of these cases, the MV has an organic lesion and a MR eccentric jet that is oriented towards the opposite side of the most abnormal leaflet.

Last, Type III of MV dysfunction is characteristic for a restricted leaflet movement pattern. Type III includes a broad group of MV diseases and can be split in three main subgroups. In the IIIa MR type the leaflets have reduced movements in systole and in diastole. It is caused by organic lesions of leaflets and/or the chordae that cause retraction of the structures and severe limitations of the movement pattern. The most frequent cause is rheumatic disease, but it is possible for many other diseases including carcinoid syndrome, lesions due to radiotherapy, lupus erythematosus, muccopolysaccharidosis or the hypereosiniophlic syndrome. The valve affectation can be irregular, like the origin or the direction of the MR jet.

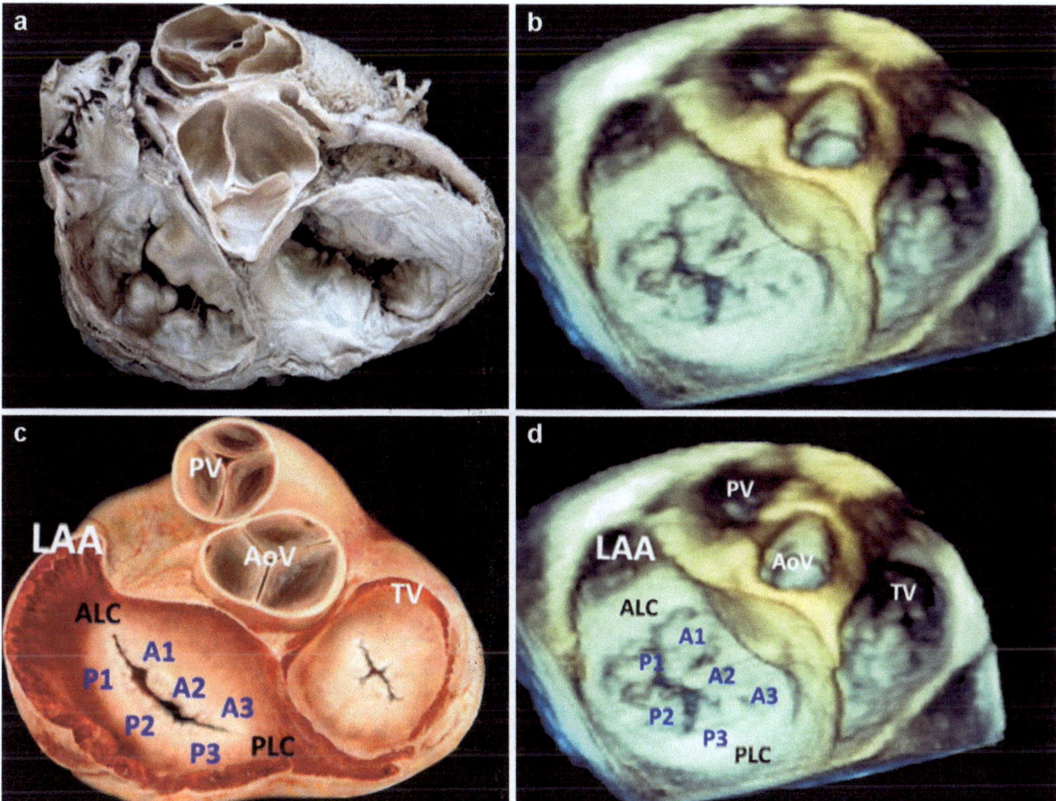

Fig. 16.6 Comparison between anatomy and 3D TEE in mitral valve study. See the nice correlation between the anatomical specimen (**a**) and the 3D TEE image (**b**). (**c**, **d**) Shows diagrams and labels. *MV* mitral valve, *LAA* left atrial appendage, *PV* pulmonary valve, *Ao* aortic valve, *TV* tricuspid valve, *AL* anterior leaflet, *A1 A2 A3* anterior leaflet scallops, *PL* posterior leaflet, *P1 P2 P3* posterior scallops, *ALC* anterolateral commissure, *PMC* posteromedial commissure, *ALP* anterolateral papillary muscle, *PMP* posteromedial papillary muscle

The IIIb dysfunction type is the symmetrical reduction of the movement of both leaflets only in systole. MV is anatomically normal but has a functional anomaly with restriction of the closure movement caused by mechanical traction from the papillary muscles that are out its normal position due to left ventricular enlargement. This is another mechanism that can be involved in the MR of patients with dilated cardiomyopathy. Strength forces move the leaflets coaptation point far to the annulus plane and cause an increase of the area comprised between the leaflets and the valve ring (the "tenting" area), a coaptation defect of the leaflets along all the closure line and a centrally oriented MR jet.

Type IIIc MR is caused by a functional reduction of the movement of only one of the leaflets or tethering. This is the mechanism of the MR in ischemic heart disease. Typically the affected leaflet is the posterior one. In this case there is a eccentric MR oriented towards the same side than the abnormal leaflet.

Evaluation of Severity

There are many echocardiographic tools that have been proposed to assess the severity of MR. The existence of many techniques gives multiple options to work with for the echocardiographer but unfortunately it also means that none is perfect. It

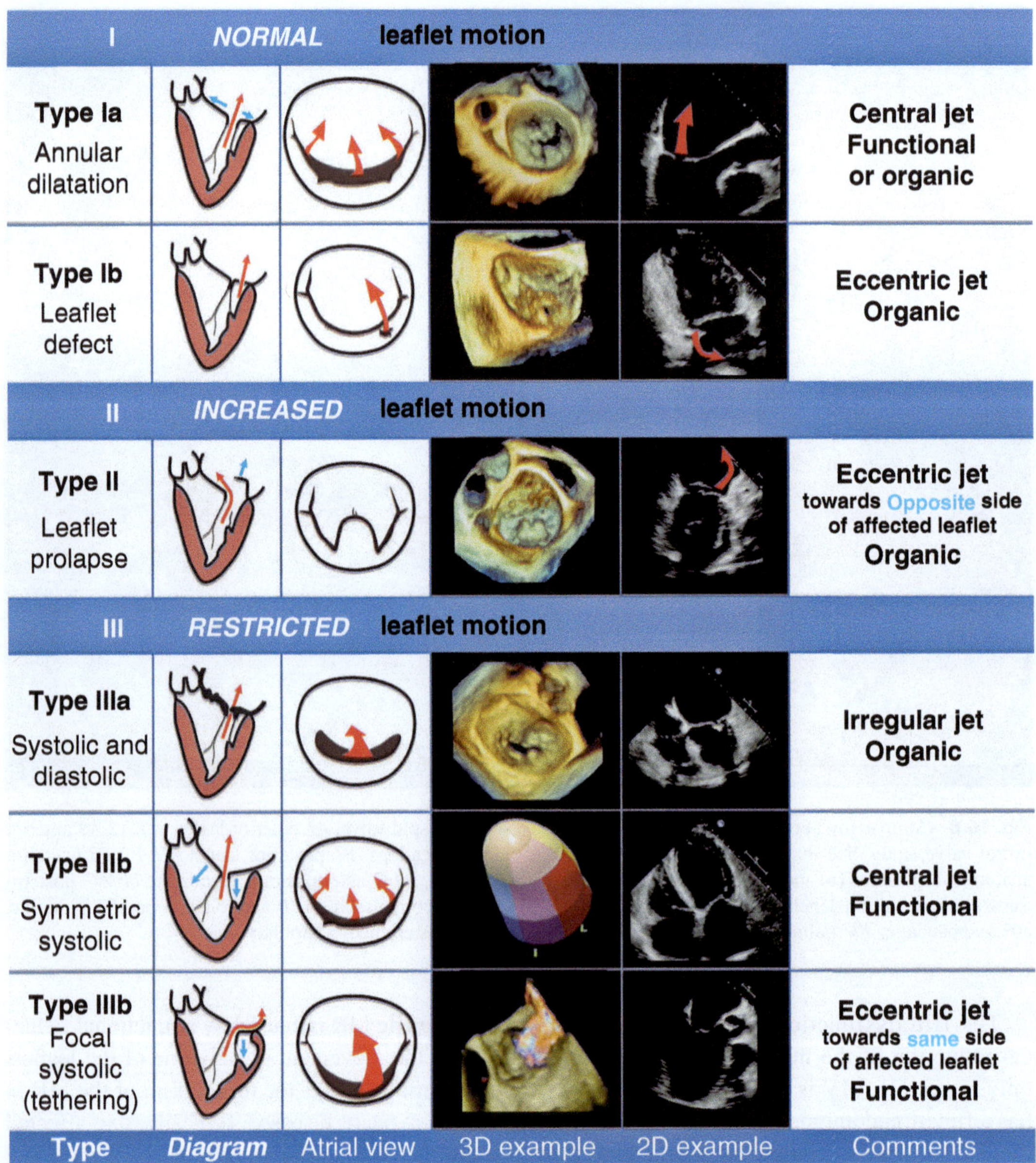

Fig. 16.7 Carpentier classification of mechanisms of mitral valve regurgitation

is recommended to use many of them, depending of the characteristics of every case, and join the information to make a final decision (Fig. 16.8).

Color Doppler is the basic tool to start the MV evaluation. The color pattern is the most useful technique to make a fast screening for MR and to distinguish the subjects that will need a more in deep study. The size of the jet has a good correlation with the severity of MR and there are measurements like the jet area or the vena contracta width (the width of the jet in its narrowest point) that allow a quantification of the disease. However, Doppler patterns are strongly dependent of the machine settings and the loading conditions of the patient and they should not be used alone to make an accurate evaluation.

One of the most useful tools is the evaluation of the flow pattern in pulmonary veins, because

Evaluation of MR severity

Parameter	Pro / CONs	Criteria for severe MR
Jet area	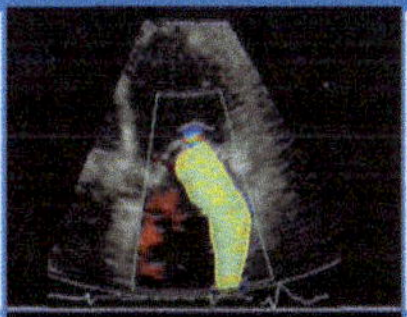 Pro: Fast and intuitive CONs: Affected by: Patient load conditions System settings Direction of the jet (coanda effect)	Jet area >8 cm^2 Jet area >40% of LA area
Vena contracta	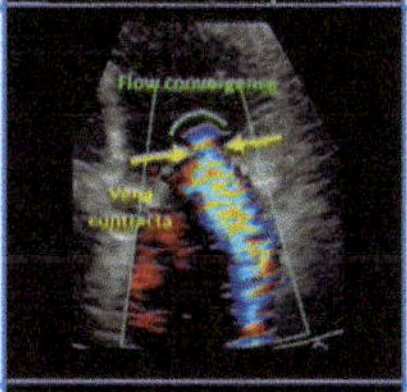 Pro: Fast and intuitive CONs: Affected by: Patient load conditions System settings Multiple jets Non circular regurgitant orifice	Width > 7 mm
Pulmonary vein flow	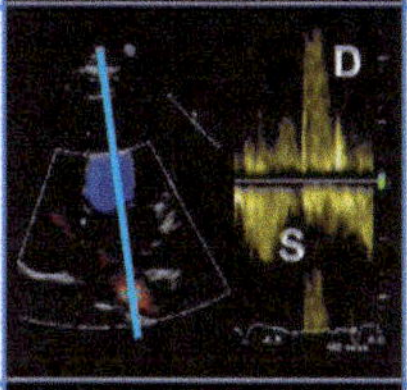 Pro: Systolic reversal of flow is very specific for severe MR CONs: Low sensibility Most of cases need of TEE	Systolic reversal
Regurgitant volume	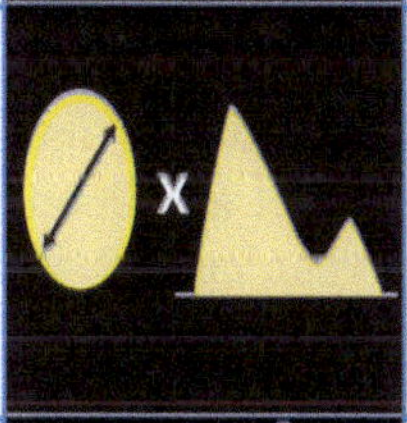 Pro: Not affected by jet/orifice shape CONs: Less useful in case of Irregular cardiac rythm Aortic regurgitant Not reliable evaluation of aortic annulus Very sensitive to accuracy of annulus measurements	Regurg volume > 60 ml Regurg fraction > 50%
ERO by PISA	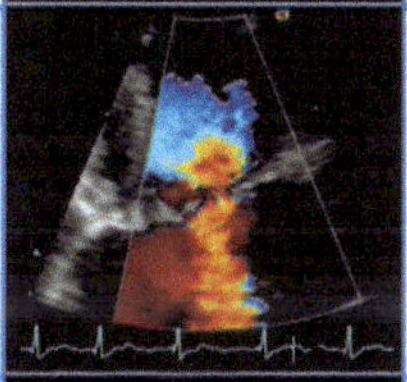 Pro: Less affected by load Not affected by associated valvular disease CONs: Low accuracy for no circular orifices	ERO > 0.4 cm^2 (ischemic MR > 0.2 cm^2)
ERO by 3D	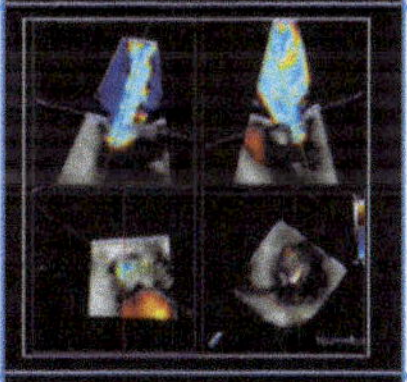 Pro: Not affected by orifice shape Not affected by jet shape Not affected by associated valvular disease CONs: Still low clinical experience	ERO > 0.4 cm^2 (ischemic MR > 0.2 cm^2)
Annulus/ leaflets measurements	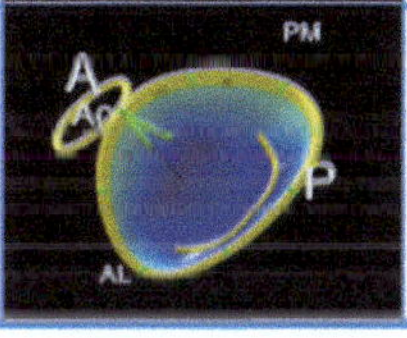 Pro: Exact modelling of annulus and leaflets Hundreds of possible variables CONs: Under clinical research	Work in progress

Fig. 16.8 Echocardiographic techniques for MR severity evaluation and criteria for severe MR. *ERO* effective regurgitant orifice

the reversal of the systolic wave is synonymous of severe MR. This finding is very specific, but has a lower sensitivity. Although the pattern can be studied by TTE, it is easier to achieve in TEE.

The third main tool in the MR severity evaluation is the computation of the regurgitant volume and the regurgitant fraction by means of the hemodynamic evaluation with Doppler. The technique is based in the possibility to compute the flow in a cardiac structure as the product of the cross-sectional area by the integral of the pulsed Doppler signal of the flow. The regurgitant volume is computed as the difference between the total flow volume passing for the mitral valve and the effective anterograde flow that equals the flow in aortic valve. The methodology is elegant, but can be imprecise because small mistakes in the measurements of the valve annulus can cause big changes in the final result.

The most used quantitative parameter in MR evaluation in the clinical setting could be the computation of the effective regurgitant orifice by PISA. This method is based on the flow acceleration that can be seen when blood moves towards the orifice that causes the regurgitation and takes advantage of the color Doppler pattern of the flow to measure an hemispheric flow convergence zone that allows the computation of the orifice. This method is more robust because it is less affected by patient load conditions. However it has also limitations because the methodology has some assumptions like the orifice is circular and the flow constant, facts that can be not true.

3D echocardiography has given also some tools for MR severity evaluation. The easiest one is to use the 3D acquisition to achieve a view with a perfect parallel orientation to the regurgitant orifice that can be used to measure the orifice area in spite of the orifice shape. There are also many new possibilities with 3D technique because the images can be used to construct complex models of the valve and the leaflets and to get all kind of measurements including area and length of the diseased segments. All of this group or new parameters are under extensive clinical research.

Evaluation of Reparability

There are many features of mitral valve disease in the literature that have been linked to the failure of the valve repair surgery (Lancellotti et al. 2010; Michelena et al. 2010) (Fig. 16.9). Most of them are indicatives of a wider extension or severity of the disease. Their evaluation is also very important because they can be useful not only to make the decision of the repair suitability, but also about where to send the patient for the surgery, because obviously the most complex cases should be treated by the most experienced surgical teams.

Timing to Surgical Intervention for Mitral Valve Regurgitation

The timing of intervention for mitral valve regurgitation is an evolving and controversial topic in the field of valvular medicine. There are two basic approaches in the literature and outlined in the ACC/AHA/ESC (Bonow et al. 2006a; Vahanian et al. 2007). Early surgery for asymptomatic patients with preserved left ventricular function (Ling et al. 1996, 1997), has been recommended by tertiary referral centers and is a Class IIa recommendation in the AHA/ACC guidelines (Bonow et al. 2006b). Early surgery may prevent left ventricular dysfunction from the chronic volume overload secondary to the mitral regurgitation. The ESC (Vahanian et al. 2007) guidelines support a more conservative strategy of watchful waiting based on careful monitoring of patients for symptoms, left ventricular dimensions, and signs of changes in clinical status. The Mayo Clinic study found that >90% of patients needed surgery within 10 years (Enriquez-Sarano et al. 2005). The study from Vienna demonstrated a much lower rate of surgical valve repair at 8 years with >50% of patients who did not meet criteria for surgical valve repair. The patient populations are different and as well as the valve lesions causing significant mitral regurgitation. This is also significant for the differences in approach as outlined in Europe as compared to the American Guidelines. The American (ACC/AHA) (Bonow et al. 2006b) guidelines, approach the patient with referral to a tertiary care center when the patient is asymptomatic with preserved ejection fraction without atrial fibrillation or pulmonary hypertension. The European (ESC) (Vahanian et al. 2007) guidelines outline a conservative approach.

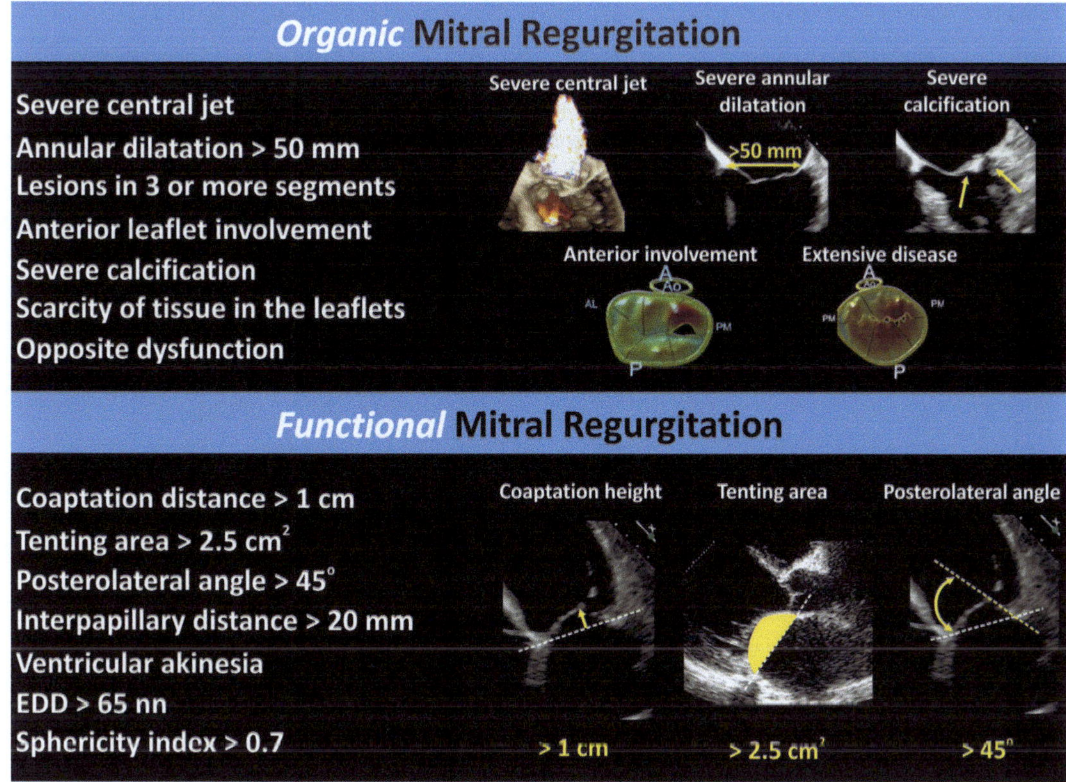

Fig. 16.9 Features linked to failure in MV repair

To obtain evidence for these approaches the Dutch AMR trial (Tietge et al. 2012) will be the first multicenter randomized trial on this topic worldwide. Two treatment strategies are compared: early surgery versus watchful waiting. The investigators anticipate that developing a foundation for the best clinical strategy for this patient population. Furthermore the results will provide solid recommendations for clinical guidelines in the future management of mitral valve disease. In addition to identification of the best treatment and evidence based medicine, it is of utmost importance to have knowledge on the cost-effectiveness of treatment. The investigators expect that the surgical strategy may be cost-effective in comparison with the strategy of watchful waiting.

The Dutch AMR investigators propose a pragmatic multicenter randomized trial in 250 adult asymptomatic patients with severe organic MV regurgitation and preserved left ventricular function. Patients who provide informed consent will be randomly assigned to either (1) watchful waiting; or (2) early MV repair. The follow-up will be 5 years. All procedures and definitions are in line with the current European Society of Cardiology (ESC) Guidelines (Vahanian et al. 2007).All asymptomatic patients (18–70 years) with severe organic MV regurgitation and preserved left ventricular function are eligible for the trial.

The exclusion criteria are: class I or IIa indications for surgery (including atrial fibrillation and pulmonary hypertension) according to the ESC guidelines (Vahanian et al. 2007). Patients should be fit to undergo surgery and the likelihood of MV repair (in contrast to replacement) should be >90%. Asymptomatic is defined as absence of subjective limitations of exercise capacity or complaints expressed by the patient and confirmed by the cardiologist. Severe organic

Table 16.1 Overview of trials monitoring the effect of early surgery in severe MR (Tietge et al. 2012)

Study	Study type	Centre	Analysis	N	Age	Outcomes	Outcomes with surgery
Ling et al. (1997)	Retrospective flail leaflets	Single	Direct comparison	221	65	Survival/CHF	79 vs. 65% at 10 years, RR=0.31/27 vs. 59% at 10 years, RR=0.38
Rosenhek et al. (2006)	Prospective flail leaflet or prolapse	Single	Time dependent	132	55	Survival/free of surgery	91±3% ns vs. expected/55±6% at 8 years
Enriquez-Sarano et al. (2005)	Prospective quantified MR	Single	Time dependent	456	63	Survival/CHF	RR=0.28 (0.14–0.55)/ RR=0.37 (0.17–0.79) at 5 years
Kang et al. (2009)	Prospective quantified MR	Single	Direct comparison	447	50	Event-free survival	99% vs. 85% at 7 years
Grigioni et al. (2008)	Retrospective flail leaflets	Multi-centre	Time dependent	394	64	Survival CVD/CHF	RR=0.42 (0.21–0.84)/ RR=0.26 (0.08–0.89) at 8 years
Chenot et al. (2009)	Prospective severe degenerative MR	Single	Time dependent	143	63	Overall/ cardiovascular survival	82±4%/90±3% at 10 years
Montant et al. (2009)	Prospective severe degenerative MR	Single	Direct comparison	192	64±15 conservative 62±12 early surgery	Survival	50±7% vs. 86±4%, at 8.5 years

Adapted from: Enriquez-Sarano and Sundt (2010). Reprinted with permission

MV regurgitation is defined as non-ischemic MV regurgitation with an organic cause (intrinsic valve lesion) as determined by consensus in reading echocardiography based on the criteria for definition of severe MR as issued by the ESC guidelines (Vahanian et al. 2007). In practice, at least two of the following items should be present on echocardiography: (1) jet characteristics (>40% of left atrial surface and/or reaching pulmonary veins); (2) vena contracta width ≥0.7 cm; (3) systolic reversal of the regurgitation jet in the pulmonary veins; (4) regurgitant volume ≥60 ml/beat; (5) effective regurgitant orifice area ≥0.40 cm^2; (6) E-wave dominant mitral inflow (E > 1.2 m/s) in the absence of MV stenosis or other causes of an elevated left atrial pressure. 'Preserved left ventricular function' is defined as left ventricular ejection fraction >60% and left ventricular end-systolic dimension <45 mm (Table 16.1).

Patient Selection

All cardiologists in the Netherlands will be asked to recruit patients for the trial (via www.dutchamr.nl and the Netherlands Society of Cardiology). They will provide written information about the trial to potential participants. They will ask patients whether they are interested in participation, and if so the referring cardiologist can contact the study centre or send the patient for a trial visit to the study centre (UMC Utrecht) to evaluate inclusion and exclusion criteria (Table 16.2). Before inclusion, the echocardiography needs to be evaluated by the core lab and the dedicated heart team (composed of dedicated cardiologists and cardiothoracic surgeons) verifying the severity of the MV regurgitation, preserved left ventricular function, the likelihood of repair and patient operability. Furthermore, 48-h ECG monitoring must

Table 16.2 Inclusion and exclusion criteria for Dutch AMR

Inclusion criteria
Age 18–70 years
Severe organic mitral regurgitation
Absence of symptoms defined as absence of subjective limitations of exercise capacity or complaints expressed by the patient and confirmed by the cardiologist
Likelihood of mitral valve repair (in contrast to replacement) should be >90%
Patients should be fit for surgery
Ejection fraction >60% and left ventricular end-systolic dimension <45 mm
Exclusion criteria
Class I or IIa indication for surgery (including atrial fibrillation and pulmonary hypertension) according to the ESC guidelines [4]
Symptoms
Ejection fraction <60% and left ventricular end-systolic dimension >45 mm
Atrial fibrillation, either on 12-lead ECG or 48-h ECG monitoring
Pulmonary hypertension (RVSP >50 mmHg on echocardiography)
Likelihood of repair <90%
Physical inability to undergo surgery
Signs of heart failure
Other life-threatening morbidity

Tietge et al. (2012). Reprinted with permission

be performed and exclude paroxysmal atrial fibrillation. If no consent is given, patients will be asked if their data can be collected in a registry. At inclusion baseline measurements will be performed: health-related quality of life questionnaires, blood sampling (brain natriuretic peptide (BNP), renal function etc.), cardiopulmonary exercise testing (including peak VO_2 consumption), cardiac MR (delayed enhancement, regurgitation quantification, function and dimensions). All measurements can be performed in the referring centre or in one of the study centers (on a one-stop base). These stringent criteria will help to promote uniformity in enrollment. Hopefully, this approach will also include the review of the pathologic mechanism of the mitral valve disease as the understanding of the biology (Caira et al. 2006) evolves in patients who present with mitral valve regurgitation. After both the patient and the physician have signed for informed consent, patients will be randomized stratified per hospital in a 1:1 ratio to (1) watchful waiting or (2) early MV repair surgery using a web-based computerized approach.

Intervention

Figure 16.10 provides the approach for the trial which includes: watchful waiting versus conservative strategy. Watchful waiting strategy will include patients will be seen by their own cardiologist in the outpatient clinic every 6 months in concordance with the ESC guidelines (Vahanian et al. 2007). Patients who reach a class I indication for surgery according to the current ESC guidelines will be referred for surgery. For patients who reach a IIa indication for surgery it is at the treating clinicians' discretion to refer the patient for surgery. The surgical strategy of MV repair will be performed in centers meeting criteria for best practice regarding MV surgery: low peri-operative mortality (<1%), repair rate of >95% in these patients, low reoperation rate after 5 years (<5%), >25 MV repair procedures/year/surgeon and >50/center (Bridgewater et al. 2006).

Conclusion

Mitral Valve Regurgitation is a complex disease process which requires expertise in imaging, evaluation and symptom management to diagnose, follow and treat this patient population. Current imaging modalities in echocardiography have vastly improved our understanding of the mechanisms of valve regurgitation, valve pathology and the natural history of this disease. DutchAMR will further help to delineate the approach and outcomes for this complex patient population and further define for physicians the timing of surgery in the future.

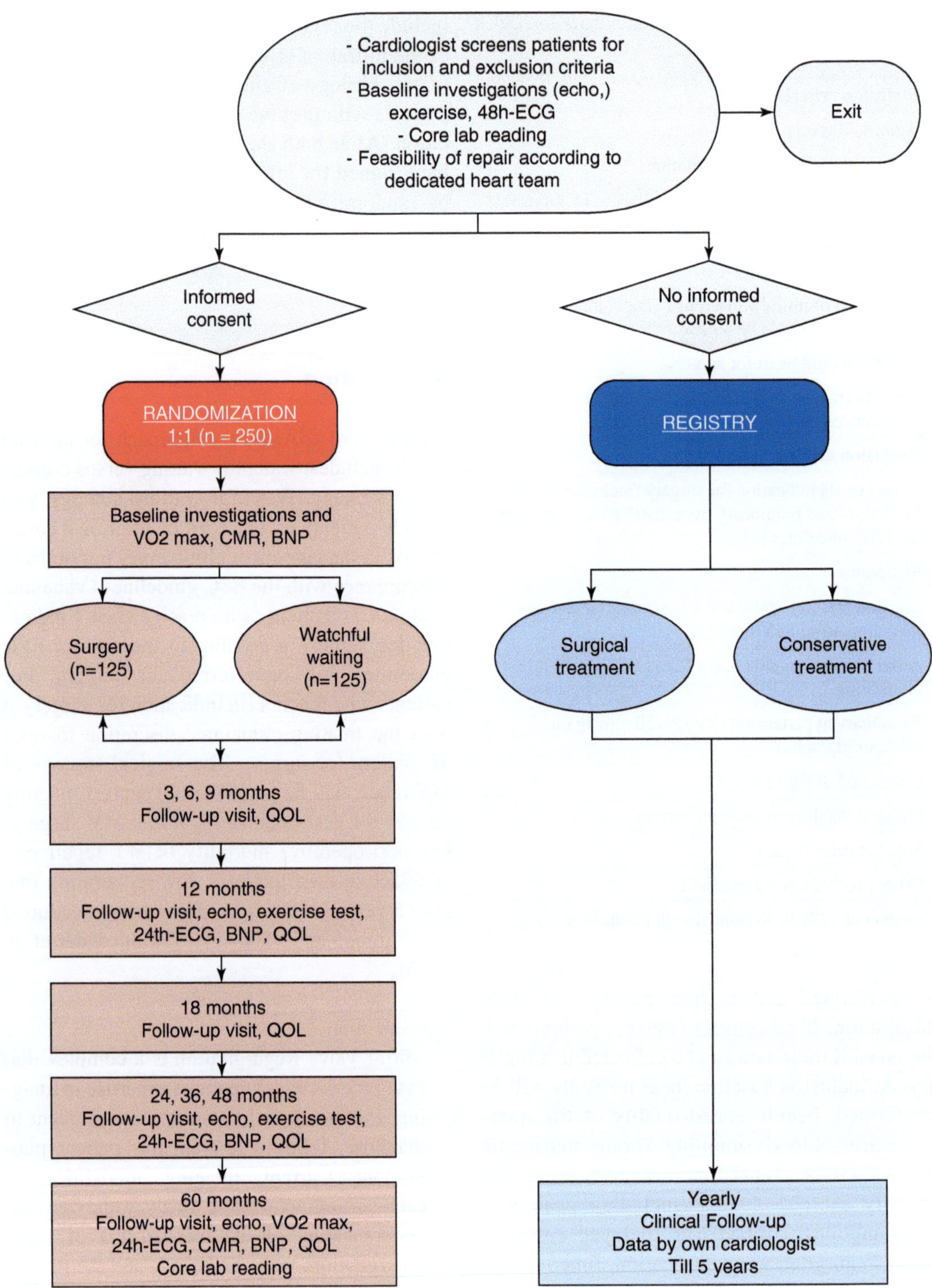

Fig. 16.10 Randomization protocol for Dutch AMR (Tietge et al. 2012. Reprinted with permission)

References

Bonow RO, Carabello BA, Kanu C, de Leon Jr AC, Faxon DP, Freed MD, Gaasch WH, Lytle BW, Nishimura RA, O'Gara PT, O'Rourke RA, Otto CM, Shah PM, Shanewise JS, Smith Jr SC, Jacobs AK, Adams CD, Anderson JL, Antman EM, Fuster V, Halperin JL, Hiratzka LF, Hunt SA, Nishimura R, Page RL, Riegel B. ACC/AHA 2006 guidelines for the management of patients with valvular heart disease: a report of the American College of Cardiology/American Heart Association Task Force on Practice Guidelines (writing committee to revise the 1998 Guidelines for the Management of Patients with Valvular Heart Disease): developed in collaboration with the Society of Cardiovascular Anesthesiologists: endorsed by the Society for Cardiovascular Angiography and Interventions and the Society of Thoracic Surgeons. Circulation. 2006a;114(5):e84–231.

Bonow RO, Carabello BA, Chatterjee K, de Leon Jr AC, Faxon DP, Freed MD, Gaasch WH, Lytle BW, Nishimura RA, O'Gara PT, O'Rourke RA, Otto CM, Shah PM, Shanewise JS, Smith Jr SC, Jacobs AK, Adams CD, Anderson JL, Antman EM, Fuster V, Halperin JL, Hiratzka LF, Hunt SA, Lytle BW, Nishimura R, Page RL, Riegel B. ACC/AHA 2006 guidelines for the management of patients with valvular heart disease: a report of the American College of Cardiology/American Heart Association Task Force on Practice Guidelines (writing Committee to Revise the 1998 guidelines for the management of patients with valvular heart disease) developed in collaboration with the Society of Cardiovascular Anesthesiologists endorsed by the Society for Cardiovascular Angiography and Interventions and the Society of Thoracic Surgeons. J Am Coll Cardiol. 2006b;48(3):e1–148.

Bridgewater B, Hooper T, Munsch C, Hunter S, von Oppell U, Livesey S, Keogh B, Wells F, Patrick M, Kneeshaw J, Chambers J, Masani N, Ray S. Mitral repair best practice: proposed standards. Heart (Br Cardiac Soc). 2006;92(7):939–44.

Caira FC, Stock SR, Gleason TG, McGee EC, Huang J, Bonow RO, Spelsberg TC, McCarthy PM, Rahimtoola SH, Rajamannan NM. Human degenerative valve disease is associated with up-regulation of low-density lipoprotein receptor-related protein 5 receptor-mediated bone formation. J Am Coll Cardiol. 2006;47(8):1707–12.

Carpentier A, Adams DH, Filsoufi F. Carpentier's reconstructive valve surgery. Maryland heights. Saunders-Elsevier, Riverport Lane, USA 2010.

Castillo JG, Solis J, Gonzalez-Pinto A, Adams DH. Surgical echocardiography of the mitral valve. Rev Esp Cardiol. 2011;64(12):1169–81.

Chenot F, Montant P, Vancraeynest D, Pasquet A, Gerber B, Noirhomme PH, El Khoury G, Vanoverschelde JL. Long-term clinical outcome of mitral valve repair in asymptomatic severe mitral regurgitation. Eur J Cardiothorac Surg. 2009;36(3):539–45.

Enriquez-Sarano M, Sundt 3rd TM. Early surgery is recommended for mitral regurgitation. Circulation. 2010;121(6):804–11; discussion 812.

Enriquez-Sarano M, Avierinos JF, Messika-Zeitoun D, Detaint D, Capps M, Nkomo V, Scott C, Schaff HV, Tajik AJ. Quantitative determinants of the outcome of asymptomatic mitral regurgitation. N Engl J Med. 2005;352(9):875–83.

Grigioni F, Tribouilloy C, Avierinos JF, Barbieri A, Ferlito M, Trojette F, Tafanelli L, Branzi A, Szymanski C, Habib G, Modena MG, Enriquez-Sarano M. Outcomes in mitral regurgitation due to flail leaflets a multicenter European study. JACC Cardiovasc Imaging. 2008;1(2):133–41.

Iung B, Vahanian A. Epidemiology of valvular heart disease in the adult. Nat Rev. 2011;8(3):162–72.

Kang DH, Kim JH, Rim JH, Kim MJ, Yun SC, Song JM, Song H, Choi KJ, Song JK, Lee JW. Comparison of early surgery versus conventional treatment in asymptomatic severe mitral regurgitation. Circulation. 2009;119(6):797–804.

Lancellotti P, Moura L, Pierard LA, Agricola E, Popescu BA, Tribouilloy C, Hagendorff A, Monin JL, Badano L, Zamorano JL. European Association of Echocardiography recommendations for the assessment of valvular regurgitation. Part 2: mitral and tricuspid regurgitation (native valve disease). Eur J Echocardiogr. 2010;11(4):307–32.

Lancellotti P, Magne J, O'Connor K, Pierard LA. Mitral valve disease. The EAE textbook of echocardiography. Oxford University Press; New York, USA 2011.

Ling LH, Enriquez-Sarano M, Seward JB, Tajik AJ, Schaff HV, Bailey KR, Frye RL. Clinical outcome of mitral regurgitation due to flail leaflet. N Engl J Med. 1996;335(19):1417–23.

Ling LH, Enriquez-Sarano M, Seward JB, Orszulak TA, Schaff HV, Bailey KR, Tajik AJ, Frye RL. Early surgery in patients with mitral regurgitation due to flail leaflets: a long-term outcome study. Circulation. 1997;96(6):1819–25.

Michelena HI, Bichara VM, Margaryan E, Forde I, Topilsky Y, Suri R, Enriquez-Sarano M. Progress in the treatment of severe mitral regurgitation. Rev Esp Cardiol. 2010;63(7):820–31.

Montant P, Chenot F, Robert A, Vancraeynest D, Pasquet A, Gerber B, Noirhomme P, El Khoury G, Vanoverschelde JL. Long-term survival in asymptomatic patients with severe degenerative mitral regurgitation: a propensity score-based comparison between an early surgical strategy and a conservative treatment approach. J Thorac Cardiovasc Surg. 2009;138(6):1339–48.

Rosenhek R, Rader F, Klaar U, Gabriel H, Krejc M, Kalbeck D, Schemper M, Maurer G, Baumgartner H. Outcome of watchful waiting in asymptomatic severe mitral regurgitation. Circulation. 2006;113(18):2238–44.

Tietge WJ, de Heer LM, van Hessen MW, Jansen R, Bots ML, van Gilst W, Schalij M, Klautz RJ, Van den Brink RB, Van Herwerden LA, Doevendans PA, Chamuleau SA, Kluin J. Early mitral valve repair versus watchful waiting in patients with severe asymptomatic organic mitral regurgitation; rationale and design of the Dutch AMR trial, a multicenter, randomised trial. Neth Heart J. 2012;20(3):94–101.

Vahanian A, Baumgartner H, Bax J, Butchart E, Dion R, Filippatos G, Flachskampf F, Hall R, Iung B, Kasprzak J, Nataf P, Tornos P, Torracca L, Wenink A. Guidelines on the management of valvular heart disease: the task force on the management of valvular heart disease of the European Society of Cardiology. Eur Heart J. 2007;28(2):230–68.

Biology of Mitral Valve Disease

17

Elena Aikawa and K. Jane Grande-Allen

Introduction

Understanding the biology of the mitral valve is becoming increasing important as surgical valve repair, percutaneous techniques and potential medical therapies are becoming important in this disease process. The mitral valve's structure, anatomy and function are quite complex making it a difficult valve lesion to treat with interventions and medical therapies. The pathology has many classifications in terms of degrees of valve severity and disease pathology. As the science in the field of mitral valve biology evolves so will our understanding towards treatment options for these patients. This chapter will discuss the scientific understanding of valve biology to date and approaches for future studies.

Normal Mitral Valve Structure, Function and Biomechanics

The coordinated opening and closing of the heart valves occurs approximately three billion times in an average human life span and is required for unidirectional blood flow. Normal mitral valve (MV) function depends on the complex interactions of all the components of MV apparatus: leaflets, chordae tendinae and papillary muscle. The MV has two leaflets, the anterior below the aortic valve and the posterior composed of three scallops. An understanding of MV disease requires understanding of normal MV structural morphology. Similar to aortic valves, normal MV leaflets have three well-defined tissue layers: ventricularis/fibrosa, spongiosa and atrialis, each containing cells and characteristic extracellular matrix (ECM) composition (Rabkin et al. 2001). The fibrosa is composed predominantly of densely packed and microscopically crimped collagen fibers arranged parallel to the free edge of the leaflet. This layer arises from the mitral annulus and faces the high-pressure left ventricle. The collagen of the fibrosa permits maximum leaflet coaptation during closure (e.g., prevent leaflet prolapse) and is essential for the maintenance of valve durability. The centrally located spongiosa is rich in chondroitin sulfate proteoglycans that provide a compressible ECM that have a cushioning and shear absorbing function. The atrialis contains lamellar collagen and elastin sheets, which contribute to leaflet recoil during uploading (Schoen 2008). At the leaflet edges, the collagen-rich chordae tendineae expand from the fibrosa to link the leaflets to the papillary muscles. The coordinated movements of the mitral apparatus are required for complete leaflet coaptation in the closed phase.

The mechanical environment and extracellular matrix composition of the diverse components of

E. Aikawa (✉)
Department of Medicine, Cardiovascular Medicine, Brigham and Women's Hospital, Harvard Medical School, Boston, MA, USA
e-mail: eaikawa@partners.org

K.J. Grande-Allen
Department of Bioengineering, Rice University, Houston, TX, USA

N.M. Rajamannan (ed.), *Cardiac Valvular Medicine*,
DOI 10.1007/978-1-4471-4132-7_17,

the mitral valve are critical to understanding their biomechanical behavior. The anterior leaflet has a very heterogeneous anatomy in which the tissue layers, described above, vary considerably in thickness from the mitral annulus to the free edge (Kunzelman et al. 1993; Stephens et al. 2010a). The region closest to the annulus is predominantly a thick fibrosa with very thin spongiosa and atrialis layers. Because this region does not have any basal attachments of chordae beneath it, it is sometimes described as the "clear zone" as opposed to the "rough zone" of the remainder of the anterior leaflet, which is supported by numerous basal and marginal chordae (Ranganathan et al. 1970). This structure allows the "clear zone" to withstand the high-pressure load when the valve is closed. The relative thicknesses of the layers change towards the middle of the leaflet, approaching the upper border of coaptation with the posterior leaflet: the fibrosa begins to demonstrate its characteristic corrugated appearance and comprises about one-third of the total leaflet thickness with the spongiosa and atrialis becoming considerably thicker. This arrangement facilitates the curvature of the closed leaflet in this region; moreover, the unfolding of the corrugated fibrosa layer contributes to the radial extensibility of the leaflet. Towards the free edge of the anterior leaflet, the thickness of the spongiosa increases profoundly, which promotes compressive load bearing in the region of coaptation.

The complex microstructure of the leaflets leads to a pronounced nonlinear anisotropic mechanical behavior (Grashow et al. 2006a, b; May-Newman and Yin 1995; Kunzelman and Cochran 1992; Liao et al. 2007; Stephens et al. 2010b). Both the anterior and posterior leaflets have a higher elastic modulus, a measure of the valve stiffness, and are less extensible in the circumferential direction compared to the radial direction. Furthermore, the posterior leaflet generally has greater extensibility and lower tensile elastic modulus, which might be attributed to the larger number of chordal attachments beneath the posterior leaflet, which provide additional mechanical support (May-Newman and Yin 1995). There is also heterogeneity of mechanical behavior throughout individual leaflets (Chen et al. 2004; Sacks et al. 2006); for example, the anterior leaflet clear zone has a circumferential tensile elastic modulus that is 30–200% higher than in the rough zone of the same leaflet (Kunzelman and Cochran 1992; Stephens et al. 2010b). Mitral valve leaflets also show a rather unique combination of viscoelastic characteristics, being remarkably independent of strain rates (Grashow et al. 2006a), while exhibiting significant stress relaxation (Grashow et al. 2006b; Stephens et al. 2010b), but negligible creep *ex vivo* (Grashow et al. 2006b) and *in vivo* (Sacks et al. 2006). The elastic modulus of chordae tendinae is roughly an order of magnitude stiffer than for the mitral leaflets (Kunzelman and Cochran 1992; Grande-Allen et al. 2005a).

Recent studies have highlighted unique features of valvular endothelial (VEC) and interstitial cells (VIC). A continuous endothelial cell layer on both atrial and ventricular aspects covers the leaflets. While VEC resemble endothelial cells elsewhere in the circulation, they have important differences and distinctive phenotype that reflects the valvular endothelium embryonic history, and potential to maintain integrity and function over a life span of dynamic mechanical stress (Bischoff and Aikawa 2011). A well-studied property that sets VEC apart is the ability to undergo an epithelial to a mesenchymal transition (EMT) (Markwald et al. 2010). In addition, recent report by Wylie-Sears et al. suggested that VEC mesenchymal differentiation potential can be redirected towards osteogenic, chondrogenic and adipogenic phenotypes (Wylie-Sears et al. 2011). This multi-lineage differentiation potential of VEC combined with a robust capacity for self-renewal strongly suggests that VEC are progenitor cells.

The deeper leaflet layers contain VIC, a constellation of a diverse, dynamic and highly plastic population of resident cells (Aikawa et al. 2006; Rabkin-Aikawa et al. 2004). Adult heart valve VIC have characteristic of quiescent non-contractile, alpha-smooth muscle actin-negative, vimentin-positive fibroblast-like cells that continuously contribute to homeostatic ECM remodeling with relatively low turnover (Aikawa et al. 2006). During conditions that required a rapid tissue remodeling (e.g., valve development, disease, abrupt changes in the mechanical stress, surgical intervention), VIC transition to an activated myofibroblast-like phenotype, expressing smooth muscle contractile proteins, matrix remodeling enzymes and cytokines (Rabkin et al. 2001). As suggested by Rabkin et al. through such mechanisms, in healthy valves, VIC plasticity contributes to adaptation to the dynamic valve environment, and to repair of functional ECM damage. In contrast, ongoing and progressive mechanical stress, when adaptation to a new environment condition is not possible, can lead to mitral valve disease (Rabkin et al. 2001).

Mitral Valve Development

There is increasing evidence that the regulatory mechanisms governing normal valve development also contribute to mitral valve disease. During early valve development, in response to myocardially-derived signals that include TGFβ1-3, BMP2-4 and Notch1-4, the endocardial cells of the embryonic heart undergo EMT and initiate endocardial cushion formation (Combs and Yutzey 2009). Post-EMT valve development involves cell migration and proliferation associated with periostin, cadherin, MMP2 and cathepsin K, RANKL, NFAT and VEGF expression. This early remodeling phase, characterized by gradual thinning and elongation of pre-valvular tissue, is concomitant with the differentiation of the cushion mesenchymal cells into VEC and VIC. Embryonic VEC possess an activated phenotype throughout fetal development (VCAM-1, ICAM-1), and VIC show a myofibroblast-like phenotype (α-smooth muscle actin, vimentin, desmin), abundant embryonic myosin (SMemb) and MMP-expression, indicating an immature/activated phenotype engaged in rapid matrix remodeling versus a quiescent fibroblast-like VIC in adults (Aikawa et al. 2006). In addition, VIC density, proliferation and apoptosis are significantly higher in fetal than adult valves. In human valves, a tri-laminar architecture appears by 36 weeks of gestation, but remains rudimentary compared with that of adult valves. Collagen content increases from early to late fetal stages, but is subsequently unchanged, while elastin significantly increases post-natally. Additionally, collagen fibers are more aligned in adult than fetal valves. Collectively, these findings from Aikawa E et al. indicate that fetal VIC and VEC activation occurs throughout development, suggesting that the analogous molecular mechanisms may direct both physiological and pathological cell activation.

Degenerative Mitral Valve Disease

Degenerative mitral valve disease (MVD) may lead to MV incompetence with dilatation of the mitral annulus, excess of valvular tissue resulting in billowing floppy leaflets (usually more prominent in the posterior leaflet), or rupture of the chordae tendineae resulting in a flail leaflet (Fornes et al. 1999). Mechanically, the diseased leaflets are roughly one-third less stiff and twice as extensible as normal leaflets (Barber et al. 2001a). The chordae tendinae are even more mechanically compromised, being about two-thirds less stiff and 75% less strong than normal chordae (Barber et al. 2001b), thus promoting the potential for chordal rupture. In the 1980s, Carpentier made a clear distinction between myxomatous MVD, now called Barlow's disease, and fibroelastic deficiency (FED) based on clinical patterns, echocardiographic findings and gross pathology (Carpentier et al. 1980). Two decades later the histopathologic features of these two entities were described (Fornes et al. 1999) followed by studies attempting to address the mechanisms of degenerative MVD (Rabkin et al. 2001).

Patients with Barlow's disease are usually younger compared to patients with FED, and present at operation after a long previous clinical history of mitral valve regurgitation. Grossly, the leaflets in myxomatous MVD are often thickened with a soft, gelatinous consistency, while the extreme thinning is observed in MVD associated with FED. There is the higher percentage of ruptured chordae in FED patients compared to Barlow's (90% vs. 64%, respectively) (Fornes et al. 1999). Microscopically, myxomatous MVD

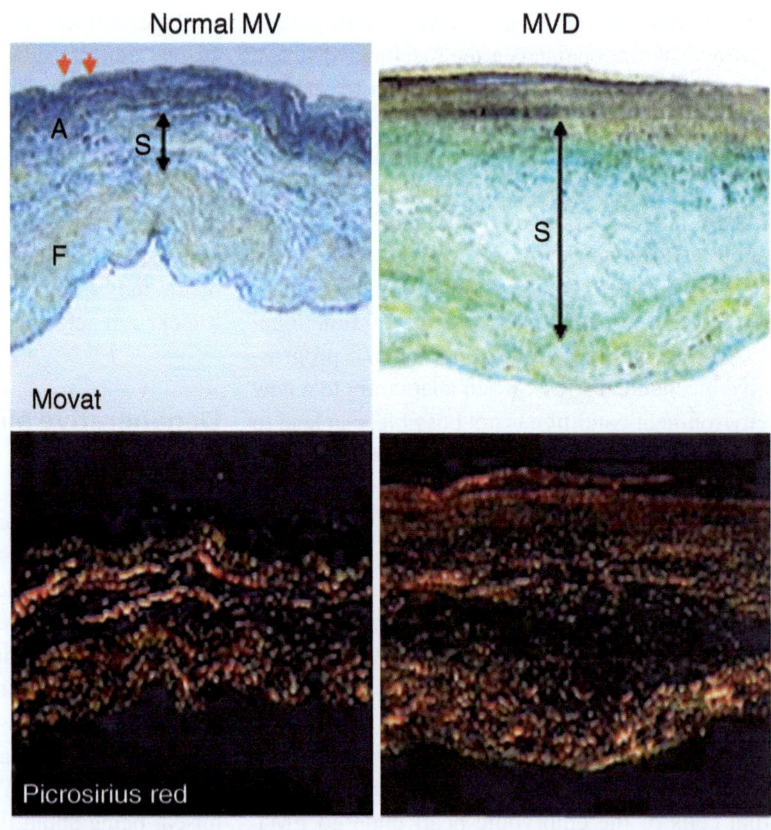

Fig. 17.1 Morphological features of normal and diseased (*MVD*) mitral valves. MVD leaflets have an altered layered architecture: loose collagen in fibrosa/ventricularis, expanded spongiosa strongly positive for proteoglycans, and distrupted elastin in atrialis, *Top*, Movat pentachrome stain (collagen stains *yellow*; proteoglycans, *blue-green*; elastin, *black*). *Bottom*, Picrosirius red staining viewed under polarized light detected disruption and lower birefringence of collagen fibers in MDV leaflets. *A* atrialis, *S* spongiosa, *F* fibrosa. Original magnification ×100 (Adapted from Rabkin et al. 2001)

is characterized by expansion of the spongiosa by accumulation of amorphous glycosaminoglycans (GAGs) and proteoglycans (Fig. 17.1). Collagen in the fibrosa is fragmented and appears less dense due invasion of proteoglycans and the GAG-hyaluronan (Grande-Allen et al. 2003; Gupta et al. 2009a). Picrosirius red staining under polarized light further shows that individual collagen fibers are disoriented, disrupted and coiled. Elastic fibers are fragmented, granulated and twisted and often appeared as clusters identified well by Movat pentachrome staining as accumulation of black amorphous clumps. These pathological patterns of elastin fiber lesions are more often present in Barlow's disease and to a lesser extend in FED patients. The myxomatous degeneration of the collagen core of chordae is frequently found and likely represents the background of the chordae rupture. Myxomatous valves often have a layer of superficial plaque characterized by the accumulation of stellate and spindle-shaped cells, particularly on the ventricular aspect of the leaflet. In more advanced disease superficial fibrosis is noted on the ventricular surface and the chordae. Owing to both expansion of the spongiosa and superficial plaque formation/fibrosis, myxomatous leaflets are thicker than normal (2.3 vs. 0.9 mm, respectively, $p<0.0001$), and have increased cell density (Rabkin et al. 2001).

Immunohistochemistry demonstrated that in normal valves VIC are quiescent, while in the early stages of MVD, VIC possess characteristics of activated myofibroblasts identified by expression of alpha-smooth muscle actin (α-SMA) and vimentin, but not SM1 or SM2, markers of differentiated smooth muscle cells. Spindle-shaped and stellate myofibroblasts are dispersed randomly in the myxomatous matrix, which is composed mainly of proteoglycans and sparse collagen. VIC in MVD express high levels of proteolytic enzymes (metalloproteinases: MMP-1, MMP-2, MMP-9, MMP-13) and elastolytic cathepsins participating in matrix degradation while collagen synthesis (procollagen-I mRNA expression) remained unchanged (Rabkin et al. 2001). These observations demonstrate an important role for excessive levels of collagenolytic and elastolytic enzymes expressed by activated VIC, as opposed to decreased collagen synthesis, in the distorted layered leaflet architecture and structural abnormalities of collagen and other connective tissue components, and suggest that these structural alterations could cause functional abnormalities in patients with MVD. A recent study by Caira et al., investigating chondrogenic and osteogenic remodeling in diseased aortic and mitral valve, demonstrated hypertrophic chondrocytes in regions of human myxomatous mitral valves that were stained strongly for bone sialoprotein. Protein and/or gene level analysis also showed greatly elevated expression of Lrp5, Cbfa 1, SOX 9, cyclin, osteocalcin, and osteopontin compared with control valves, suggesting a role for chondrogenic differentiation or process resembling the early cartilage phenotype in the development of this disease (Caira et al. 2006).

While accurate diagnosis of the two entities (Barlow's and FED) is extremely important because they require different surgical planning, it is also challenging because it relies on qualitative evaluation of mitral valve gross pathology by a surgeon and echocardiography by an imaging specialist. As a result these difficulties could affect pre-surgical planning and decision-making and could lead to either unsuccessful repair or replacement with poor outcome in patients with complex valvular disease. While the surgeon's diagnosis based on clinical examination, echocardiographical findings, and operative macroscopic examination of the entire mitral valve apparatus remains the gold standard, the histological findings should be taken into consideration as far as prognosis is concerned. In addition, 3D echocardiographic analysis can be successfully used to assess a spectrum of pathomorphological abnormalities in MVD and differentiate Barlow's disease form FED patients (Chandra et al. 2011). This analysis may facilitate not only the conformation of etiology, but also demonstrates quantitatively anatomic differences between Barlow's disease and FED, and provides a framework for pre-operative assessment of the complexity of repair (Chandra et al. 2011). As quantification tools become more automated and less reliant on expertise, they may be used to support clinical decision-making. Until then genetic and histomorphological studies followed by careful immunohistochemical and biochemical analyses are needed to address potentially different mechanisms involved in the development of these two entities.

MV Remodeling in Human Heart Failure and Impact on Mechanics

In addition to the mitral regurgitation (MR) caused by myxomatous MVD, the other most common incidence of MR is in patients with ischemic or idiopathic dilated cardiomyopathy resulting in congestive heart failure (CHF) (Blondheim et al. 1991; Smolens et al. 2000). Because the mitral valve in these patients often appears normal on echocardiographic or gross pathologic examination, this MR has often been generally considered to be a functional consequence of alterations in the cardiac geometry (abnormal ventricular wall motion, annular dilatation, reorientation of the papillary muscles (He et al. 1999; Levine et al. 2002; Tibayan et al. 2003)) and hence was termed functional mitral regurgitation (FMR) of an apparently normal mitral valve. However, the altered cardiac geometry as well as altered blood chemistry associated with heart failure change the mechanical and chemical environment experienced by the valve tissues, which likely drives cell-mediated remodeling. Grande-Allen et al. investigated the mitral valves from patients with congestive heart failure (CHF) using biochemical assays for cells and extracellular matrix, echocardiographic measures of heart and valve anatomy and function, and mechanical testing to assess tissue strength, stiffness, and extensibility (Grande-Allen et al. 2005a, b). The mitral valves of patients with CHF contained significantly more DNA (indicating greater cell density), more glycosaminoglycans, and more collagen, and were slightly but significantly less hydrated than age-matched normal mitral valves. In addition, many of these deranged biochemical measures of the leaflet and chordal tissues were significantly associated with the echocardiographic valve measurements, such as an absence of anterior leaflet redundancy, annular diameter, and left atrial diameter, all characteristics of the annular dilatation commonly found in FMR. With respect to the mechanical behavior of the tissues, the mitral anterior leaflets were profoundly stiffer, both radially and circumferentially, compared to age-matched control valves. The viscous behavior in the radial direction was also reduced, as was overall leaflet extensibility. The chordae for CHF patients were also stiffer. This remodeling is very different from the type of ECM and mechanical behavior changes reported in myxomatous MVD.

These findings provide evidence for the hypothesis that loading conditions contribute to matrix remodeling, and indicate that the functional MR that develops secondary to ischemic or dilated cardiomyopathy is associated with distinctive and abnormal structural changes in the valves. The altered proportions of ECM, particularly collagen, in these mitral valves from patients with CHF indicate that the tissue has become heavily fibrotic, a finding supported by the greater stiffness and reduced tissue extensibility. This fibrosis may represent a tissue adaptation to provide additional tensile strength, particularly in patients with CHF, who have higher than normal plasma and ventricular levels of proteolytic enzymes (Yamazaki et al. 2004) and disruptions of the normal renin-angiotensin system (Sun and Weber 2003). The excess GAGs in these tissues may also be related to fibrosis, because certain GAGs, via their association with proteoglycans, have roles in collagen fibril organization (Grande-Allen et al. 2004). It is proposed that the annular and subvalvular dilation causes the leaflet to become more stretched than normal across the mitral orifice, resulting in a loss of coaptation. This leaflet extension and stretching applies high tensile and membrane loads to the posterior leaflet and the free edge of the anterior leaflet, which are regions of the valve that would normally experience compressive stress relief during

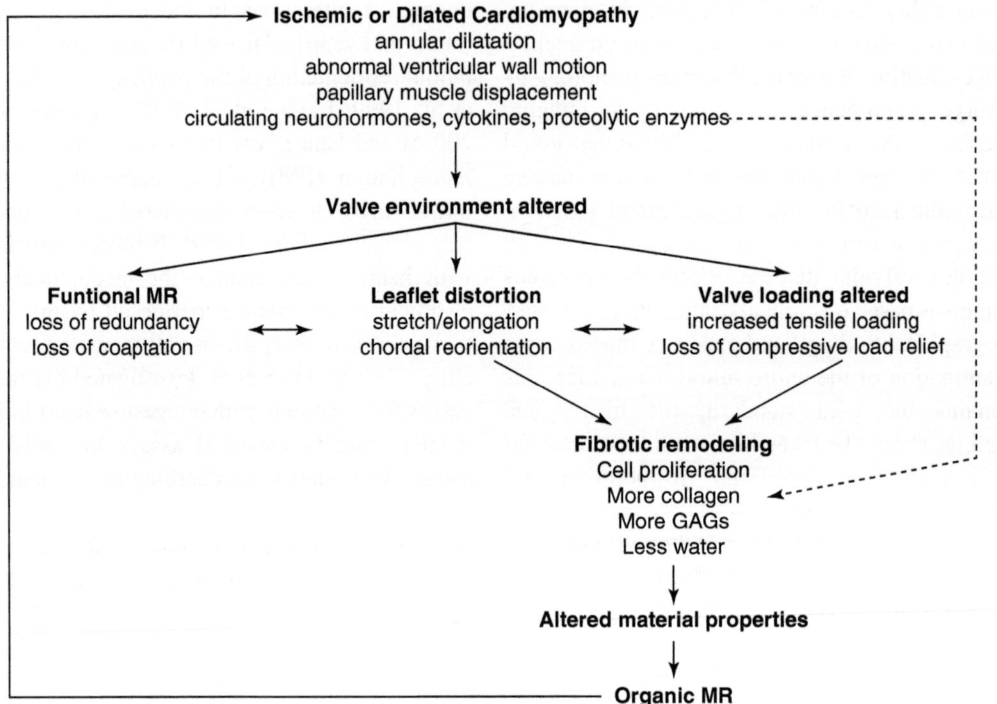

Fig. 17.2 Proposed mechanism for secondary valvular remodeling. *GAGs* glycosaminoglycans, *MR* mitral regurgitation (Adapted from Grande-Allen et al. 2005b)

leaflet coaptation. Indeed, these regions exhibited greater magnitude changes in tissue composition than the chordae and the center of the anterior leaflet, which normally experience high tensile loads. As a result of these altered loading conditions and ECM remodeling, the mitral valve tissues become significantly stiffer and less able to stretch sufficiently to cover the valve orifice, which perpetuates the mitral regurgitation (Fig. 17.2). Recognizing that the presence of FMR worsens the prognosis of CHF, numerous surgeons are performing mitral annuloplasty on these patients to reduce morbidity and mortality while awaiting heart transplantation surgery (Smolens et al. 2000).

Animal Models of Mitral Valve Disease

Animal models fill an important niche in the investigation of mitral valve remodeling. These models can provide more information on the development of the valve dysfunction and changes, since that rarely accompanies the analysis of clinical valve samples, which are most commonly segments of tissue excised during surgical repair or replacement procedures. The sheep is the most common animal model for investigations of mitral regurgitation. There is a long history of employing sheep and other large animal models to examine how mitral regurgitation, generated through various approaches such as tachycardia-induced dilatation, volume overload, coronary artery occlusion, or transection of one of the valve leaflets leads to remodeling of the valve anatomy and myocardium (Nguyen et al. 2008; Timek et al. 2001; Goetz et al. 2003; Tsutsui et al. 1994; Tamura et al. 2000; Ryan et al. 2007). More recently, there has been a focus on evaluating the changes in the mitral leaflet that result from these MR models. For example, it was found that tachycardia-induced cardiomyopathy, which mimics some aspects of heart failure, induced collagen and elastic fiber turnover throughout the mitral valve leaflets (Stephens et al. 2009). Coronary artery ligation resulting in abnormal ventricular wall motion produced a comparable effect, in that there was an increase in the amount of procollagen within the mitral leaflets (Kunzelman et al. 1998). This finding of active extracellular matrix remodeling within mitral valve leaflets was also shown in a model of isolated MR without heart dysfunction (Stephens et al. 2008), which suggests that the MR alone can promote mitral leaflet remodeling. Tamura et al. used a scalpel to cut through a segment of the mitral anterior leaflet and then observed a robust wound-healing response involving abundant production of glycosaminoglycans (Tamura et al. 2000). Another model in which the papillary muscle tips were displaced downwards, thus imposing additional stretch on the valve leaflets, resulted in a profound thickening of the leaflet tissues (largely due to an increase in the thickness of the spongiosa), increased expression of α-SMA by VIC and VEC (the latter case due to endothelial-to-mesenchyme transdifferentiation; EMT), and reduced collagen fiber organization (Dal-Bianco et al. 2009) (Fig. 17.3). Finally, the utility of small animal models in the study of mitral valve remodeling should be noted. Rabbits in particular have been employed to investigate mechanistic aspects of numerous valve diseases, such as the suppression of the anti-angiogenic glycoprotein chondromodulin in infective endocarditis (Grammer et al. 2007), the transport of large macromolecules into the valve leaflets of hyperlipidemic rabbits (Zeng et al. 2007), and the ability of statins to blunt calcific remodeling in hypercholesterolemic rabbits (Makkena et al. 2005).

Genetic Mutations and Disease Pathways

MV prolapse and leaflet thickening occure in several connective tissue disorders, including Marfan syndrome, Ehlers-Danlos syndrome, aneurysm-osteoarthritis syndrome, and Loeys-Dietz syndrome. Affected people often have elongated MV leaflets with thickening similar to the morphology in Barlow disease (Carpentier et al. 1980). Echocardiographic studies found that MV dysfunction occurs in up to 50% of Marfan patients (Pyeritz and Wappel 1983). Marfan syndrome is caused by mutations in

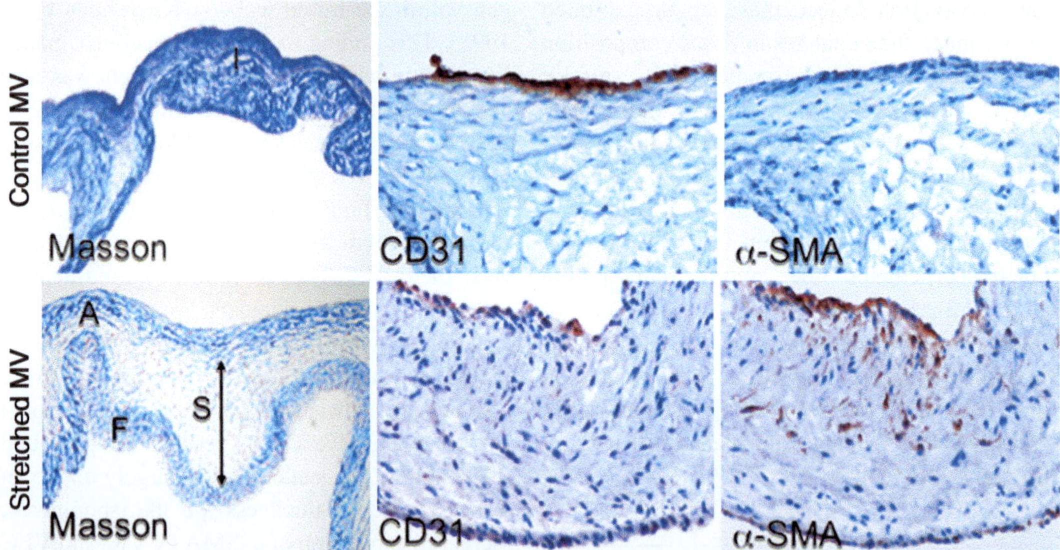

Fig. 17.3 ECM changes and EMT in a Stretched MV model. Masson staining (*left*) in the normal and stretched sheep MV demonstrates increased spongiosa layer stretched model similar to MVD. Original magnification ×40. Unstretched MV (*top panels*) shows negative α-SMA staining along the CD31 positive endothelium. Stretched MV (*bottom panels*) shows α-SMA staining in the atrial CD31- positive endothelium with nest of α-SMA-positive cells appearing to penetrate the interstitium suggesting leaflet repopulation with new cells via EMT process. *A* trialis, *S* spongiosa, *F* fibrosa. Original magnification ×200 (Adapted from Dal-Bianco et al. 2009)

FBN1, the gene encoding fibrillin-1, the principal component of the extracellular matrix microfibril (Dietz et al. 1991). In addition, several lines of evidence suggest that excessive signaling by the transforming growth factor-β (TGF-β) may cause many features of Marfan syndrome. Fibrillin-1 is similar to the latent TGF-β -binding proteins. Studies of mice harboring mutations in *Fbn1* have demonstrated longer and thicker MV compared to control mice (Ng et al. 2004). Of note, neutralizing antibodies to TGF-β prevented the MV elongation and thickening (Ng et al. 2004). Since many features of Marfan syndrome could be treated by TGF-β antagonism in mice, investigations on related human phenotypes focused on this pathway (Ng et al. 2004; Neptune et al. 2003; Habashi et al. 2006). The other disorder leading to MV prolapse, known as Loeys-Dietz syndrome, is characterized by aortic aneurysm and dissection, and long bone overgrowth (Loeys et al. 2005). This condition is caused by mutations in the genes encoding TGF-β receptors (*TFGBR1* and *TGFBR2*). A similar condition, termed aneurysm-osteoarthritis syndrome, is caused by mutations in *MADH3*, encoding Smad3, a TGF-β associated protein (van de Laar et al. 2011). Examination of tissues affected in these three disorders consistently shows increased activation of the TGF-β family (Ng et al. 2004). While the function of TGF-β is confirmed in murine models of Marfan syndrome, its role needs further investigation for aneurysm-osteoarthritis and Loeys-Dietz disorders.

Mutations in the Filamin-A gene were recently shown by genetic studies to cause an X-linked form of myxomatous valve degeneration in humans (Kyndt et al. 2007). Emerging evidence suggests that Filamin-A expression is upregulated in activated myofibroblasts of human myxomatous valves, reflecting an altered cell phenotype. In addition, Filamin-A participates in matrix compaction and collagen deposition, both of which associate with the biomechanical properties of the cardiac valves. In one study Norris et al. proposed that Filamin-A mutations result in defects in the molecular machinery essential for TGF-β-mediated signaling, collagen deposition and matrix remodeling, ultimately affecting the biomechanical stability of MV (Norris et al. 2010). The generation of point mutation knock-in mouse models will test this hypothesis and provide mechanistic insights into pathways governing valvular diseases.

In Vitro and Cell Biology Approaches

The insight into mitral valve biology and disease gained from human and animals studies has been profoundly enhanced by numerous in vitro and cell biology investigations employing a wide range of experimental approaches. One of the most significant class of tools in this regard has been the use of flow loops and bioreactor systems to apply mechanical stimulation to mitral valve tissues or cultured cells and then observe their resulting deformation or behavior. Some of these systems are non-sterile, such as those developed by Yoganathan and colleagues, which were used to assess the effects of papillary muscle position and annular reinforcement on the strain patterns in the mitral leaflet and chordae, as well as on the nature of the mitral regurgitant jet (Jimenez et al. 2003; Nielsen et al. 1999; He et al. 2003). For example, they have reported that the misalignment of papillary muscles increases the chordal tethering force, resulting in restricted leaflet mobility, a tented leaflet configuration, and greater forces applied to the anterior leaflet coaptation area (Nielsen et al. 1999). Papillary muscle repositioning also impacts the timing of mitral valve closure (He et al. 2003). Gheewala et al. developed a variation on this system that allows for the sterile organ culture of mitral valves for up to 3 weeks, during which time a variety of mechanical loading conditions can be implemented (Gheewala and Grande-Allen 2011). The organ culture approach also offers the potential to adding chemicals to the culture medium in order to determine how cellular responses to altered biochemical environments, as well as mechanical environments, translate into changes in valve structure and function. This chemical approach was employed by Barzilla et al. who cultured segments of mitral valve tissues within a small rotating bioreactor to model conditions leading to fenfluramine-mediated valvulopathy (Barzilla et al. 2010). After 2 weeks of culture, this model was able to differentiate the cellular and extracellular matrix remodeling caused by norfenfleuramine from that caused by serotonin, and intriguingly even resulted in the formation of plaques atop the leaflet surfaces. Valves that have been organ cultured for shorter time periods (hours to less than a week) have provided information about the viability and migration patterns of VIC and VEC (Lester and Gotlieb 1988) as well as the functional coupling of VIC with collagen fibers via α2β1 integrins connections to the actin cytoskeleton (Stephens et al. 2010b). In this latter case, it was found that KCl-stimulated isometric force generation by the mitral VIC in situ could be blocked either by blocking the α2β1 integrins with antibodies or blocking actin polymerization via cytochalasin.

Several other in vitro studies have examined the behavior of mitral VIC and VEC by culturing them in 2D monolayers or in 3D using an engineered tissue approach. Gotlieb and colleagues have performed numerous scrape-wounding assays on mitral VIC to observe their migration and proliferative behavior (Liu and Gotlieb 2008; Gotlieb et al. 2002). They have shown that mitral VIC treated with transforming growth factor-β (TGF-β) increased proliferation (Liu and Gotlieb 2008), which interestingly is opposite of the response by aortic VIC (Walker et al. 2004). Moreover, the actively migrating mitral VIC in an *in vitro* scratch wound model upregulate fibroblast growth factor-2 (FGF-2) and fibroblast growth factor receptor 1 (Gotlieb et al. 2002) as well as greater expression of TGF-β and α-SMA and phosphorylation of Smad2/3 (Liu and Gotlieb 2008). In one of several elegant studies of VEC, Flanagan et al. showed that VEC readily synthesized the basement membrane components laminin and type IV collagen, but not type I collagen and chondroitin sulfate (Flanagan et al. 2006a). VEC were also found to synthesize endothelial nitric oxide synthase (NOS) both *in vivo* and *in vitro*, in contrast with VIC, for which only a minority of cells expressed neuronal NOS *in vitro* (Flanagan et al. 2006a). These same authors found that growing mitral VEC atop collagen-chondroitin sulfate scaffolds promoted a more *in vivo* like phenotype than did culture on collagen-only scaffolds (Flanagan et al. 2006b). Finally, several studies by Gupta et al. in which mitral VIC were cultured within 3D collagen gels and subjected to mechanical loading, showed that the stretching conditions modulated the synthesis and deposition of GAGs and proteoglycans by the VIC in a manner that reflected the tissue source of the cells (leaflets or chordae), presence and magnitude of stretch, and time course of applied stretch (Gupta et al. 2008, 2009b).

Summary and Future Directions

Despite remarkable progress in understanding the pathogenesis of mitral valve disease, many questions still remain unanswered. Future research needs to focus on understanding the mechanisms of MVD, including the role of EMT and dysregulation of growth factors, development of small animal models, genetic analysis of patient populations, understanding of the influence of biomechanical stress on the pathogenesis of MVD, and development of new technologies for early diagnosis and imaging of MVD. These efforts will lead to novel therapies to improve MVD without surgery.

References

Aikawa E, Whittaker P, Farber M, Mendelson K, Padera RF, Aikawa M, Schoen FJ. Human semilunar cardiac valve remodeling by activated cells from fetus to adult: implications for postnatal adaptation, pathology, and tissue engineering. Circulation. 2006;113(10):1344–52.

Barber JE, Kasper FK, Ratliff NB, Cosgrove DM, Griffin BP, Vesely I. Mechanical properties of myxomatous mitral valves. J Thorac Cardiovasc Surg. 2001a;122(5):955–62.

Barber JE, Ratliff NB, Cosgrove 3rd DM, Griffin BP, Vesely I. Myxomatous mitral valve chordae. I: mechanical properties. J Heart Valve Dis. 2001b;10(3):320–4.

Barzilla JE, Acevedo FE, Grande-Allen KJ. Organ culture as a tool to identify early mechanisms of serotonergic valve disease. J Heart Valve Dis. 2010;19(5):626–35.

Bischoff J, Aikawa E. Progenitor cells confer plasticity to cardiac valve endothelium. J Cardiovasc Transl Res. 2011;4(6):710–9.

Blondheim DS, Jacobs LE, Kotler MN, Costacurta GA, Parry WR. Dilated cardiomyopathy with mitral regurgitation: decreased survival despite a low frequency of left ventricular thrombus. Am Heart J. 1991;122(3 Pt 1):763–71.

Caira FC, Stock SR, Gleason TG, McGee EC, Huang J, Bonow RO, Spelsberg TC, McCarthy PM, Rahimtoola SH, Rajamannan NM. Human degenerative valve disease is associated with up-regulation of low-density lipoprotein receptor-related protein 5 receptor-mediated bone formation. J Am Coll Cardiol. 2006;47(8):1707–12.

Carpentier A, Chauvaud S, Fabiani JN, Deloche A, Relland J, Lessana A, D'Allaines C, Blondeau P, Piwnica A, Dubost C. Reconstructive surgery of mitral valve incompetence: ten-year appraisal. J Thorac Cardiovasc Surg. 1980;79(3):338–48.

Chandra S, Salgo IS, Sugeng L, Weinert L, Tsang W, Takeuchi M, Spencer KT, O'Connor A, Cardinale M, Settlemier S, Mor-Avi V, Lang RM. Characterization of degenerative mitral valve disease using morphologic analysis of real-time three-dimensional echocardiographic images: objective insight into complexity and planning of mitral valve repair. Circ Cardiovasc Imaging. 2011;4(1):24–32.

Chen L, McCulloch AD, May-Newman K. Nonhomogeneous deformation in the anterior leaflet of the mitral valve. Ann Biomed Eng. 2004;32(12):1599–606.

Combs MD, Yutzey KE. Heart valve development: regulatory networks in development and disease. Circ Res. 2009;105(5):408–21.

Dal-Bianco JP, Aikawa E, Bischoff J, Guerrero JL, Handschumacher MD, Sullivan S, Johnson B, Titus JS, Iwamoto Y, Wylie-Sears J, Levine RA, Carpentier A. Active adaptation of the tethered mitral valve: insights into a compensatory mechanism for functional mitral regurgitation. Circulation. 2009;120(4):334–42.

Dietz HC, Cutting GR, Pyeritz RE, Maslen CL, Sakai LY, Corson GM, Puffenberger EG, Hamosh A, Nanthakumar EJ, Curristin SM, et al. Marfan syndrome caused by a recurrent de novo missense mutation in the fibrillin gene. Nature. 1991;352(6333):337–9.

Flanagan TC, Black A, O'Brien M, Smith TJ, Pandit AS. Reference models for mitral valve tissue engineering based on valve cell phenotype and extracellular matrix analysis. Cells Tissues Organs. 2006a;183(1):12–23.

Flanagan TC, Wilkins B, Black A, Jockenhoevel S, Smith TJ, Pandit AS. A collagen-glycosaminoglycan co-culture model for heart valve tissue engineering applications. Biomaterials. 2006b;27(10):2233–46.

Fornes P, Heudes D, Fuzellier JF, Tixier D, Bruneval P, Carpentier A. Correlation between clinical and histologic patterns of degenerative mitral valve insufficiency: a histomorphometric study of 130 excised segments. Cardiovasc Pathol. 1999;8(2):81–92.

Gheewala N, Grande-Allen KJ. Design and mechanical evaluation of a physiological mitral valve organ culture system. Cardiovasc Eng Technol. 2011;1(2):123–31.

Goetz WA, Lim HS, Pekar F, Saber HA, Weber PA, Lansac E, Birnbaum DE, Duran CM. Anterior mitral leaflet mobility is limited by the basal stay chords. Circulation. 2003;107(23):2969–74.

Gotlieb AI, Rosenthal A, Kazemian P. Fibroblast growth factor 2 regulation of mitral valve interstitial cell repair in vitro. J Thorac Cardiovasc Surg. 2002;124(3):591–7.

Grammer JB, Eichinger WB, Bleiziffer S, Benz MR, Lange R, Bauernschmitt R. Valvular chondromodulin-1 expression is downregulated in a rabbit model of infective endocarditis. J Heart Valve Dis. 2007;16(6):623–30; discussion 630.

Grande-Allen KJ, Griffin BP, Ratliff NB, Cosgrove DM, Vesely I. Glycosaminoglycan profiles of myxomatous mitral leaflets and chordae parallel the severity of mechanical alterations. J Am Coll Cardiol. 2003;42(2):271–7.

Grande-Allen KJ, Calabro A, Gupta V, Wight TN, Hascall VC, Vesely I. Glycosaminoglycans and proteoglycans in normal mitral valve leaflets and chordae: association with regions of tensile and compressive loading. Glycobiology. 2004;14(7):621–33.

Grande-Allen KJ, Barber JE, Klatka KM, Houghtaling PL, Vesely I, Moravec CS, McCarthy PM. Mitral valve stiffening in end-stage heart failure: evidence of an organic contribution to functional mitral regurgitation. J Thorac Cardiovasc Surg. 2005a;130(3):783–90.

Grande-Allen KJ, Borowski AG, Troughton RW, Houghtaling PL, Dipaola NR, Moravec CS, Vesely I, Griffin BP. Apparently normal mitral valves in patients with heart failure demonstrate biochemical and structural derangements: an extracellular matrix and echocardiographic study. J Am Coll Cardiol. 2005b; 45(1):54–61.

Grashow JS, Yoganathan AP, Sacks MS. Biaixal stress-stretch behavior of the mitral valve anterior leaflet at physiologic strain rates. Ann Biomed Eng. 2006a;34(2):315–25.

Grashow JS, Sacks MS, Liao J, Yoganathan AP. Planar biaxial creep and stress relaxation of the mitral valve anterior leaflet. Ann Biomed Eng. 2006b;34(10):1509–18.

Gupta V, Werdenberg JA, Lawrence BD, Mendez JS, Stephens EH, Grande-Allen KJ. Reversible secretion of glycosaminoglycans and proteoglycans by cyclically stretched valvular cells in 3D culture. Ann Biomed Eng. 2008;36(7):1092–103.

Gupta V, Barzilla JE, Mendez JS, Stephens EH, Lee EL, Collard CD, Laucirica R, Weigel PH, Grande-Allen KJ. Abundance and location of proteoglycans and hyaluronan within normal and myxomatous mitral valves. Cardiovasc Pathol. 2009a;18(4):191–7.

Gupta V, Tseng H, Lawrence BD, Grande-Allen KJ. Effect of cyclic mechanical strain on glycosaminoglycan and proteoglycan synthesis by heart valve cells. Acta Biomater. 2009b;5(2):531–40.

Habashi JP, Judge DP, Holm TM, Cohn RD, Loeys BL, Cooper TK, Myers L, Klein EC, Liu G, Calvi C, Podowski M, Neptune ER, Halushka MK, Bedja D, Gabrielson K, Rifkin DB, Carta L, Ramirez F, Huso DL, Dietz HC. Losartan, an AT1 antagonist, prevents aortic aneurysm in a mouse model of Marfan syndrome. Science. 2006;312(5770):117–21.

He S, Lemmon Jr JD, Weston MW, Jensen MO, Levine RA, Yoganathan AP. Mitral valve compensation for annular dilatation: in vitro study into the mechanisms of functional mitral regurgitation with an adjustable annulus model. J Heart Valve Dis. 1999;8(3):294–302.

He Z, Sacks MS, Baijens L, Wanant S, Shah P, Yoganathan AP. Effects of papillary muscle position on in-vitro dynamic strain on the porcine mitral valve. J Heart Valve Dis. 2003;12(4):488–94.

Jimenez JH, Soerensen DD, He Z, He S, Yoganathan AP. Effects of a saddle shaped annulus on mitral valve function and chordal force distribution: an in vitro study. Ann Biomed Eng. 2003;31(10):1171–81.

Kunzelman KS, Cochran RP. Stress/strain characteristics of porcine mitral valve tissue: parallel versus perpendicular collagen orientation. J Card Surg. 1992;7(1):71–8.

Kunzelman KS, Cochran RP, Murphree SS, Ring WS, Verrier ED, Eberhart RC. Differential collagen distribution in the mitral valve and its influence on biomechanical behaviour. J Heart Valve Dis. 1993;2(2):236–44.

Kunzelman KS, Quick DW, Cochran RP. Altered collagen concentration in mitral valve leaflets: biochemical and finite element analysis. Ann Thorac Surg. 1998;66(6 Suppl):S198–205.

Kyndt F, Gueffet JP, Probst V, Jaafar P, Legendre A, Le Bouffant F, Toquet C, Roy E, McGregor L, Lynch SA, Newbury-Ecob R, Tran V, Young I, Trochu JN, Le Marec H, Schott JJ. Mutations in the gene encoding filamin A as a cause for familial cardiac valvular dystrophy. Circulation. 2007;115(1):40–9.

Lester WM, Gotlieb AI. In vitro repair of the wounded porcine mitral valve. Circ Res. 1988;62(4):833–45.

Levine RA, Hung J, Otsuji Y, Messas E, Liel-Cohen N, Nathan N, Handschumacher MD, Guerrero JL, He S, Yoganathan AP, Vlahakes GJ. Mechanistic insights into functional mitral regurgitation. Curr Cardiol Rep. 2002;4(2):125–9.

Liao J, Yang L, Grashow J, Sacks MS. The relation between collagen fibril kinematics and mechanical properties in the mitral valve anterior leaflet. J Biomech Eng. 2007;129(1):78–87.

Liu AC, Gotlieb AI. Transforming growth factor-beta regulates in vitro heart valve repair by activated valve interstitial cells. Am J Pathol. 2008;173(5):1275–85.

Loeys BL, Chen J, Neptune ER, Judge DP, Podowski M, Holm T, Meyers J, Leitch CC, Katsanis N, Sharifi N, Xu FL, Myers LA, Spevak PJ, Cameron DE, De Backer J, Hellemans J, Chen Y, Davis EC, Webb CL, Kress W, Coucke P, Rifkin DB, De Paepe AM, Dietz HC. A syndrome of altered cardiovascular, craniofacial, neurocognitive and skeletal development caused by mutations in TGFBR1 or TGFBR2. Nat Genet. 2005;37(3):275–81.

Makkena B, Salti H, Subramaniam M, Thennapan S, Bonow RH, Caira F, Bonow RO, Spelsberg TC, Rajamannan NM. Atorvastatin decreases cellular proliferation and bone matrix expression in the hypercholesterolemic mitral valve. J Am Coll Cardiol. 2005;45(4):631–3.

Markwald RR, Norris RA, Moreno-Rodriguez R, Levine RA. Developmental basis of adult cardiovascular diseases: valvular heart diseases. Ann N Y Acad Sci. 2010;1188:177–83.

May-Newman K, Yin FC. Biaxial mechanical behavior of excised porcine mitral valve leaflets. Am J Physiol. 1995;269(4 Pt 2):H1319–27.

Neptune ER, Frischmeyer PA, Arking DE, Myers L, Bunton TE, Gayraud B, Ramirez F, Sakai LY, Dietz HC. Dysregulation of TGF-beta activation contributes to pathogenesis in Marfan syndrome. Nat Genet. 2003;33(3):407–11.

Ng CM, Cheng A, Myers LA, Martinez-Murillo F, Jie C, Bedja D, Gabrielson KL, Hausladen JM, Mecham RP, Judge DP, Dietz HC. TGF-beta-dependent pathogenesis of mitral valve prolapse in a mouse model of Marfan syndrome. J Clin Invest. 2004;114(11):1586–92.

Nguyen TC, Itoh A, Carlhall CJ, Bothe W, Timek TA, Ennis DB, Oakes RA, Liang D, Daughters GT, Ingels Jr NB, Miller DC. The effect of pure mitral regurgitation on mitral annular geometry and three-dimensional saddle shape. J Thorac Cardiovasc Surg. 2008;136(3):557–65.

Nielsen SL, Nygaard H, Fontaine AA, Hasenkam JM, He S, Andersen NT, Yoganathan AP. Chordal force distribution determines systolic mitral leaflet configuration and severity of functional mitral regurgitation. J Am Coll Cardiol. 1999;33(3):843–53.

Norris RA, Moreno-Rodriguez R, Wessels A, Merot J, Bruneval P, Chester AH, Yacoub MH, Hagege A, Slaugenhaupt SA, Aikawa E, Schott JJ, Lardeux A, Harris BS, Williams LK, Richards A, Levine RA, Markwald RR. Expression of the familial cardiac valvular dystrophy gene, filamin-A, during heart morphogenesis. Dev Dyn. 2010;239(7):2118–27.

Pyeritz RE, Wappel MA. Mitral valve dysfunction in the Marfan syndrome. Clinical and echocardiographic study of prevalence and natural history. Am J Med. 1983;74(5):797–807.

Rabkin E, Aikawa M, Stone JR, Fukumoto Y, Libby P, Schoen FJ. Activated interstitial myofibroblasts express catabolic enzymes and mediate matrix remodeling in myxomatous heart valves. Circulation. 2001;104(21):2525–32.

Rabkin-Aikawa E, Farber M, Aikawa M, Schoen FJ. Dynamic and reversible changes of interstitial cell phenotype during remodeling of cardiac valves. J Heart Valve Dis. 2004;13(5):841–7.

Ranganathan N, Lam J, Wigle E, Silver M. Morphology of the human mitral valve. II. The valve leaflets. Circulation. 1970;41:459–67.

Ryan LP, Jackson BM, Parish LM, Plappert TJ, St John-Sutton MG, Gorman 3rd JH, Gorman RC. Regional and global patterns of annular remodeling in ischemic mitral regurgitation. Ann Thorac Surg. 2007;84(2):553–9.

Sacks MS, Enomoto Y, Graybill JR, Merryman WD, Zeeshan A, Yoganathan AP, Levy RJ, Gorman RC, Gorman 3rd JH. In-vivo dynamic deformation of the mitral valve anterior leaflet. Ann Thorac Surg. 2006;82(4):1369–77.

Schoen FJ. Evolving concepts of cardiac valve dynamics: the continuum of development, functional structure, pathobiology, and tissue engineering. Circulation. 2008;118(18):1864–80.

Smolens IA, Pagani FD, Bolling SF. Mitral valve repair in heart failure. Eur J Heart Fail. 2000;2(4):365–71.

Stephens EH, Nguyen TC, Itoh A, Ingels Jr NB, Miller DC, Grande-Allen KJ. The effects of mitral regurgitation alone are sufficient for leaflet remodeling. Circulation. 2008;118(14 Suppl):S243–9.

Stephens EH, Timek TA, Daughters GT, Kuo JJ, Patton AM, Baggett LS, Ingels NB, Miller DC, Grande-Allen KJ. Significant changes in mitral valve leaflet matrix composition and turnover with tachycardia-induced cardiomyopathy. Circulation. 2009;120(11 Suppl):S112–9.

Stephens EH, de Jonge N, McNeill MP, Durst CA, Grande-Allen KJ. Age-related changes in material behavior of porcine mitral and aortic valves and correlation to matrix composition. Tissue Eng Part A. 2010a;16(3):867–78.

Stephens EH, Durst CA, Swanson JC, Grande-Allen KJ, Ingels NB, Miller DC. Functional coupling of valvular interstitial cells and collagen via alpha2beta1 integrins in the mitral leaflet. Cell Mol Bioeng. 2010b;3(4):428–37.

Sun Y, Weber KT. RAS and connective tissue in the heart. Int J Biochem Cell Biol. 2003;35(6):919–31.

Tamura K, Jones M, Yamada I, Ferrans VJ. Wound healing in the mitral valve. J Heart Valve Dis. 2000;9(1):53–63.

Tibayan FA, Lai DT, Timek TA, Dagum P, Liang D, Zasio MK, Daughters GT, Miller DC, Ingels Jr NB. Alterations in left ventricular curvature and principal strains in dilated cardiomyopathy with functional mitral regurgitation. J Heart Valve Dis. 2003;12(3):292–9.

Timek TA, Dagum P, Lai DT, Liang D, Daughters GT, Ingels Jr NB, Miller DC. Pathogenesis of mitral regurgitation in tachycardia-induced cardiomyopathy. Circulation. 2001;104(12 Suppl 1):I47–53.

Tsutsui H, Spinale FG, Nagatsu M, Schmid PG, Ishihara K, DeFreyte G, Cooper Gt, Carabello BA. Effects of chronic beta-adrenergic blockade on the left ventricular and cardiocyte abnormalities of chronic canine mitral regurgitation. J Clin Invest. 1994;93(6):2639–48.

van de Laar IM, Oldenburg RA, Pals G, Roos-Hesselink JW, de Graaf BM, Verhagen JM, Hoedemaekers YM, Willemsen R, Severijnen LA, Venselaar H, Vriend G, Pattynama PM, Collee M, Majoor-Krakauer D, Poldermans D, Frohn-Mulder IM, Micha D, Timmermans J, Hilhorst-Hofstee Y, Bierma-Zeinstra SM, Willems PJ, Kros JM, Oei EH, Oostra BA, Wessels MW, Bertoli-Avella AM. Mutations in SMAD3 cause a syndromic form of aortic aneurysms and dissections with early-onset osteoarthritis. Nat Genet. 2011;43(2):121–6.

Walker GA, Masters KS, Shah DN, Anseth KS, Leinwand LA. Valvular myofibroblast activation by transforming growth factor-beta: implications for pathological extracellular matrix remodeling in heart valve disease. Circ Res. 2004;95(3):253–60.

Wylie-Sears J, Aikawa E, Levine RA, Yang JH, Bischoff J. Mitral valve endothelial cells with osteogenic differentiation potential. Arterioscler Thromb Vasc Biol. 2011;31(3):598–607.

Yamazaki T, Lee JD, Shimizu H, Uzui H, Ueda T. Circulating matrix metalloproteinase-2 is elevated in patients with congestive heart failure. Eur J Heart Fail. 2004;6(1):41–5.

Zeng Z, Nievelstein-Post P, Yin Y, Jan KM, Frank JS, Rumschitzki DS. Macromolecular transport in heart valves. III. Experiment and theory for the size distribution of extracellular liposomes in hyperlipidemic rabbits. Am J Physiol Heart Circ Physiol. 2007;292(6):H2687–97.

Mitral Valve Devices

18

M.J. Swaans and J.A.S. van der Heyden

Introduction

Mitral valve regurgitation (MR) is an important clinical issue as MR represents >30% of native valve diseases (Enriquez-Sarano et al. 2009). Patients with symptomatic MR not only experience a low quality of life, but also have a poor prognosis with a 5% annual mortality rate in the absence of surgery (Alvarez et al. 1996; Mirabel et al. 2007). Optimal medical management can improve symptoms of heart failure but does not affect survival (Carabello 2008). Therefore, surgery is recommended by the current guidelines for patients with symptomatic severe MR or asymptomatic severe MR with evidence of left ventricular (LV) dysfunction or dilatation (Bonow et al. 2008; Vahanian et al. 2007). Studies have shown that despite a severe MR and symptoms up to 50% of the patients are not considered to be eligible for surgery. Reasons for denying surgery include impaired left ventricular ejection fraction, a high operative risk, multiple comorbidities or advanced age (Mirabel et al. 2007). When surgery is performed, mitral valve repair, rather than replacement, has become the preferred surgical treatment for severe MR since mitral valve repair has improves patients outcome, preserves the left ventricular function and eliminates the need for chronic anticoagulation therapy. However the benefit of repair over replacement in patients with a functional MR is less certain (Enriquez-Sarano et al. 1995; Gillinov et al. 2001).

The fact that a significant proportion of patients with a symptomatic MR is considered not suitable for surgery has led to the desire to develop less invasive treatment options to avoid cardiopulmonary bypass. This has driven to the development of transcatheter techniques that mimic surgical approaches. The target of these novel transcatheter techniques is to provide results similar to those of conventional surgery in terms of efficacy, safety, and durability, but with a lower periprocedural risk for the patient. Over the last years various technologies have emerged and are at different stages of investigation. The large amount of devices is due to the fact that the mitral valve apparatus is a complex structure. The mitral valve apparatus consists of the mitral annulus, anterior and posterior leaflets, chordae tendineae, the left atrium, the left ventricle and the papillary muscles (Fig. 18.1). Mitral regurgitation may occur when a disease affects one of more of these components (Otto 2001). The percutaneous devices can be classified according to their mechanism of action on the mitral valve apparatus components (Chiam and Ruiz 2011). This chapter provides an overview of these emerging approaches of transcatheter valve repair/implantation procedures.

M.J. Swaans, M.D. (✉) • J.A.S. van der Heyden, M.D., PhD.
Department of Cardiology, St. Antonius Hospital,
Koekoekslaan, Nieuwegein, The Netherlands
e-mail: m.swaans@antoniusziekenhuis.nl

N.M. Rajamannan (ed.), *Cardiac Valvular Medicine*,
DOI 10.1007/978-1-4471-4132-7_18, © Springer-Verlag London 2013

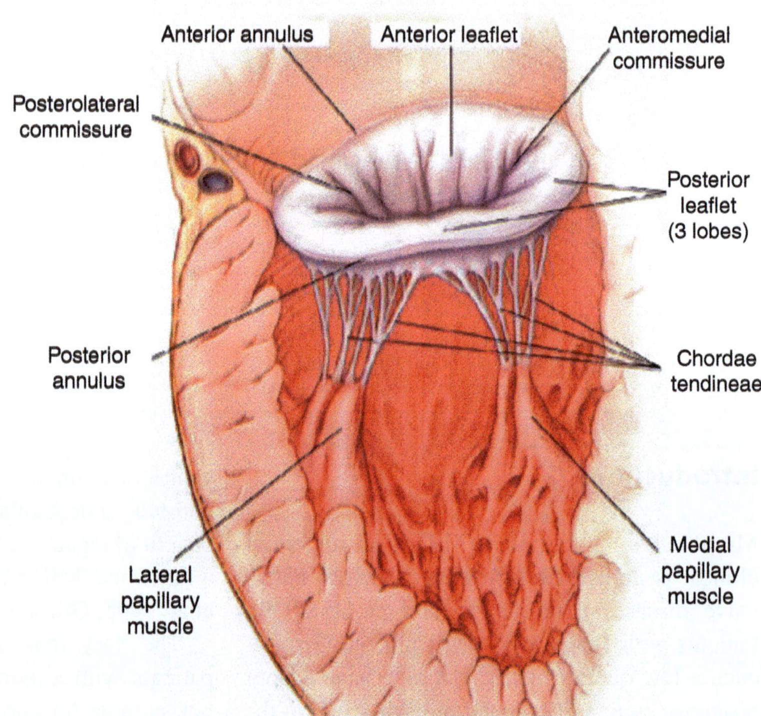

Fig. 18.1 Anatomy of the mitral valve (From Otto CM: Clinical practice. Evaluation and management of chronic mitral regurgutation. N Engl J Med. 2001 Sep 6;345(10): 740-6, with permission.)

Leaflets

Edge-to-Edge Leaflet Repair

Principle

The transcatheter edge-to-edge MV repair mimics a simple surgical technique for mitral valve repair introduced by Alfieri in 1991. It involves the placement of a surgical suture in the mid portion of the anterior en posterior leaflets, creating a double-orifice mitral valve that is not stenotic and effectively reduces MR. This technique ensures a fixed area of coaptation during systole, without disturbing the subvalvular and annular function, preserving left ventricular function (Alfieri et al. 2001; Maisano et al. 1998).

Mitraclip (Abbott Vascular, Santa Clara, California)

The Mitraclip system (Fig. 18.2a, e) uses a transseptal approach to deliver a steerable catheter into the left atrium. On this steerable catheter is a clip which is advanced into the LV and retracted during systole, grasping the MV leaflets, resulting in permanent leaflet approximation to create a double-orifice (Swaans et al. 2009). The EVEREST I study (Endovascular Valve Edge-to-Edge Repair) was the first to demonstrate the safety and feasibility of the MitraClip device (Feldman et al. 2009). The data of the EVEREST II trial have been recently published, providing the largest volume of evidence of the efficacy of this therapy (Feldman et al. 2011). Two hundred and seventy-nine patients were randomized in a 2:1 fashion to MitraClip (n = 184) or surgical repair (n = 95). The study showed an efficacy of 72.4% and 87.8% defined as freedom from mitral regurgitation >2+, freedom from cardiac surgery for valve dysfunction, and freedom from death at 12 months in the device and surgical group respectively, meeting the noninferiority hypothesis. The safety endpoint was superior in the device group, although mainly due to the higher amount of blood transfusions in the surgical group. It is important to note that, based on the results of the EVEREST I and II trials, the feasibility of surgical mitral valve repair in patients requiring mitral valve surgery after an attempt of MitraClip placement was 84%. This indicates that this procedure would not limit future options of surgical valve repair if needed (Feldman et al. 2011; Rogers et al. 2009a).

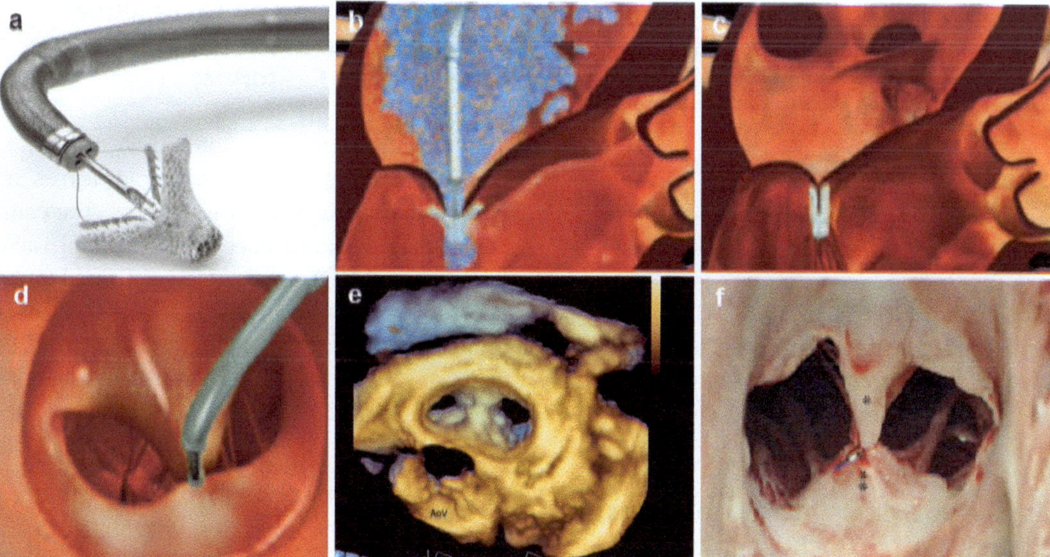

Fig. 18.2 Edge-to-Edge leaflet repair. (**a**) the Mitraclip device. (**b**) The mitraclip in the left ventricle at the site of the largest regurgitant jet before leaflet grasping (**c**) the mitraclip after grasping the leaflets and deployment from the delivery catheter. (**d**) the double orifice created by the mitraclip after grasping the A2 and P2 segment of the mitral valve. (**e**) 3DTEE image of the mitral valve after placement of a Mitraclip showing the double orifice. (**f**) The double orifice after suturing the A2 and P2 segment of the mitral valve with the Mobius device (Single black asterisk represents the anterior mitral valve leaflet and double black asterisks represent posterior mitral valve leaflet). (Courtesy to Abbott Vascular, Santa Clara, California and from Swaans MJ, Van den Branden BJ, Van der Heyden JA, et al.: Three-dimensional transoesophageal echocardiography in a patient undergoing percutaneous mitral valve repair using the edge-to-edge clip technique. Eur J Echocardiogr. 2009 Dec;10(8):982-3, with permission of Oxford University Press and Naqvi TZ, Buchbinder M, Zarbatany D et al.: Beating-heart percutaneous mitral valve repair using a transcatheter endovascular suturing device in an animal model. Catheter Cardiovasc Interv. 2007 Mar 1;69(4):525-31, with permission of John Wiley and Sons.)

Mitraflex (TransCardiac Therpeutics, Atlanta, Georgia)

This mitral valve repair system is designed for direct thoracoscopic approach to deliver a clip (and if necessary an artificial chordae tendineae) through the apex of a beating heart. This clip captures and connects the mid portions of the leaflets creating a double-orifice. This device is in the pre-clinical testing phase.

Mobius (Edwards Life Sciences, Irving, California)

This device used a transseptal puncture to deliver a catheter across the mitral orifice. Suction through this catheter lumen was used to pull the edge of the anterior or posterior mitral leaflet against the catheter, and a needle and suture were passed through the leaflet. The device then was then rotated, and the procedure was repeated against the other mitral leaflet, with tensioning and cutting of the suture to maintain the edge-to-edge approximation (Fig. 18.2f). Feasibility was shown in an animal study, but the program was abandoned due to technical difficulties and suture dehiscence in the initial human experience (Maisano et al. 2009; Naqvi et al. 2007).

Limitations

Major limitation of this technique is that most patients treated with the surgical "Alfieri-stitch" also needed an annuloplasty. The surgical literature suggests that the absence of a ring is associated with suboptimal results and the frequent need for reoperation in patients with more severe MR, especially in patients with a functional MR (Bhudia et al. 2004; Maisano et al. 2003). Although the tissue overgrowth and the formation of fibrous tissue bridge over time which prevents annular dilatation may mimic the effects of an annuloplasty with the Mitraclip system

(Ladich et al. 2011). Another limitation is the possibility of causing an iatrogenic mitral stenosis (MS).

Space Occupier

Principle

An implant acting like a "buoy" is positioned across the MV orifice will provide a sealing surface for the leaflets of the mitral valve, thereby reducing or eliminating MR.

Percu-Pro System (Cardiosolutions, Stoughton, Massachusetts)

The Percu-Pro device consists of a polyurethane-silicone polymer space-occupying buoy that is anchored at the apex through the mitral valve, acting as a spacer in the mitral orifice. A transseptal or transapical approach is required to implant the anchor in the apex. The device does not alter the mitral valve in any way that would preclude a patient from having open valve repair or replacement surgery at a future time. It is undergoing phase 1 trial.

Limitations

Possible limitations of this device are that the restricted ventricular inflow may cause iatrogenic MS, Further limitations are the possibility of thrombus formation on the device and the inability to treat residual MR.

Leaflet Ablation

Principle

The application of radiofrequency energy to mitral valve leaflet(s) and their associated structures with an ablation catheter causes controlled damage that leads to fibrotic scarring and contracture of valve leaflets and surrounding structures in patients with degenerative MR.

Thermocool Irrigated Tip Ablation Catheter (Biosense Webster Inc., Diamond Bar, California)

This radiofrequency ablation (RFA) catheter is placed into the left ventricle retrograde across the aortic valve via femoral artery access. The catheter is placed into contact with the mitral valve leaflet(s), and RFA is selectively delivered to the leaflet(s) until structural (fibrosis) and/or functional (reduced motions) alterations are seen. A proof-of-concept study was performed in animals (Williams et al. 2008).

Limitations

This first limitation of this technique is that is can only be used in patients with degenerative MR. Secondly the chronic effects of RFA on the mitral valve leaflet(s) and their associated structures is unknown. Thirdly, the application of RFA might not be precise and leaflet perforation or damage to the adjacent cardiac structures might occur and finally, too-long or too-short application of RF-energy might result in residual or even worsening of MR.

Mitral Valve Annulus

The mainstay of surgical repair is annuloplasty, especially in patients with a functional MR. Annular dilatation due to dilatation of the left ventricle and geometric distortion of the mitral apparatus is the mechanism of MR in this group of patients. The devices in this paragraph mimic the surgical annuloplasty without the need for cardiopulmonary bypass.

Indirect Annuloplasty: Coronary Sinus Approach

Principle

The coronary sinus (CS) runs from the lateral LV wall medially to the right atrium. This approach uses the fact that the coronary sinus encircles about

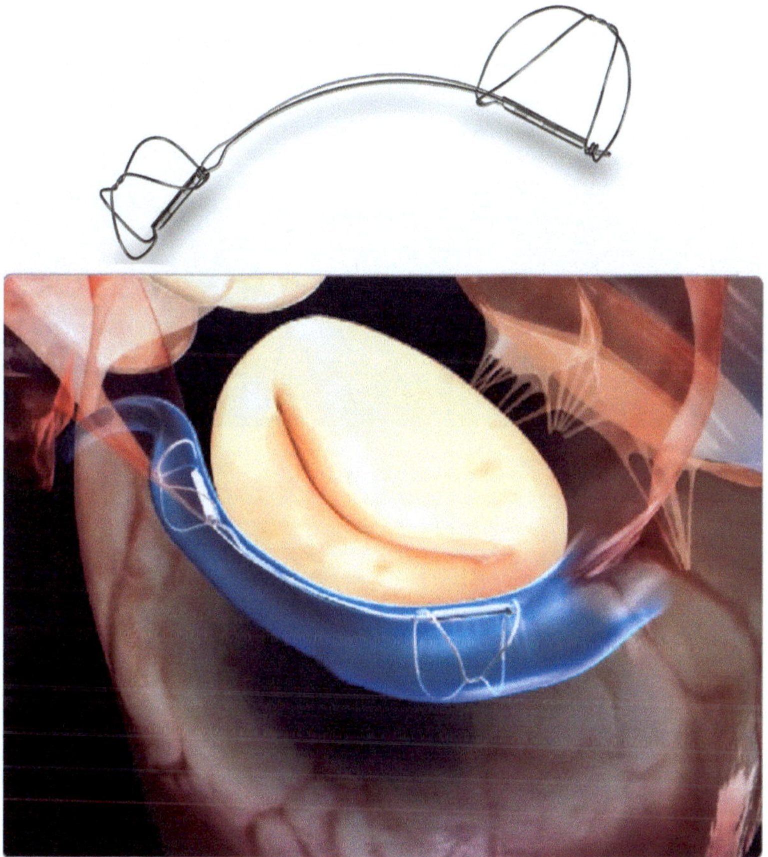

Fig. 18.3 The CARILLON Mitral Contour System is a fixed length, double-anchor, nitinol device designed to be positioned within the coronary sinus/great cardiac vein to reduce functional mitral valve regurgitation. The arc of the nitinol ribbon, which connects the 2 anchors, serves to orient the device automatically during deployment. (Courtesy to Cardiac Dimension Inc., Kirkland, Washington.)

two-thirds of the mitral annulus and its course is roughly parallel to the posterior mitral annulus. The devices in this approach are placed in the CS which creates tension or a constricting force transmitted to the MV and the mitral annulus, pushing the posterior annulus anteriorly with a reduction of the septal-lateral (anterior posterior) dimension and ideally have improved coaptation of the posterior and anterior mitral valve leaflets as a result. Several approaches to the coronary sinus annuloplasty have been developed and are in clinical testing.

Carillon Mitral Contour System (Cardiac Dimension Inc., Kirkland, Washington)

The implant consists of two self-expendable anchors made of nitinol loops that are connected by a nitinol bridge and is placed in the great cardiac vein and proximal CS via a catheter-based system (Fig. 18.3). After the distal anchor is deployed, tension is applied via the delivery system until a satisfactory acute effect is demonstrated. The proximal anchor is then deployed and locked in the proximal coronary sinus. The first generation of the device was challenged by difficulty in anchoring. This problem was rapidly corrected with improvements in engineering, and some first-in-human experience has been successfully achieved. The AMADEUS (Carillon Mitral Annuloplasty Device European Union Study)-trial, a multicentre human safety and feasibility study including 48 patients was completed. Successful device implantation was achieved in 60% of the patients (30/48). In 18 patients implantation could not be achieved due

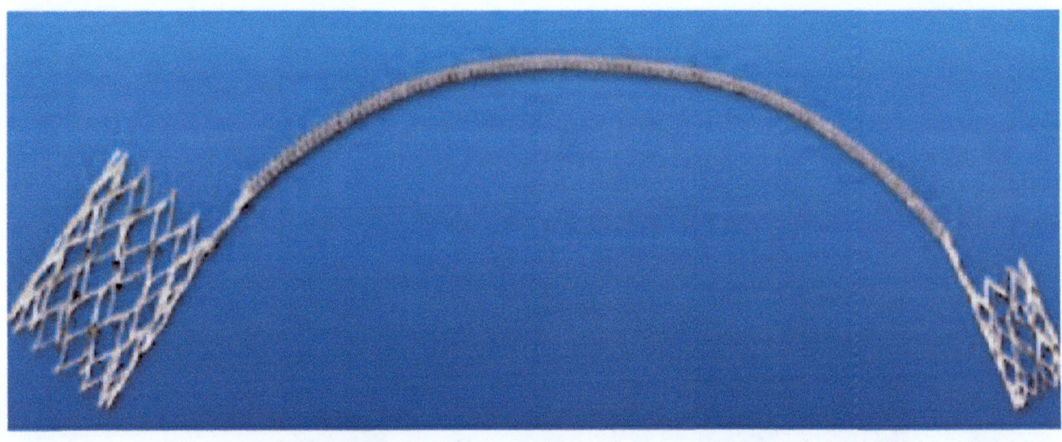

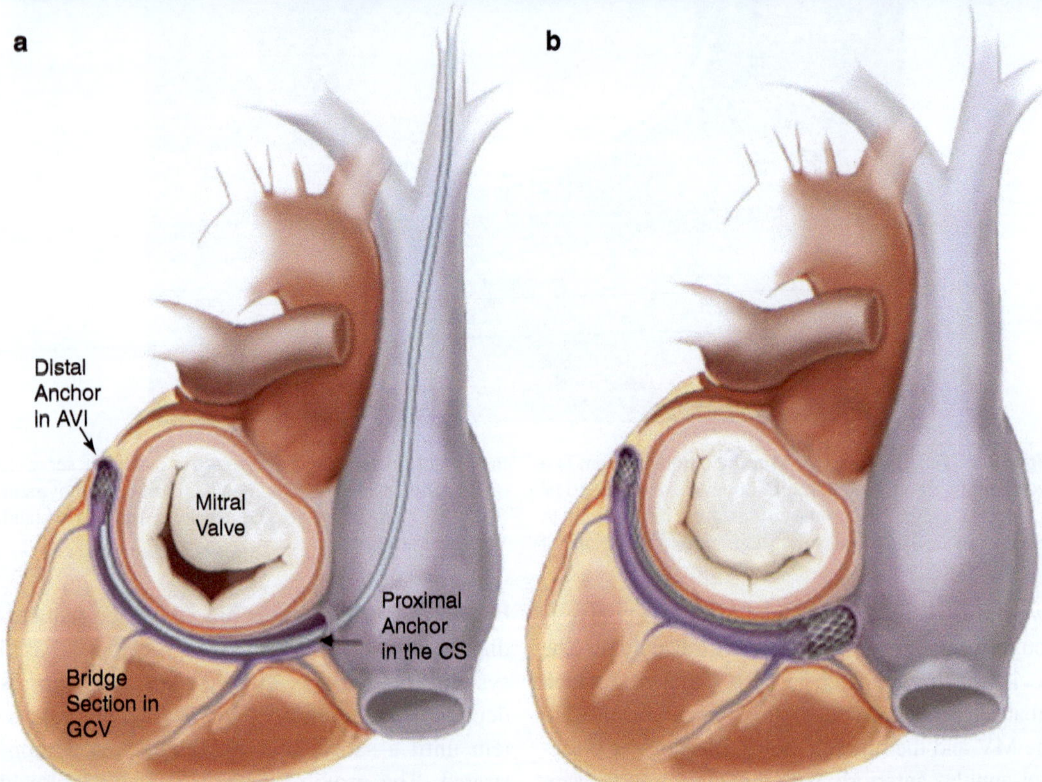

Fig. 18.4 The Monarc device. The Monarc device encircles the posterior leaflet of the mitral valve in systole at implant (**a**) and in its activated state (**b**). The small distal anchor is positioned in the anterior interventricular vein, the springlike bridge section is positioned in the great cardiac vein, and the large proximal anchor is positioned in the ostium of the coronary sinus. The bridge section shortens during the first month after implantation. The putative mechanism of action is a reduction of the septal-lateral diameter of the mitral annulus with improved coaptation of the leaflets and a reduction in mitral regurgitation. AIV = anterior interventricular vein; CS = coronary sinus; GCV = great cardiac vein. (From Harnek J, Webb JG, Kuck KH, et al.: Transcatheter implantation of the MONARC coronary sinus device for mitral regurgitation: 1-year results from the EVOLUTION phase I study (Clinical Evaluation of the Edwards Lifesciences Percutaneous Mitral Annuloplasty System for the Treatment of Mitral Regurgitation). J Am Coll Cardiol Intv 2011;4:115-122, with permission of Elsevier.)

to access issues (CS dissection/perforation), insufficient MR reduction, and coronary artery compression. The major adverse event rate was not trivial, with seven events (13%) at 30 days in 48 patients. There was a statistically significant reduction in severity of mitral regurgitation at 6 months with an increase in 6 min walk distance (Schofer et al. 2009).

Monarc (Viking) System (Edwards Lifesciences, Irving, California)

The device consists of a distal self-expanding stent-like anchor, a spring-like bridge, and a proximal stent anchor (Fig. 18.4). The distal anchor is delivered into the anterior interventricular vein, and the proximal anchor is placed near the coronary sinus ostium. Thus, this device captures a greater part of the circumference of the mitral annulus than does the Carillon device. The bridge between the anchors has a biodegradable suture that acts as a temporary spacer to hold the spring open. The suture material dissolves over 3–4 weeks after implantation, and the bridge shortens and displaces the posterior annulus. The device was tested in the EVOLUTION (Clinical Evaluation of the Edwards Lifesciences Percutaneous Mitral Annuloplasty System for the Treatment of Mitral Regurgitation) trial, a multicenter feasibility and safety study performed in Europe and Canada. Of the 72 patients included in the study, 59 patients (82%) had the device implanted. Reasons for not implanting the device were tortuous anatomy or inappropriate coronary sinus dimension. Three myocardial infarctions occurred due to coronary compression. At 2 years follow-up, mitral regurgitation severity reduced in ≥1 grade in 54% of patients. Event-free survival was 81%, 72% and 64% at 1 year and 2 and 3 years, respectively. Despite these favorable preliminary results the development of this device has been stopped by the sponsor due to slow enrollment in the EVOLUTION II (Harnek et al. 2011).

Viacor Percutaneous Transvenous Mitral Annuloplasty (PTMA) System (Viacor Inc., Wilmington, Massachusetts)

The PTMA system includes three stiff stainless rods that are inserted into a multilumen catheter positioned in the CS. These stiff nitinol rods are passed through the lumens of the catheter to apply pressure to the central part of the posterior mitral leaflet and compress the septolateral dimension, rather than to encircle and constrict or cinch the mitral annulus. Rods of varying stiffness may be used. During the implant process, a sequence of rods may be placed through the lumens to determine the optimal amount of compression of the posterior annulus to result in a reduction in MR. The preliminary results of the PTOLEMY (Percutaneous TransvenOus Mitral AnnuloplastY) trial, involving 27 patients showed that temporary implantation of the PTMA devices was feasible. The diagnostic PTMA was effective in 13 patients, but only in 9 patients the PTMA implants were successfully placed. Four devices were removed uneventfully, 3 for annuloplasty surgery due to observed PTMA device migration and/or diminished efficacy. Although no procedure or device-related major adverse events with permanent sequela were observed further development of this device is also halted (Sack et al. 2009; Dubreuil et al. 2007).

Limitations

The coronary sinus approach has several limitations. Although this approach exploits the fact that the CS is located near the MA, but the coronary sinus is an atrial structure and is frequently not in the same plane as the mitral valve annulus (Fig. 18.5). The distance between the coronary sinus and the posterior mitral annulus increases with chronic ischemic MR because of structural chamber remodeling (Tops et al. 2007; Choure et al. 2006). Furthermore, the circumflex coronary

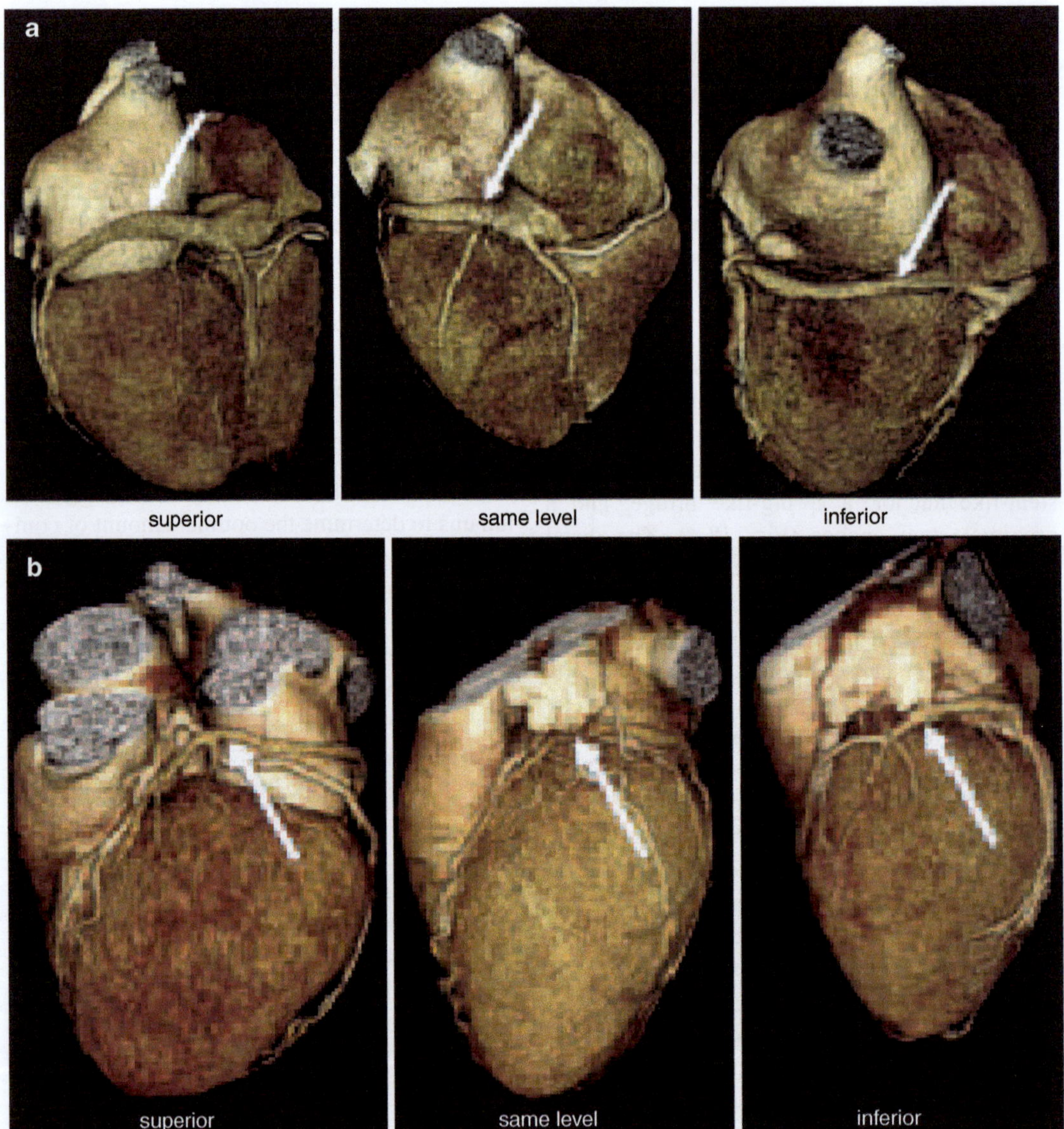

Fig. 18.5 Volume-rendered 3-dimensional reconstructions were used to assess the position of the coronary sinus (*white arrow*) in relation to the mitral valve annulus. At the proximal coronary sinus (**a**) and at the distal coronary sinus (**b**), the relative position (superior/same level/inferior) of the coronary sinus was determined. (From Tops LF, Van de Veire NR, Schuijf JD, et al.: Noninvasive evaluation of coronary sinus anatomy and its relation to the mitral valve annulus: implications for percutaneous mitral annuloplasty. Circulation. 2007 Mar 20;115(11):1426-32, with permission of Wolters Kluwer Health)

artery or its numerous branches may lie between the mitral annulus and the coronary sinus and might be compressed by the device (Fig. 18.6). Other limitations include severe annulus calcification, the risk of perforating the CS, difficulty or impossibility to place device with the presence of CS pacing leads and it might jeopardize future cardiac resynchronization devices.

Indirect Annuloplasty: Asymmetrical Approach

Principle

This approach uses also the proximity of the CS to the mitral valve annulus to try to reshape the annulus, but in addition exert traction force on

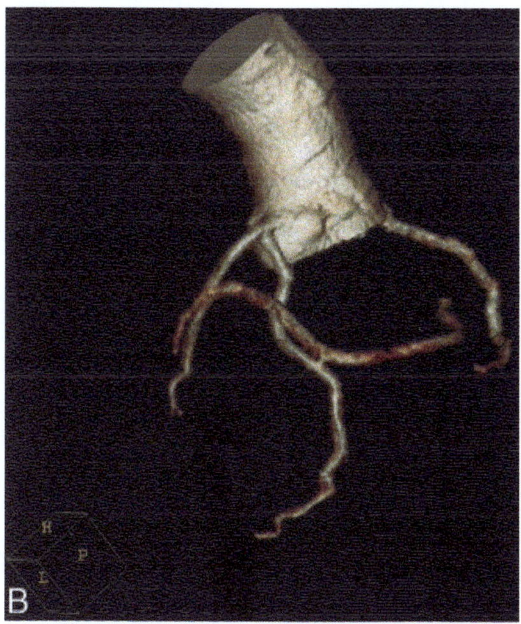

Fig. 18.6 Reconstructed 3-dimensional image showing the left circumflex coronary artery crossing "under (or deep to)" the coronary sinus. (From Choure AJ, Garcia MJ, Hesse B, et al.: In vivo analysis of the anatomical relationship of coronary sinus to mitral annulus and left circumflex coronary artery using cardiac multidetector computed tomography: implications for percutaneous coronary sinus mitral annuloplasty. J Am Coll Cardiol. 2006 Nov 21;48(10):1938-45, with permission of Elsevier.)

another part of the left or right atrium, resulting in asymmetrical forces. Hereby it reduces the anterior-posterior (septal-lateral) dimension of the mitral valve annulus to improve leaflet coaptation and reducing MR.

Percutaneous Septal Sinus Shortening (PS3) System (Ample Medical, Foster City, California)

This atrium based device creates a transatrial bridge. A T-shaped anchor is first placed in the CS behind the posterior leaflet and a tether is placed across the left atrium and through an atrial septal anchor (Amplatzer PFO occluder [AGA Medical, Plymouth, Minnesota]). This tether is then shortened, thereby pulling the posterior annulus toward the interatrial septum with shortening of the septal-lateral dimension of the mitral valve and reducing MR (Figs. 18.7 and 18.8). Although an animal study showed long-term durability and safety with a significant decreased septal-lateral diameter and MR reduction further device development was stopped (Palacios et al. 2007; Rogers et al. 2009b).

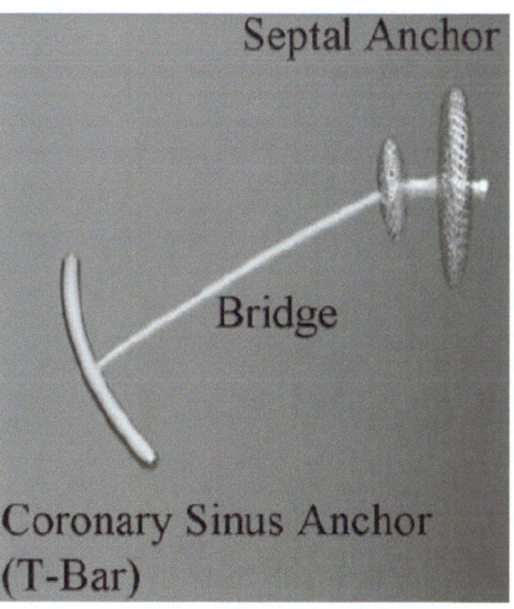

Fig. 18.7 The Percutaneous Septal Sinus Shortening (PS3) Device. The device consists of an atrial septal occluder device and T-bar element that act as anchors in the interatrial septum and coronary sinus, respectively. (From Piazza N, Asgar A, Ibrahim R, et al.: Transcatheter mitral and pulmonary valve therapy. J Am Coll Cardiol. 2009 May 19;53(20):1837-51, with permission of Elsevier.)

National Institutes of Health (NIH) Cerclage

For this technique a guidewire loop is created around the mitral annulus and left ventricular outflow tract, and then exchanged for a suture. The guidewire traverses the coronary sinus and the proximal great cardiac vein into the first septal perforator vein towards the basal interventricular septum. It is then directed across a short segment of myocardium to re-enter a right heart chamber where it is ensnared and exchanged for a suture and tension-fixation device (Fig. 18.9). An initial animal study showed promising results in reducing the MR acutely (Kim et al. 2009).

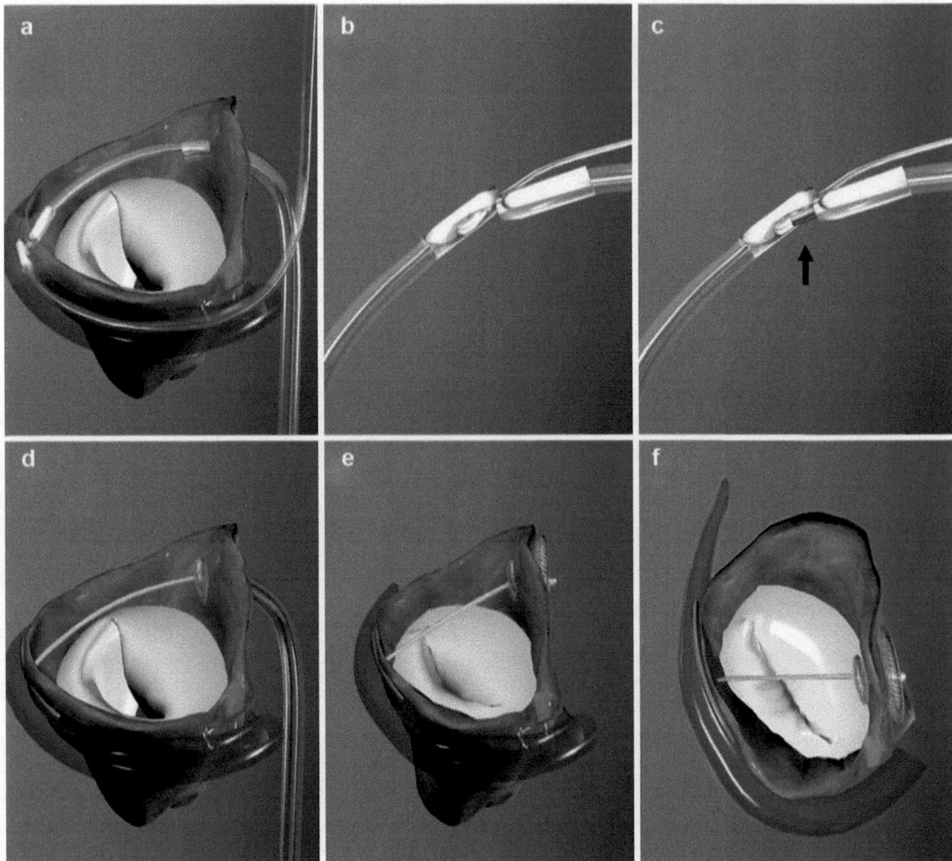

Fig. 18.8 The PS3 system implantation procedure. (**a**) Great cardiac vein (GCV) and LA MagneCaths in position and magnetically linked. (**b**) Close-up of magnetically linked LA and GCV MagneCaths. (**c**) Coring catheter (*arrow*) in position to allow passage of the loop glide wire from the LA to GCV (the loop wire allows the bridge element to be pulled back across the LA). (**d**) The PS3 system in place before tensioning. (**e**) Tensioning the bridge results in precise shortening and elimination of functional mitral valve regurgitation; the final position is secured with a suture lock. (**f**) Superior view of the PS3 system. Because the interatrial septal anchor passes through the fossa ovalis, the angle of the bridge element is ~20° to 30° posterior to a true anteroposterior orientation. (From Rogers JH, Macoviak JA, Rahdert DA, et al.: Percutaneous septal sinus shortening: a novel procedure for the treatment of functional mitral regurgitation. Circulation. 2006 May 16;113(19):2329-34, with permission of Wolters Kluwer Health.)

St. Jude Percutaneous Mitral Annuloplasty (PMVR) Device (St. Jude Medical, Minneapolis, Minnesota)

The PMVR device is designed to reduce the area of the valve annulus in a manner analogous to open surgical ring annuloplasty. The PMVR device consists of four helical anchors, two loading spacers, a tether rope, and a locking mechanism (Fig. 18.10). Using endovascular techniques, the implant system is delivered to the mitral annulus via the coronary sinus and right atrium. The distal pair of anchors is first implanted into the ventricular myocardium near the P2 segment of the mitral leaflet from the coronary sinus. The proximal pair of anchors subsequently is implanted near the posteromedial trigone at the coronary sinus from the right atrium. Between these two pairs of anchors, a connecting polyester tether is used to shorten the annular distance, thereby effecting favorable change in mitral annular geometry while lessening the risk of lateral coronary obstruction. Dynamic shortening of mitral annular distance can be performed manually and reversibly to ascertain the degree of reduction in regurgitation

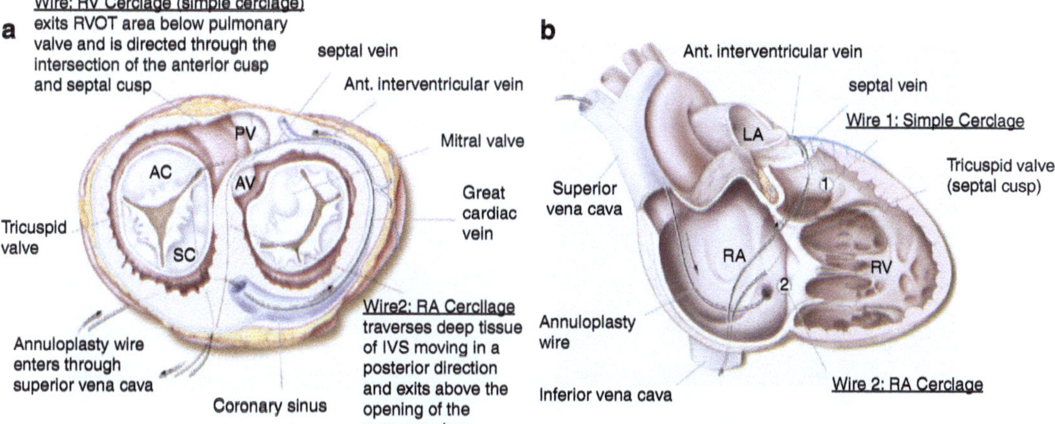

Fig. 18.9 Mitral cerclage annuloplasty. (**a**) shows the mitral annulus from the cardiac apex and (**b**) shows with the free walls of the right atrium and ventricle removed. A guidewire through the coronary sinus enters a basal septal perforator vein and traverses a short distance of septal myocardium. Wire 1 follows a right ventricular (RV) cerclage trajectory into the right ventricular outflow tract, and Wire 2 a longer trajectory to re-enter the right atrium directly. The guidewire is replaced with a suture, and tension is applied to both ends and fixed near the coronary sinus ostium. (From Kim JH, Kocaturk O, Ozturk C, et al.: Mitral cerclage annuloplasty, a novel transcatheter treatment for secondary mitral valve regurgitation: initial results in swine. J Am Coll Cardiol. 2009 Aug 11;54(7):638-51, with permission of Elsevier)

and untoward effects on the coronary sinus or adjacent coronary arteries. The final locking mechanism of the PMVR device is a self-retracting, nitinol structure that maintains the cinched load (Sorajja et al. 2008).

Limitations

There is little clinical experience with these devices and like with the indirect annuloplasty with the coronary sinus approach the CS might not be in the same plane as the mitral valve annulus which might reduce the effect of these techniques. The long term effects of the tension on the CS and left atrium are unknown. There is also a theoretical risk of device erosion of fracture and possible thrombus formation on the connecting cable. Further coronary compression, tricuspid dysfunction and entrapment of the conduction system are limitations of the NIH cerclage technique. Although for the coronary compression a rigid-arch protection device was created to displace compressive forces away from an entrapped coronary artery. This protection device is positioned over the cerclage suture where it crosses the coronary artery, identified by selective coronary arteriography.

Direct Annuloplasty

Principle

This group of devices reshapes the mitral annulus directly without using the CS and might overcome the limitations of the indirect annuloplasty devices. The annulus can be approached from the left atrium of left ventricle side. The technologies in this group have been developed in an effort to reproduce the effects of surgical mitral annuloplasty using suture-, anchor-, or (RF) energy-based circumferential reduction of the mitral annulus. Surgical closed-ring mitral annuloplasty is currently considered the gold standard for treating functional MR. Before the advent of open and closed rigid rings, suture-based annuloplasty, based on the prior work by Burr et al. had been used (1977). This technique has been shown to reduce the septal-lateral diameter in patients undergoing adjunctive annuloplasty in the setting of degenerative leaflet repair or repair of functional MR.

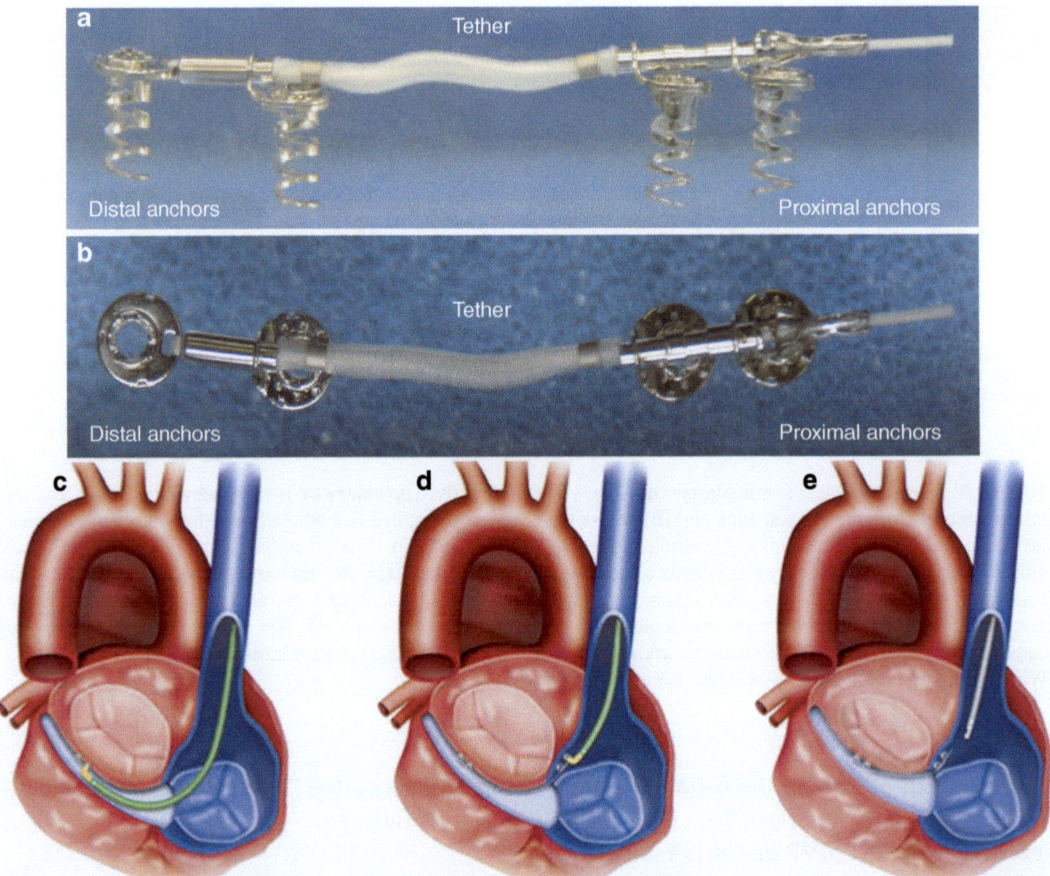

Fig. 18.10 The PMVR device. (**a**) Side view of PMVR device showing 4 helical stainless steel screw anchors connected by a biocompatible tether. (**b**) Top view of PMVR device. (**c**) The articulating guide catheter is used to implant 2 anchors near the P2 segment of the mitral valve. (**d**) Two anchors are then implanted into the posteromedial trigone. (**e**) The device is then cinched and released by a set of cutters. (From Sorajja P, Nishimura RA, Thompson J, et al.: A novel method of percutaneous mitral valve repair for ischemic mitral regurgitation. JACC Cardiovasc Interv. 2008 Dec;1(6):663-72, with permission of Elsevier)

Accucinch Ventriculoplasty System (Guided Delivery Systems, Santa Clara, California)

This device is focused on reducing the diameter of the base of the left ventricle to improve leaflet coaptation and improve left ventricular function. It uses a retrograde percutaneous femoral artery access to deliver a series of anchors in the subannular myocardium to directly modify the geometry of the mitral apparatus in order to reduce MR (Fig. 18.11). The LV RESTORE (A Study of Percutaneous Left Ventricular REShaping of Mitral Apparatus to Reduce FuncTiOnal Mitral REgurgitation and Improve LV Function Using the Accucinch® System) is ongoing.

Mitralign Percutaneous Annuloplasty (Mitralign, Tewksbury, Massachusetts)

This device mimics the focal/segmental surgical suture annuloplasty. The system consists of bident catheter delivering two pairs of surgical pledgets on the P1 and P3 site of the posterior annulus via a retrograde transaortal approach (Fig. 18.12). Radiofrequency wires are used to penetrate the mitral annulus and gain access to the left atrial side of the annulus. The pledgets of each pair are pulled together and locked from the ventricular site of the annulus with a small stainless steel lock, reducing the posterior annulus by approximately 15 mm.

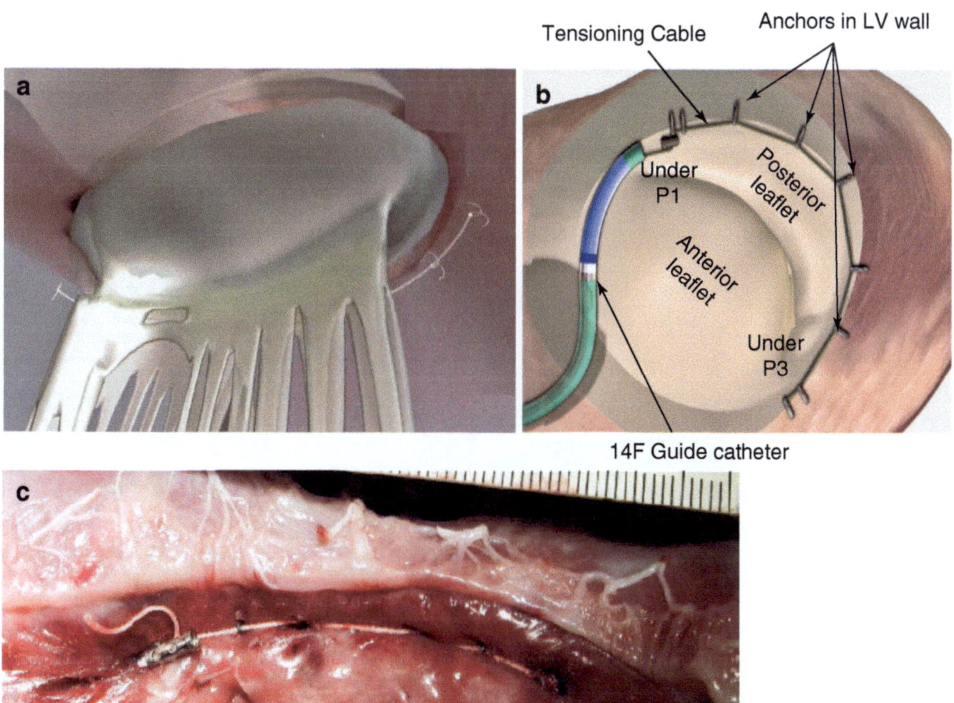

Fig. 18.11 Accucinch Ventriculoplasty System (**a**) and (**b**) Sub-valvular placement of anchors and a tensioning cable along the LV free wall via a retrograde trans-femoral approach. (**c**) Acute result in ovine study (leaflet and chordae resected). (Courtesy to Guided Delivery Systems, Santa Clara, California.)

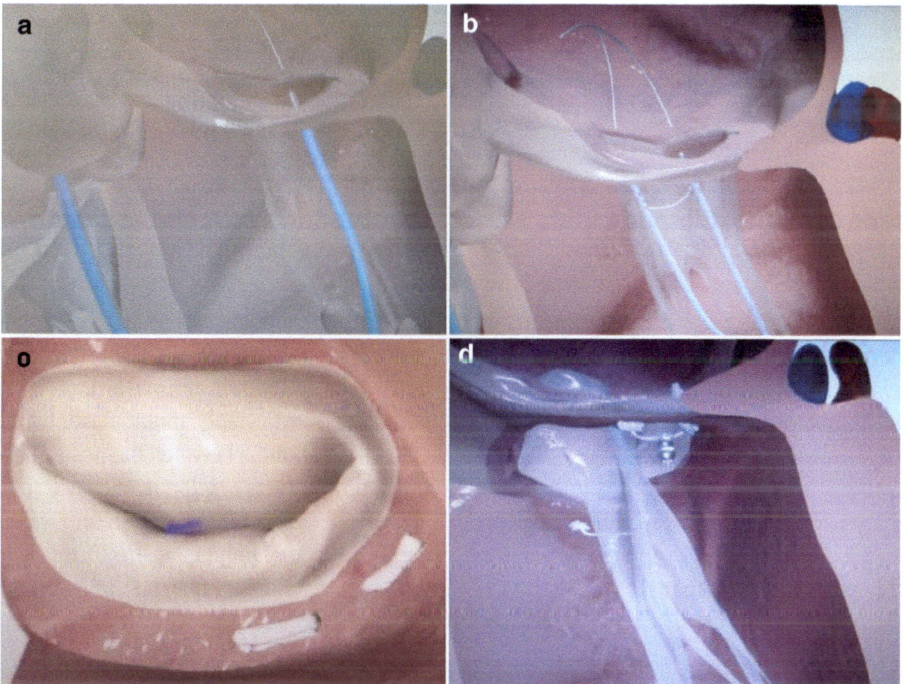

Fig. 18.12 Mitralign Percutaneous Annuloplasty (**a**) Wire crossing to left atrium by RF-energy (**b**) Placement of bident catheter and second wire delivery (**c**) Anchors are placed on the posterior mitral annulus and connected with a suture (**d**) Plication and lock at P1 and P3. (Courtesy to Mitralign, Tewksbury, Massachusetts.)

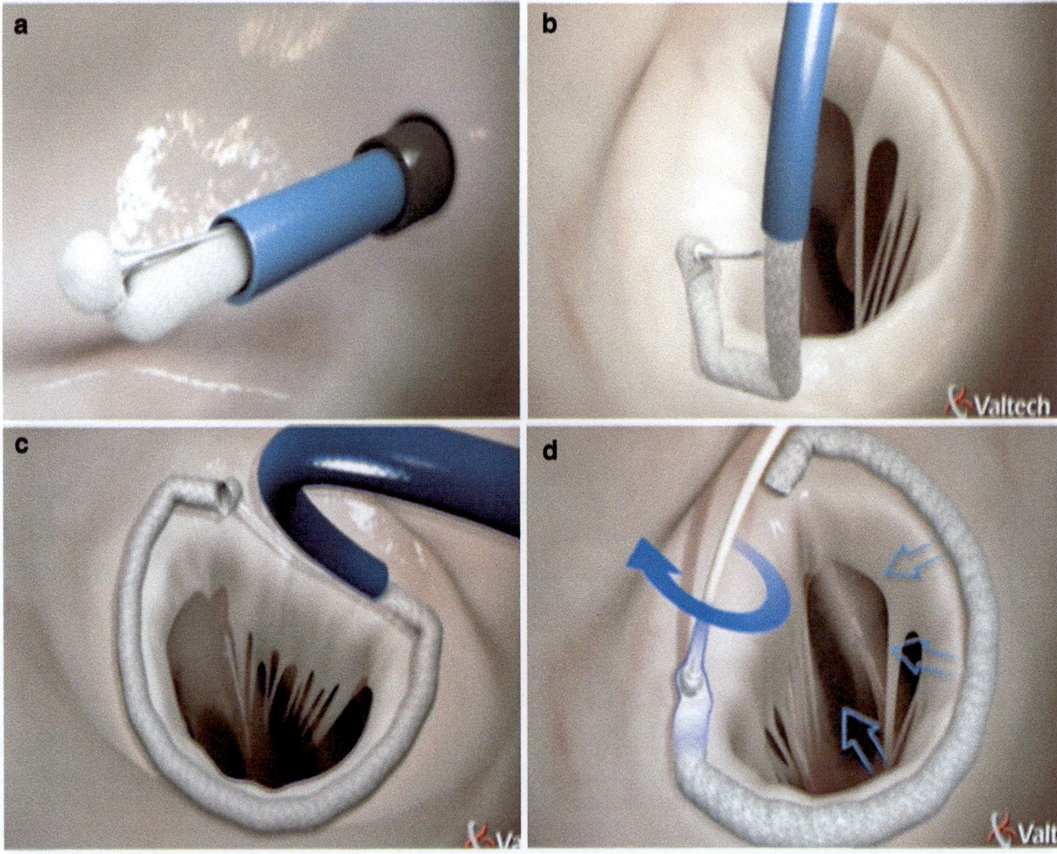

Fig. 18.13 The Valtech Cardioband. (**a**) A flexible catheter is introduced in the left atrium through a transseptal puncture. (**b**) and (**c**) an adjustable annuloplasty band is delivered to the annulus between the posterior and anterior commissures with helical fixation elements. (**d**) The annuloplasty ring is adjusted to reduce the intercommissural and septolateral dimension. (Courtesy to Valtech Cardio Ltd, Or Yehuda, Israel.)

Millepede System (Millepede LCC., Ann Arbor, Michigan)

This is a ring originally designed to treat tricuspid regurgitation and involves the placement of a novel self-expanding, self-centering annular ring with an unique attachment system via either minimally invasive surgical or percutaneous methods to restore the native mitral annular shape and diameter. The device is currently under preclinical development, is repositionable and retrievable prior to deployment.

Cardioband (Valtech Cardio Ltd, or Yehuda, Israel)

The Cardioband mimics a semi-circular surgical annuloplasty. Through a flexible catheter, that is introduced in the left atrium through a transseptal puncture, an adjustable annuloplasty band is delivered to the annulus between the posterior and anterior commissures, without the use of sutures. Helical fixation elements were systematically deployed in the annular wall (4.5 mm gaps) from the central lumen of the transcatheter band

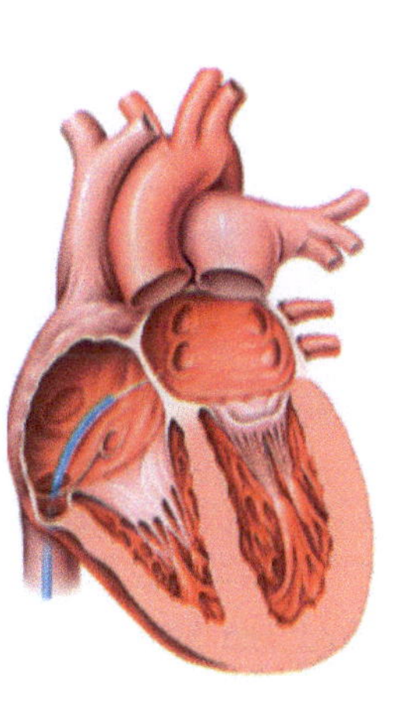
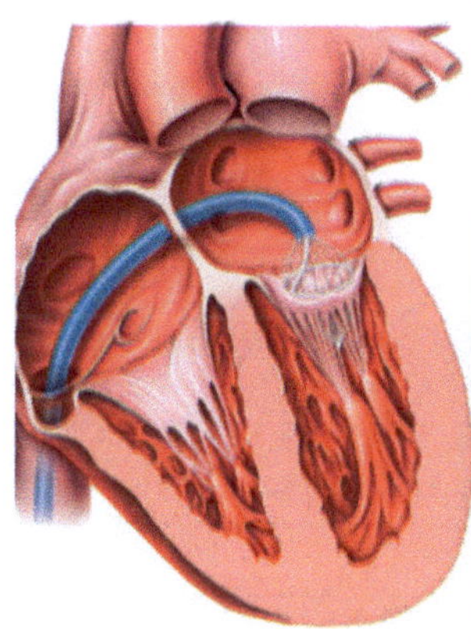
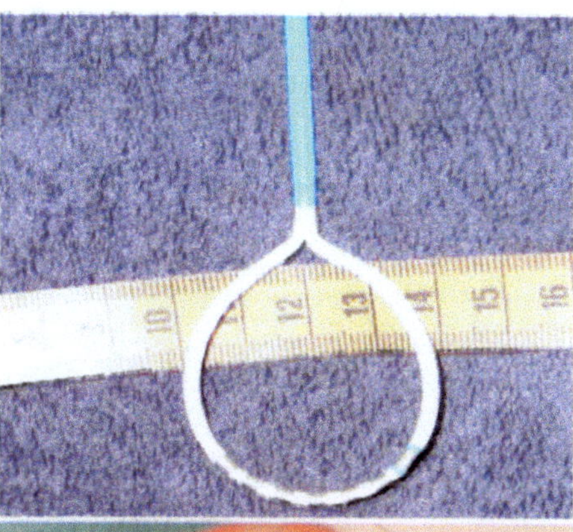

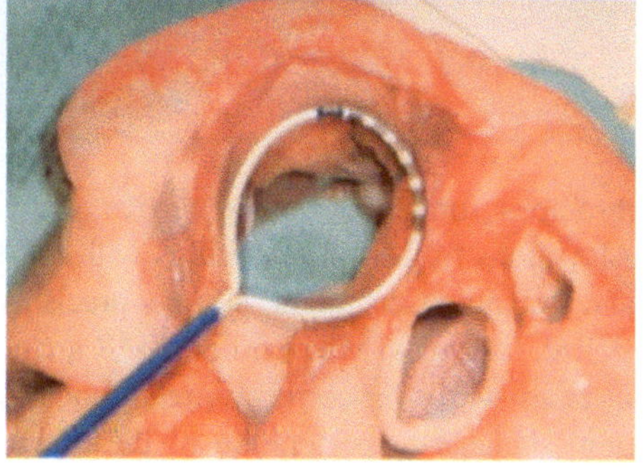

Fig. 18.14 The QuantumCor device (From Piazza N, Asgar A, Ibrahim R, et al.: Transcatheter mitral and pulmonary valve therapy. J Am Coll Cardiol. 2009 May 19;53(20):1837-51 , with permission of Elsevier.)

implantation tool (Fig. 18.13). Subsequent to implantation, the band length was adjusted on the beating heart to reduce the intercommissural and septolateral dimension. This technique is already surgically tested and animal studies are performed.

QuantumCor (QuantumCor, Lake Forrest, California)

Based on the concept of thermal remodeling of collagen. Because the mitral valve annulus has a high collagen content, catheter-based application of RF energy at subablative temperatures to the mitral annulus will heat and contract the collagen fibers, thereby reducing mitral annular circumference (Fig. 18.14). This technology has been proven to reduce mitral annular dimensions and MR in an animal model (Goel et al. 2009; Heuser et al. 2008).

ReCor (ReCor, Paris, France)

Ultrasonic energy is delivered by a steerable balloon catheter positioned via a transseptal puncture in the region of the posterior mitral valve annulus. Heating of the collagen causes shrinking and therefore reduction of the annulus and MR. The Saturn I (Safety and performance Assessment of Therapeutic Ultrasound for the treatment of mitral RegurgitatioN) is ongoing (Jilaihawi et al. 2010).

Limitations

Only a posterior annuloplasty is performed with using the Mitralign, the Accucinch and the Cardioband and may not lead to optimal results. The Millepede system creates a complete annuloplasty, but this approach has only limited data and

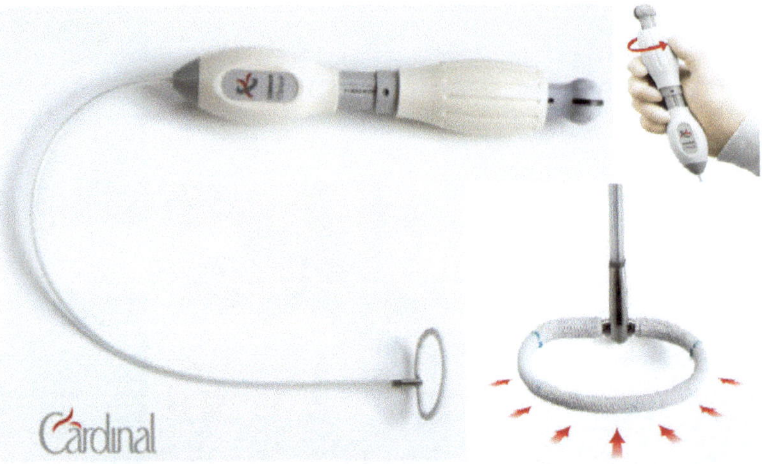

Fig. 18.15 Cardinal adjustable annuloplasty ring. (Courtesy to Valtech Cardio Ltd, Or Yehuda, Israel.)

thrombus formation on the device may occur. Alterations to the mitral annulus with the ReCor and QuantumCor might not be precisely controlled. Iatrogenic MS or residual MR are possible in cases with over-correction resp. under-correction. Damage or perforation of the mitral valve leaflets or adjacent cardiac structures might occur.

Direct Annuloplasty: Hybrid Approach

Principle

An annuloplasty ring is implanted surgically implanted and can be adjusted or reshaped intra-operatively or at a later date upon recurrence of MR with minimal invasive of percutaneous techniques.

Mechanical Adjustable Annuloplasty Ring

The adjustable annuloplasty Ring (MitralSolutions, Fort Lauderdale, Florida) and the Cardinal ring (Valtech Cardio Ltd, Or Yehuda, Israel) are surgically implanted and can be adjusted by a mechanical rotating cable attached to the annuloplasty ring (Fig. 18.15). In the MAARS (Mitral Adjustable Annuloplasty Ring Feasibility and Safety Study for Treatment of Patients with Mitral Valve Regurgitation in Open Surgical Repair) study the MitralSolutions ring is tested and also for the Cardinal ring the FIM results are presented and is ongoing further clinical testing.

Radiofrequency Adjustable Annuloplasty Ring

The Dynamic annuloplasty ring/enCor system (MiCardia Inc., Irving, California) can be reshaped following surgical implantation using radiofrequency. This annuloplasty ring is tested in the DYANA (Dynamic Annuloplasty Activation) study.

Limitations

The major limitation of this approach is that initially a surgical implantation is required with the patient on cardiopulmonary bypass. These devices might evolve to full percutaneous techniques.

Chordae Tendineae

Principle

Artificial chords or sutures are implanted via transapical or transseptal approach to treat subvalvular chordal damage/rupture. The chords are anchored onto the leaflet at one end, and the LV myocardium at the other. The length of the chord adjusted to achieve optimal leaflet coaptation and reduce MR. This approach is mainly for patients with degenerative MR.

Transapical Chordal Implantation

There are currently three devices in development that use a left-lateral mini-thoracotomy and a transapical access to implant the artificial chords: the Mitraflex system (TransCardiac Therapeutics, Atlanta, Georgia), the Neochord device (Neochord Inc., Minnetonka, Minnesota) and the V-chordal system (Valtech Cardio Ltd, Or Yehuda, Israel) (Fig. 18.16). This artificial chord is than anchored in the inner LV myocardium (the Mitraflex and Neochord device) or in the head of the papillary muscle (V-chordal system). The Neochord device is tested in the clinical setting in the TACT (Transapical Artificial Chordae Tendinae)-trial, a multicenter, prospective, single arm study (Maisano et al. 2009; Seeburger et al. 2012).

Transapical-Transseptal Chordal Implantation

The transapical-transseptal approach is used for implantation of the Babic device. With this device two continuous suture tracks from LV apex through the target leaflet are created and are exteriorized via the transseptal route. A pledget is anchored onto the atrial side of the leaflet and a custom-made polymer elastic tube interposed between leaflet and LV wall. The sutures are pulled and released until a good coaptation of the prolapsed/flail segment is achieved and secured to the epicardial surface (Panic et al. 2009).

Limitations

This approach is not suitable for patients with a FMR. Further proper tensioning of the artificial chords is crucial: if the artificial chord is too long a residual leaflet prolapse and when the chord is too short a restricted leaflet will persist with the possibility of a residual MR.

Left Ventricle

Principle

A device is used to reduce the anterior-posterior dimensions of the left ventricle. By remodeling the LV geometry it indirectly decreases the septal to lateral distance, it stabilizes the sub-mitral structures and also brings the papillary muscles closer to the leaflets for improved leaflet coaptation and decrease of MR. These devices are mainly suitable for patients with a FMR in which the combined annular and ventricular deformities are the cause of the MR.

Coapsys/Icoapsys System (Myocor, Maple Grove, Minnesota)

The concept of moving the ventricle, rather than the annulus, to increase leaflet coaptation and eliminate functional MR led to the development of the surgical Coapsys device. This device employs a transventricular splint with pads on the outer surface of the left ventricle in an open chest; this can be placed without cardiopulmonary bypass under direct echocardiographic guidance. Pads attached to each end of the splint are tightened gently to pull the ventricle into the region of the papillary muscles and also to move the posterior leaflet to better coapt with the anterior leaflet. The iCoapsys was based on this surgical Coapsys system and performs the same role but can be delivered in a minimally invasive procedure with fluoroscopic guidance (Fig. 18.17). The concept of surgical ventricular reshaping was tested in the RESTOR-MV (Randomized Evaluation of a Surgical Treatment for Off-pump Repair of the Mitral Valve) trial. This trial randomized 165 patients with coronary artery disease and ischemic mitral regurgitation to traditional open coronary artery bypass grafting (CABG) and mitral repair to CABG and Coapsys device placement. The data showed an improved survival and a significant decrease in major adverse outcomes in the group treated with the Coapsys device (Grossi et al. 2010). The safety and feasibility of the percutaneous iCoapsys was

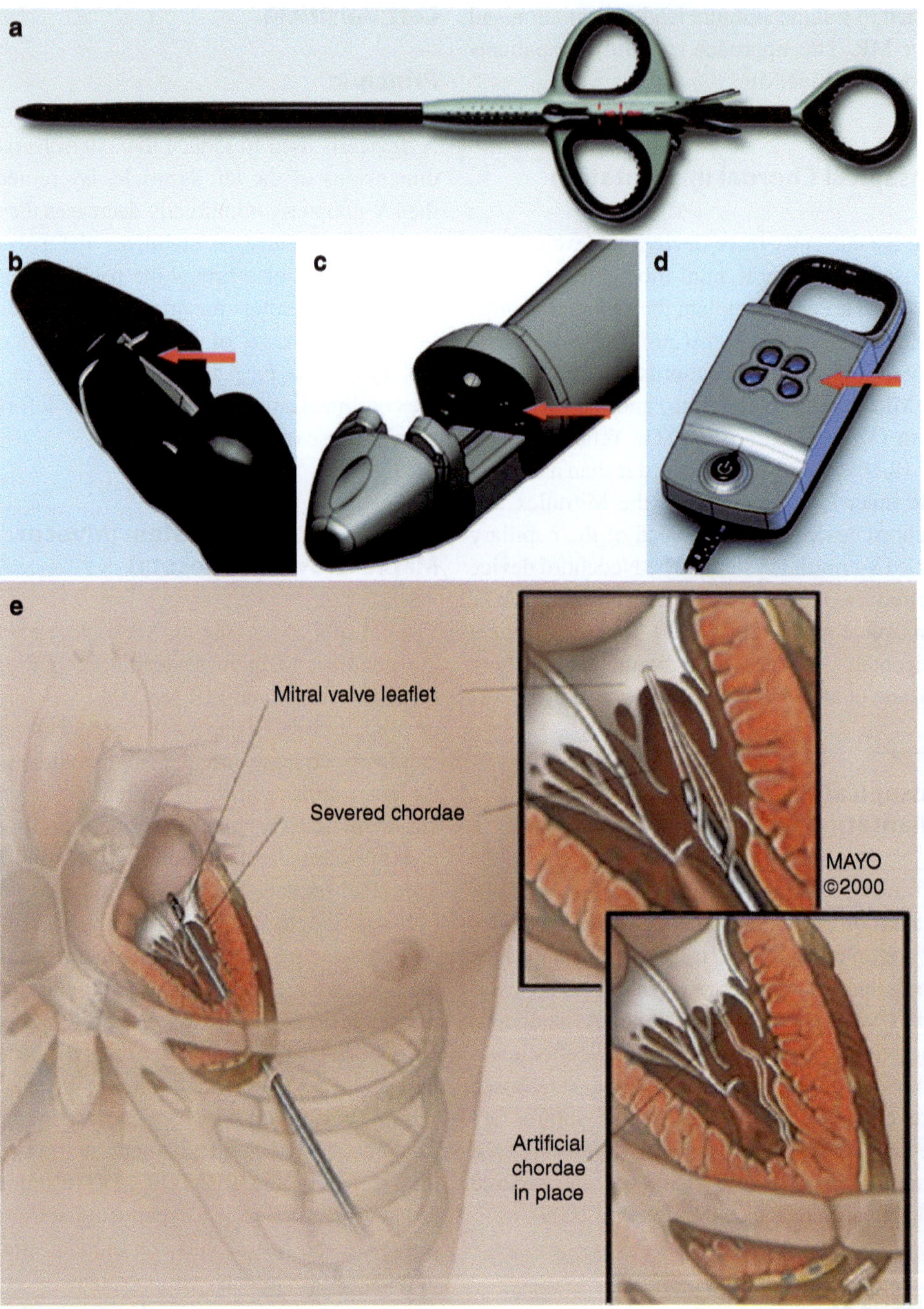

Fig. 18.16 The NeoChord system. (**a**) for transapical implantation of neochordae to the MV has the following technical features: a tip with 2 adjustable jaws to grasp the leaflet, which includes a dull needle to puncture the leaflet segment and retract the neochord through the device exteriorly (**b**), and 4 fiber-optic spots that are distributed in a symmetrically on the proximal grasping jaw (**c**), each of which relates to a signal light on the devoice monitor (**d**) to confirm adequate tissue grasping. (**e**) The grasping and transapical placement of neochordae with the NeoChord system. (Courtesy to Neochord Inc., Minnetonka, Minnesota and from Seeburger J, Borger MA, Tschernich H, et al: Transapical beating heart mitral valve repair. Circ Cardiovasc Interv. 2010 Dec;3(6):611-2, with permission of Wolters Kluwer Health.) At the time of publication, the NeoChord device is an investigational device and is not available for commercial use.)

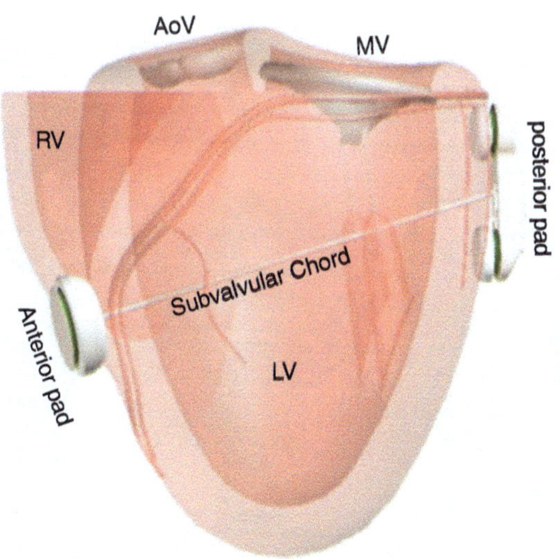

Fig. 18.17 Implanted iCoapsys device. AoV = aortic valve; MV = mitral valve; RV = right ventricle; LV = left ventricle. (From Pedersen WR, Block P, Leon M, et al.: iCoapsys mitral valve repair system: Percutaneous implantation in an animal model. Catheter Cardiovasc Interv. 2008 Jul 1;72(1):125-31, with permission of John Wiley and Sons.)

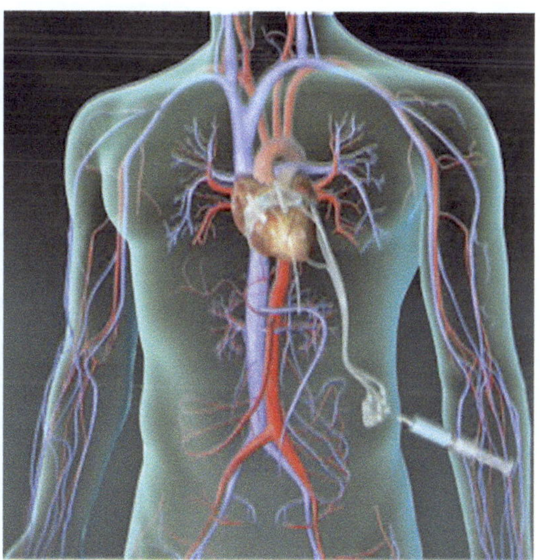

Fig. 18.18 Mardil-Bace device. (From Raman J, Jagannathan R, Chandrashekar P, et al.: Can we repair the mitral valve from outside the heart? A novel extra-cardiac approach to functional mitral regurgitation. Heart Lung Circ. 2011 Mar;20(3):157-62, with permission of Elsevier.)

tested in an animal model and although the device was successfully implanted without complications device development has been stopped (Pedersen et al. 2008).

BACE (Basal Annuloplasty of the Cardia Externally) Device (Mardil Inc., Morrisville, North Carolina)

The BACE Device consists of a silicone band assembly with inflatable silicone chambers that is placed via a mini-thoracotomy (Fig. 18.18). This band is slipped around the base of the heart and positioned at the level of the atrio-ventricular (AV) groove and the adjacent ventricular muscle. The device is held in place with sutures attached to the exterior surface of the heart through tabs on the polyester belt loops. Chambers incorporated into the band are inflated by filling them with saline through subcutaneous ports attached via tubing to the BACE Device. The volume of saline can be adjusted peri- and post-operatively by access through the ports to provide the appropriate amount of support to the heart muscle that will produce a reduction in MR. The filled chambers apply pressure at appropriate points of the heart to re-shape the mitral valve annulus and also provide sub-annular support that allows better closure of the mitral valve. The feasibility and safety was first tested in an animal model. The proof-of-concept study was demonstrated in 12 patients with ischemic heart disease, congestive heart failure and moderate functional MR. In this study there were no perioperative complications or deaths related to the surgical procedure. The device could be placed in all patients and the post-operative was significantly improved MR and left ventricular ejection fraction which maintained 18 months post operatively. In addition to that the patients also had a significant improvement of New York Heart Association (NYHA) functional status (Raman et al. 2009, 2011).

Limitations

This approach is not suitable for patients with a DMR. There is only limited clinical data, and adverse events and long-term outcomes are unknown.

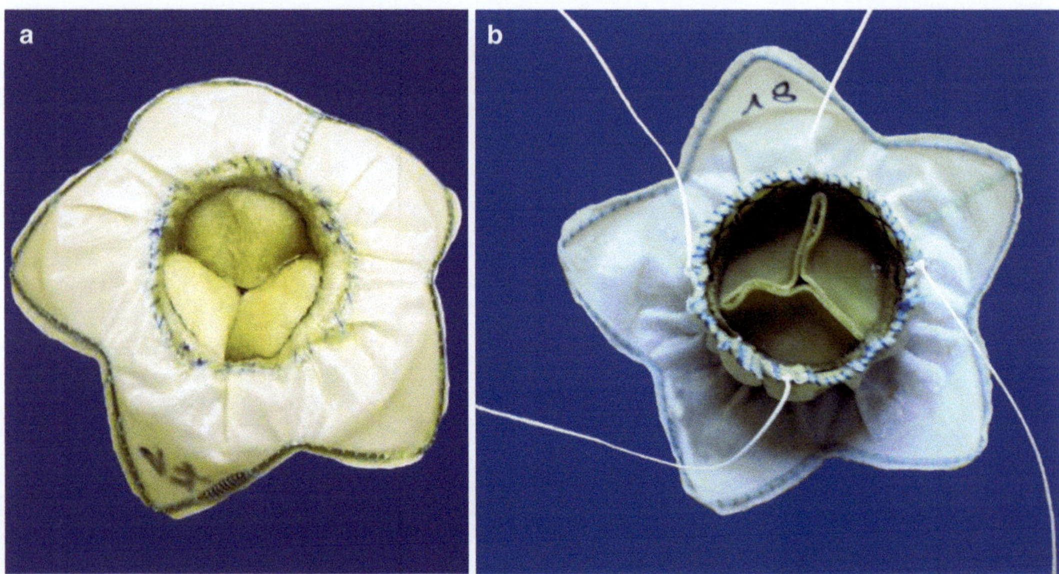

Fig. 18.19 The Lutter-Lozonschi prosthesis. (**a**) Atrial view of the prototype valved stent and (**b**) ventricular view. (From Lutter G, Quaden R, Osaki S, et al.: Off-pump transapical mitral valve replacement. Eur J Cardiothorac Surg. 2009 Jul;36(1):124-8, with permissions of Oxford University Press.)

Percutaneous Mitral Valve Replacement

Principle

Replacement of the native mitral valve with a (bio)prosthesis via right mini-thoracotomy, transapically or percutaneously.

Endovalve Prosthesis (Endovalve Inc., Princeton, New Jersey)

This folded bioprosthetic mitral valve is implanted via a minimally invasive surgical approach (right mini-thoracotomy) directly into the LA with a special delivery system and removable wires allowing contraction, repositioning, and release. The prosthesis includes a ring and bioprosthetic leaflets with a foldable tripod frame. For fixation and attachment in the beating heart it has integrated gripper features. A sewn fabric skirts provides paravalvular sealing. This approach was successfully tested in an animal model. A true percutaneous version is under development.

Lutter-Lozonschi Prosthesis

A radially self-expandable nitinol stent-valve is delivered transapically and consists of different components: a flat star-like disk (atrial fixation system), a tubular ventricular piece, which accommodates a tricuspid pericardial heart valve (diameter 25–33 mm) and a ventricular fixation system (Fig. 18.19). To guarantee the sealing, minimize paravalvular leakage, and to allow easier repositioning an ultra-thin polytetrafluoroethylene (PTFE) membrane is sutured onto the atrial springs and over the ventricular component. This was tested in an animal model (Lutter et al. 2009; Lozonschi et al. 2010).

CardiAQ Prostheses (CardiAQ Valve Technologies Inc, Irvine, California)

This system consists of a self-expanding bi-level nitinol frame with a porcine pericardial tissue valve. The effective orifice is about 30 mm with a 40-mm unique foreshortening anchoring frame designed for annular attachment without radial force (Fig. 18.20). This valve is implanted percu-

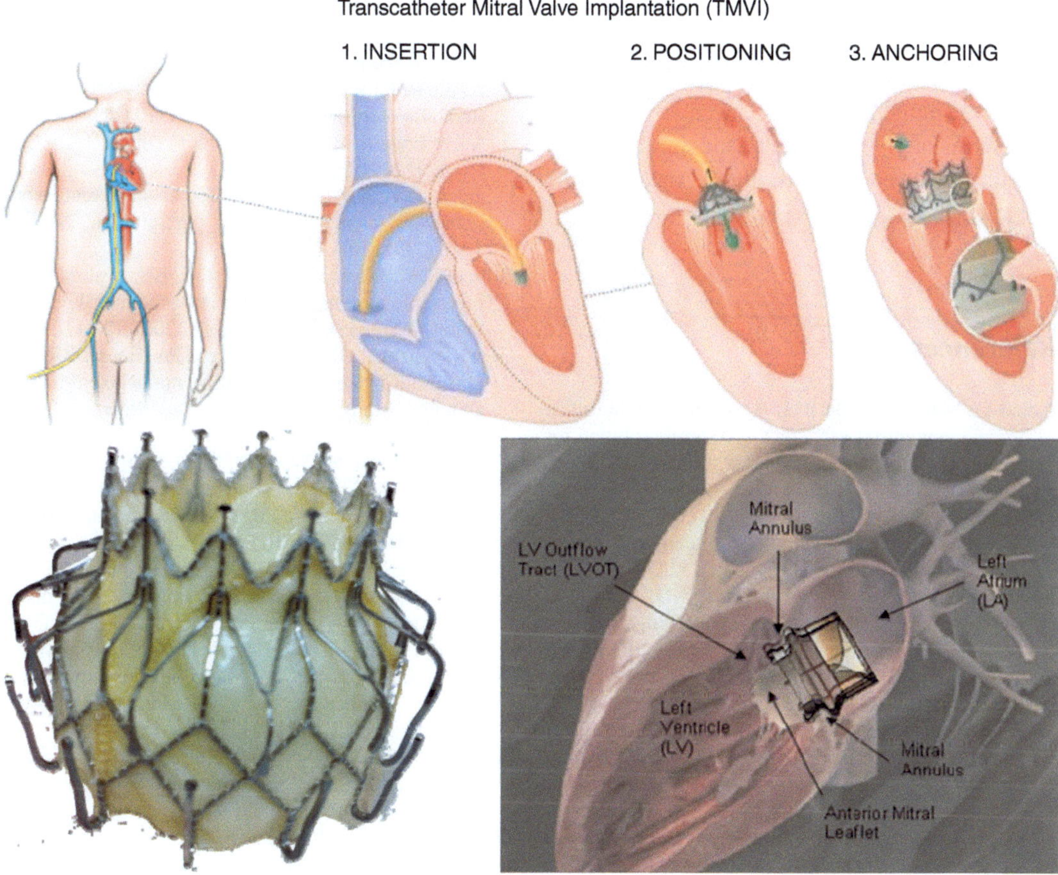

Fig. 18.20 The CardiaQ system (Courtesy to CardiAQ Valve Technologies Inc, Irvine, California.)

taneously via a venous transvenous, transseptal, antegrade approach. The system is in pre-clinical development and has only been used in an animal model.

Limitations/Challenges

The mitral valve apparatus is much more complex structure compared to the aortic valve making replacement more difficult. Compared to the aortic annulus the mitral valve annulus is saddle shaped, making anchoring more difficult. Also anchoring systems that cause radial force on the mitral valve annulus might cause further dilatation with paravalvular leakage or even valve displacement as a result. Further obstruction of the left ventricular outflow tract by the supporting structures of the implanted valve or components of the native valve most likely the AMVL should be avoided.

Conclusion

Mitral valve regurgitation (MR) is a common valvular abnormality and patients with symptomatic MR not only experience a low quality of life, but also have a poor prognosis in the absence of surgery. Although multiple studies have shown that surgery will improve symptoms en prognosis of these patients up to 50% are not considered for surgical interventions. New therapies will benefit patients with shorter hospital stays, decreased morbidity, and provide alternate options for those who are not conventional surgical candidates. This has driven to the development of transcatheter techniques that mimic surgical approaches. Currently several devices are under investigation. It is necessary that these devices provide results similar to those of conventional surgery in terms of efficacy, safety, and durability, but with a lower periprocedural risk for the patient.

References

Alfieri O, Maisano F, De BM, et al. The double-orifice technique in mitral valve repair: a simple solution for complex problems. J Thorac Cardiovasc Surg. 2001;122:674–81.

Alvarez JM, Deal CW, Loveridge K, et al. Repairing the degenerative mitral valve: ten- to fifteen-year follow-up. J Thorac Cardiovasc Surg. 1996;112:238–47.

Bhudia SK, McCarthy PM, Smedira NG, Lam BK, Rajeswaran J, Blackstone EH. Edge-to-edge (Alfieri) mitral repair: results in diverse clinical settings. Ann Thorac Surg. 2004;77:1598–606.

Bonow RO, Carabello BA, Chatterjee K, et al. 2008 Focused update incorporated into the ACC/AHA 2006 guidelines for the management of patients with valvular heart disease: a report of the American College of Cardiology/American Heart Association Task Force on Practice Guidelines (Writing Committee to Revise the 1998 Guidelines for the Management of Patients with Valvular Heart Disease): endorsed by the Society of Cardiovascular Anesthesiologists, Society for Cardiovascular Angiography and Interventions, and Society of Thoracic Surgeons. Circulation. 2008;118:e523–661.

Burr LH, Krayenbuhl C, Sutton MS. The mitral plication suture: a new technique of mitral valve repair. J Thorac Cardiovasc Surg. 1977;73:589–95.

Carabello BA. The current therapy for mitral regurgitation. J Am Coll Cardiol. 2008;52:319–26.

Chiam PT, Ruiz CE. Percutaneous transcatheter mitral valve repair: a classification of the technology. JACC Cardiovasc Interv. 2011;4:1–13.

Choure AJ, Garcia MJ, Hesse B, et al. In vivo analysis of the anatomical relationship of coronary sinus to mitral annulus and left circumflex coronary artery using cardiac multidetector computed tomography: implications for percutaneous coronary sinus mitral annuloplasty. J Am Coll Cardiol. 2006;48:1938–45.

Dubreuil O, Basmadjian A, Ducharme A, et al. Percutaneous mitral valve annuloplasty for ischemic mitral regurgitation: first in man experience with a temporary implant. Catheter Cardiovasc Interv. 2007;69:1053–61.

Enriquez-Sarano M, Schaff HV, Orszulak TA, Tajik AJ, Bailey KR, Frye RL. Valve repair improves the outcome of surgery for mitral regurgitation. A multivariate analysis. Circulation. 1995;91:1022–8.

Enriquez-Sarano M, Akins CW, Vahanian A. Mitral regurgitation. Lancet. 2009;373:1382–94.

Feldman T, Kar S, Rinaldi M, et al. Percutaneous mitral repair with the MitraClip system: safety and midterm durability in the initial EVEREST (Endovascular Valve Edge-to-Edge REpair Study) cohort. J Am Coll Cardiol. 2009;54:686–94.

Feldman T, Foster E, Glower DD, et al. Percutaneous repair or surgery for mitral regurgitation. N Engl J Med. 2011;364:1395–406.

Gillinov AM, Wierup PN, Blackstone EH, et al. Is repair preferable to replacement for ischemic mitral regurgitation? J Thorac Cardiovasc Surg. 2001;122:1125–41.

Goel R, Witzel T, Dickens D, Takeda PA, Heuser RR. The QuantumCor device for treating mitral regurgitation: an animal study. Catheter Cardiovasc Interv. 2009;74: 43–8.

Grossi EA, Patel N, Woo YJ, et al. Outcomes of the RESTOR-MV trial (randomized evaluation of a surgical treatment for off-pump repair of the mitral valve). J Am Coll Cardiol. 2010;56:1984–93.

Harnek J, Webb JG, Kuck KH, et al. Transcatheter implantation of the MONARC coronary sinus device for mitral regurgitation: 1-year results from the EVOLUTION phase I study (Clinical Evaluation of the Edwards Lifesciences Percutaneous Mitral Annuloplasty System for the Treatment of Mitral Regurgitation). JACC Cardiovasc Interv. 2011;4:115–22.

Heuser RR, Witzel T, Dickens D, Takeda PA. Percutaneous treatment for mitral regurgitation: the QuantumCor system. J Interv Cardiol. 2008;21:178–82.

Jilaihawi H, Virmani R, Nakagawa H, et al. Mitral annular reduction with subablative therapeutic ultrasound: pre-clinical evaluation of the ReCor device. EuroIntervention. 2010;6:54–62.

Kim JH, Kocaturk O, Ozturk C, et al. Mitral cerclage annuloplasty, a novel transcatheter treatment for secondary mitral valve regurgitation: initial results in swine. J Am Coll Cardiol. 2009;54:638–51.

Ladich E, Michaels MB, Jones RM, et al. Pathological healing response of explanted MitraClip devices. Circulation. 2011;123:1418–27.

Lozonschi L, Bombien R, Osaki S, et al. Transapical mitral valved stent implantation: a survival series in swine. J Thorac Cardiovasc Surg. 2010;140:422–6.

Lutter G, Quaden R, Osaki S, et al. Off-pump transapical mitral valve replacement. Eur J Cardiothorac Surg. 2009;36:124–8.

Maisano F, Torracca L, Oppizzi M, et al. The edge-to-edge technique: a simplified method to correct mitral insufficiency. Eur J Cardiothorac Surg. 1998;13:240–5.

Maisano F, Caldarola A, Blasio A, De BM, La CG, Alfieri O. Midterm results of edge-to-edge mitral valve repair without annuloplasty. J Thorac Cardiovasc Surg. 2003;126:1987–97.

Maisano F, Michev I, Rowe S, et al. Transapical endovascular implantation of neochordae using a suction and suture device. Eur J Cardiothorac Surg. 2009;36:118–22.

Mirabel M, Iung B, Baron G, et al. What are the characteristics of patients with severe, symptomatic, mitral regurgitation who are denied surgery? Eur Heart J. 2007;28:1358–65.

Naqvi TZ, Buchbinder M, Zarbatany D, et al. Beating-heart percutaneous mitral valve repair using a transcatheter endovascular suturing device in an animal model. Catheter Cardiovasc Interv. 2007;69:525–31.

Otto CM. Clinical practice. Evaluation and management of chronic mitral regurgitation. N Engl J Med. 2001;345:740–6.

Palacios IF, Condado JA, Brandi S, et al. Safety and feasibility of acute percutaneous septal sinus shortening: first-in-human experience. Catheter Cardiovasc Interv. 2007;69:513–8.

Panic G, Ristic M, Putnik S, Markovic D, Divac I, Babic UU. A novel technique for treatment of mitral valve prolapse/flail. J Thorac Cardiovasc Surg. 2009;137:1568–70.

Pedersen WR, Block P, Leon M, et al. ICoapsys mitral valve repair system: percutaneous implantation in an animal model. Catheter Cardiovasc Interv. 2008;72:125–31.

Raman J, Hare D, Storer M, Hata M. Epicardial cardiac basal annuloplasty: preliminary findings on extra-cardiac mitral valve repair. Heart Lung Circ. 2009;18:401–6.

Raman J, Jagannathan R, Chandrashekar P, Sugeng L. Can we repair the mitral valve from outside the heart? A novel extra-cardiac approach to functional mitral regurgitation. Heart Lung Circ. 2011;20:157–62.

Rogers JH, Yeo KK, Carroll JD, et al. Late surgical mitral valve repair after percutaneous repair with the MitraClip system. J Card Surg. 2009a;24:677–81.

Rogers JH, Rahdert DA, Caputo GR, et al. Long-term safety and durability of percutaneous septal sinus shortening (the PS(3) system) in an ovine model. Catheter Cardiovasc Interv. 2009b;73:540–8.

Sack S, Kahlert P, Bilodeau L, et al. Percutaneous transvenous mitral annuloplasty: initial human experience with a novel coronary sinus implant device. Circ Cardiovasc Interv. 2009;2:277–84.

Schofer J, Siminiak T, Haude M, et al. Percutaneous mitral annuloplasty for functional mitral regurgitation: results of the CARILLON Mitral Annuloplasty Device European Union Study. Circulation. 2009;120:326–33.

Seeburger J, Leontjev S, Neumuth M, et al. Trans-apical beating-heart implantation of neo-chordae to mitral valve leaflets: results of an acute animal study. Eur J Cardiothorac Surg. 2012;41:173–6.

Sorajja P, Nishimura RA, Thompson J, Zehr K. A novel method of percutaneous mitral valve repair for ischemic mitral regurgitation. JACC Cardiovasc Interv. 2008;1:663–72.

Swaans MJ, Van den Branden BJ, Van der Heyden JA, et al. Three-dimensional transoesophageal echocardiography in a patient undergoing percutaneous mitral valve repair using the edge-to-edge clip technique. Eur J Echocardiogr. 2009;10:982–3.

Tops LF, Van de Veire NR, Schuijf JD, et al. Noninvasive evaluation of coronary sinus anatomy and its relation to the mitral valve annulus: implications for percutaneous mitral annuloplasty. Circulation. 2007;115:1426–32.

Vahanian A, Baumgartner H, Bax J, et al. Guidelines on the management of valvular heart disease: The Task Force on the Management of Valvular Heart Disease of the European Society of Cardiology. Eur Heart J. 2007;28:230–68.

Williams JL, Toyoda Y, Ota T, et al. Feasibility of myxomatous mitral valve repair using direct leaflet and chordal radiofrequency ablation. J Interv Cardiol. 2008;21:547–54.

19 Anatomy and Pathology of Right-Sided Atrioventricular and Semilunar Valves

Cristina Basso, Denisa Muraru, Luigi P. Badano, and Gaetano Thiene

Normal Anatomy of Right-Sided Heart Valves

Tricuspid Valve

The atrio-ventricular (AV) valve apparatus, either left or right-sided, consists of annulus (or ring), leaflets, chordae tendineae, papillary muscles and ventricular myocardium they are attached to (Martinez et al. 2006; Sutton et al. 1995; Lamers et al. 1995; Xanthos et al. 2011; Cosío et al. 1999; Muraru et al. 2011a; Badano et al. 2009).

The tricuspid valve (TV) annulus points anteriorly, inferiorly and to the left, with an estimated circumference of 10–11.1 cm in women and 11.2–11.8 in men. The right-sided AV valve (TV) is composed of three leaflets (i.e. septal, anterior and posterior) at difference from the left-sided which is bi-leaflet (i.e. anterior or aortic and posterior or mural) (Figs. 19.1, 19.2, and 19.3). The three leaflets hang from the annulus as a veil and are separated by commissures (i.e. antero-septal, postero-septal, antero-posterior), tethered by fan-shaped chordae tendineae (Fig. 19.2). Each leaflet shows a distal rough zone, a proximal basal zone and an intermediate clear zone free of chordal insertions. The anterior (or antero-superior) leaflet is usually the longest and has a semicircular or quadrangular shape; anatomic variations include the possibility of a distinct scallop in its medial portion near the antero-septal commissure.

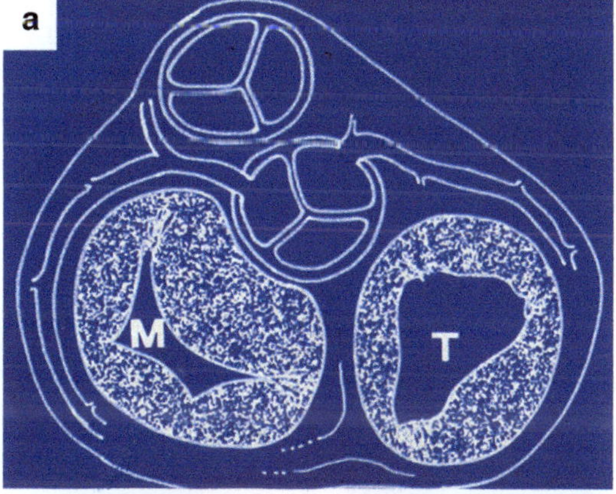

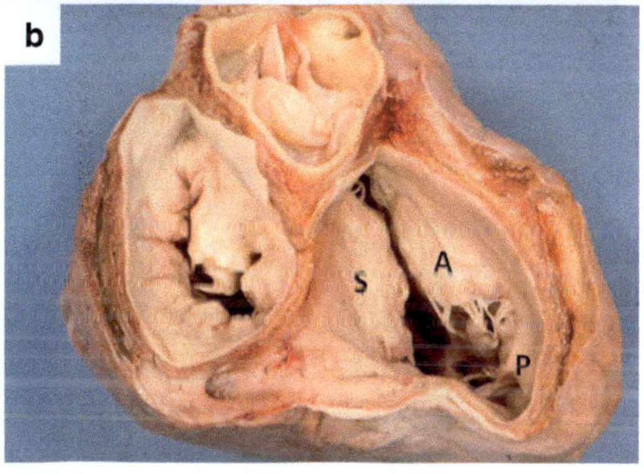

Fig. 19.1 Normal tricuspid valve. Diagram (**a**) and corresponding anatomic specimen (**b**) of the base of the heart after removal of the atrial chambers and arterial trunks at the level of the AV junctions. Note the three-leaflets structure of the right-sided AV valve as compared to the bi-leaflet structure of the left sided one

C. Basso, M.D., Ph.D. (✉) • D. Muraru, M.D.
L.P. Badano, M.D. • G. Thiene, M.D., FRCP
Department of Cardiac, Thoracic and Vascular Sciences, University of Padua, Padua, Italy
e-mail: cristina.basso@unipd.it

N.M. Rajamannan (ed.), *Cardiac Valvular Medicine*,
DOI 10.1007/978-1-4471-4132-7_19, © Springer-Verlag London 2013

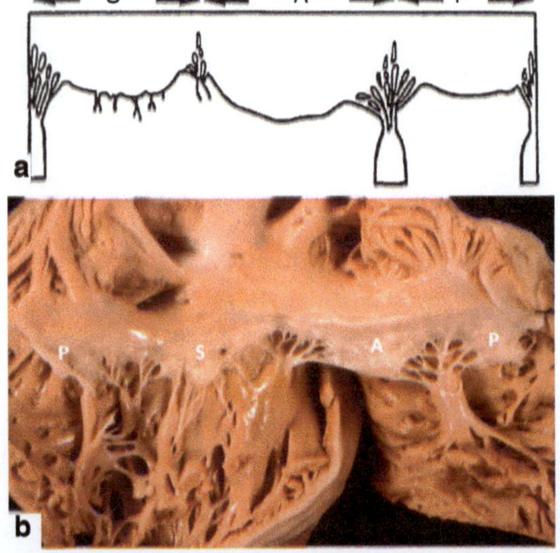

Fig. 19.2 Normal tricuspid valve. Diagram (**a**) and corresponding anatomic specimen (**b**) of the tricuspid valve after opening of the right ventricle along the acute margin: note the three leaflets (*A* anterior, *S* septal, *P* posterior), the septal attachment of the septal leaflet either direct or through the papillary muscles, and the fan-like distribution of chordate tendineae at the level of the commissures

The septal leaflet, semioval in shape, often shows a fold on the atrial surface at the point of passage from the posterior ventricular free wall to the membranous septum. The posterior (or inferior or mural) leaflet has a variable number of scallops due to clefts in its free edge, marked by fan-shaped chordae, usually two or three. Five types of chordae are found, i.e. fan-shaped, rough-zone, basal, free-edge, and deep.

A distinct small papillary muscle (PM) (the medial or conal or septal PM, also called Lancisi's PM) supports the zone of apposition between the septal and anterior leaflets; this PM may be double or multiple and arises high on the septo-marginal band. A much larger PM (the anterior PM), supports the commissure between antero-superior and inferior leaflets. The third commissure, between inferior and septal leaflet, is supported by the smaller inferior PM.

The unique feature of the TV, as opposed to the mitral valve, is the septal attachment. In particular, multiple attachments of chordae tendineae from the septal leaflet to the ventricular septum are

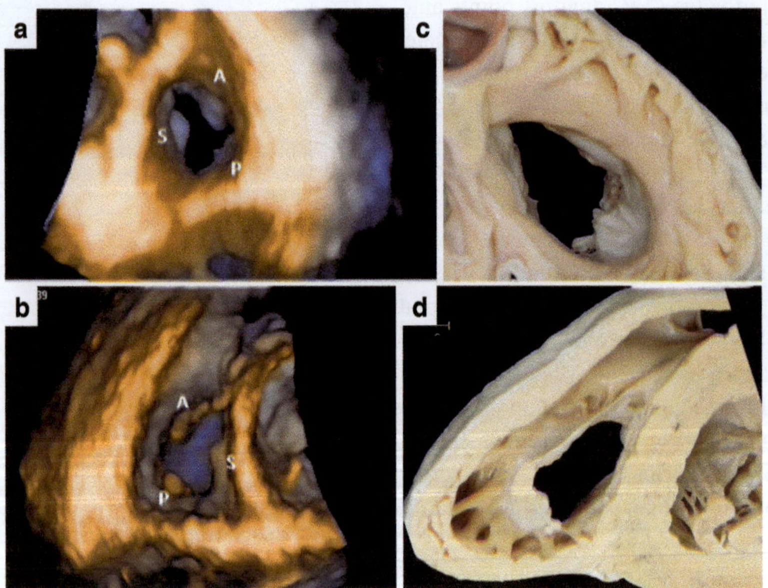

Fig. 19.3 Normal tricuspid valve: 3D transthoracic echocardiography vs. anatomy. Volume rendering display of the tricuspid valve, atrial view obtained after cropping the right atrial roof (**a**) and ventricular view obtained after cropping the right ventricle (**b**), and corresponding anatomic specimens (**c, d**). *P* posterior leaflet, *S* septal leaflet, *A* anterior leaflet

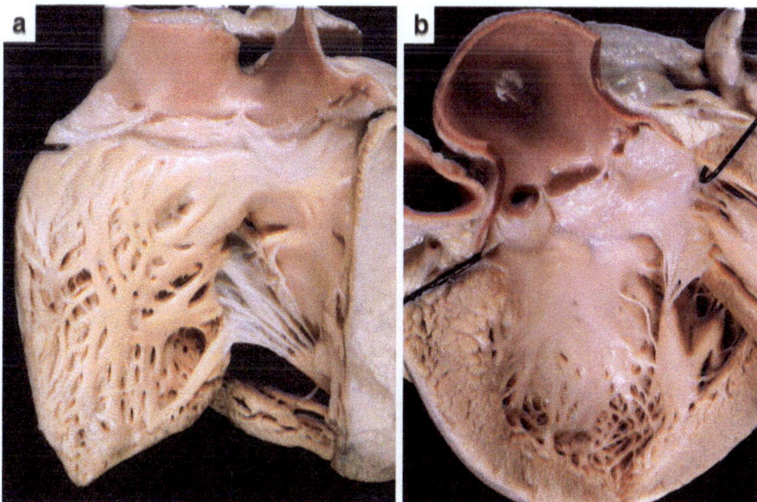

Fig. 19.4 Normal semilunar valves: pulmonary valve vs. aortic valve. (**a**) Right ventricular outflow: note the complete muscular structure of the outflow with three semilunar pulmonary cusps at the top, attached to the myocardium along their entire circumference and separated from the tricuspid valve by the supraventricular crest. (**b**) Left ventricular outflow: unlike the pulmonary valve, the three semilunar aortic cusps are not exclusively supported by ventricular myocardium. Part of the non-coronary cusp and left coronary cusp are in fibrous continuity with the aortic leaflet of the mitral valve

found, either direct or through the Lancisi's PM. Moreover, at difference from the left-sided AV valve, there is no fibrous continuity with the right-sided semilunar valve due to the interposition of the muscle of the crista supraventricularis (Fig. 19.4).

The AV valve leaflets are covered with endothelial cells and present four layers, identified as the auricularis, the spongiosa, the fibrosa and the ventricularis, respectively (Silver and Silver 2001; Veinot et al. 2001). The TV is similar to the mitral valve, with few differences, i.e. the layers are thinner and the auricularis on the posterior and septal leaflet is prominent with abundant smooth muscle cells. The auricularis covers the spongiosa on the atrial aspect of the AV leaflet closest to the annulus and is composed of collagen, elastin and smooth muscle cells. The ventricularis covers the fibrosa layer on the ventricular aspect of the AV leaflet and again not extending close to the free margin and consists mainly of small elastic fibers. Thus, the distal third of the leaflet does not present either auricularis or ventricularis.

The fibrosa is the central layer of AV valves and is composed of collagen and elastic fibers as an extension of the valvular annulus. On the ventricular aspect these connective tissue components extend into the chordae tendineae and the tip of the PM.

The spongiosa contains mainly glycosaminoglycans (such as hyaluronic acid, chondroitin sulfate B, chondroitin sulfate AC and heparin), sparse collagen and elastic fibers and connective tissue cells such as fibroblasts and primitive mesechymal cells. Both the spongiosa and the fibrosa layer extend the entire length of the leaflet.

A distinct type of cardiac interstitial cells is present in all valve layers (valvular interstitial cells, VIC) with two morphologies, elongated and cobblestone. The VIC resemble smooth muscle cells and show gap junctions and contractile elements. Their function is to secrete matrix and participate in valve repair.

The chordae tendineae appears at histology as tendon-like structure composed mainly of collagen bundles arranged in a parallel fashion with few elastic fibers, covered by a thin layer of endocardium. Sometimes, muscular components are seen in the so-called thicker chordae muscularis.

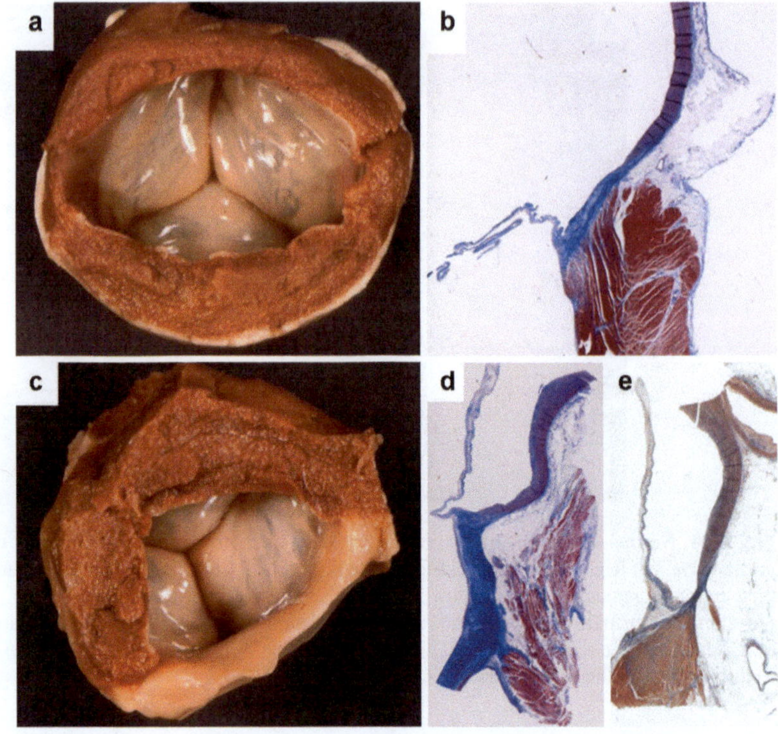

Fig. 19.5 Normal pulmonary vs. aortic root. (**a**) Excised pulmonary root showing the circumferential muscular attachment of the three semilunar cusps; (**b**) Correspond histology of a semilunar pulmonary cusp attached to the right ventricular outflow tract myocardium (Heidenhain trichrome stain); (**c**) Excised aortic root showing the attachment of the semilunar cusps to myocardium for two thirds and to fibrous tissue (mitro-aortic fibrous continuity) for one third of the circumference; (**d**) Correspond histology of a semilunar aortic cusp attached to the fibrous continuity (Heidenhain trichrome stain); (**e**) Correspond histology of a semilunar aortic cusp attached to the left ventricular outflow myocardium (Heidenhain trichrome stain)

Pulmonary Valve

The right-sided semilunar valve lies at the top of the pulmonary infundibulum (right ventricular outflow tract) and is attached to the pulmonary annulus, which points posteriorly, superiorly and to the left (Silver and Silver 2001; Veinot et al. 2001; Stamm et al. 1998). The estimated circumference of the pulmonary annulus is 5.7–7.4 cm in women and 6.0–7.5 cm in men, and it is approximately 1.5 cm higher than the aortic annulus. The distinct feature of the ventricular outflow is that it is a complete muscular structure which winds across the anterior aspect of the aortic root (Figs. 19.4 and 19.5). It supports the three cusps of the pulmonary valve in a semilunar fashion with a U-type insertion. Each cusp is attached in a way that the base is within the ventricle while the tip of the commissures is at the junction between the sinusal portion and the tubular portion of the pulmonary trunk (i.e. the most distal portion of the pulmonary fibrous annulus). This unique arrangement, which is also observed on the left side at the level of the aortic valve, explains why the use of the term "annulus" is often debated while describing the semilunar arterial valves. Three ring-like structures within the arterial valvular complexes are usually described, i.e. the sino-tubular junction, the line at the basal attachment of the semilunar cusp and the line at the sinusal portion of the arterial root, but none of them corresponds to the semilunar attachment of the cusps, i.e. the anatomic ventriculo-arterial junction which is crown-shaped.

The three cusps are named anterior, right (facing the right coronary aortic cusp) and left (facing the left coronary aortic cusp). Similarly to the aortic valve, the three pulmonary cusps demarcate shallow sinuses and are often fenestrated in the zone between the line of closure and the free edge (i.e. lunulae). Not so rarely, fibrous nodules (Morgagni nodules, the equivalent of Arantius nodules in the aortic cusps) are located centrally on the free edge of the semilunar cusps.

The histologic structure of the semilunar valves is similar to that of the AV valves (Stamm et al. 1998). Four layers are identifiable as well, named the ventricularis, the spongiosa, the fibrosa and the arterialis, respectively. The major structural component is the fibrosa, which consists mostly of collagen, elastic fibers and fibroblasts. At the base of the cusps, elastic fibers may aggregate to form a ill-defined layer, i.e. the arterialis. The spongiosa is prominent in the basal third of the cusp, not reaching the free edge. Lying between the ventricularis and the fibrosa, it consists mainly of proteoglycans, collagen, and fibroblasts. The ventricularis contains mostly elastic fibers and represents a continuation of the ventricular endocardial layer. Thus, the free edge of the pulmonary cusps consists only of two layers, the fibrosa and the ventricularis.

Pathology of Right-Sided Heart Valves

Tricuspid valve dysfunction may result from "structural" alterations (either congenital or acquired) of the valve apparatus or from an abnormal function of a structurally normal valve (Waller et al. 1995a, b, c). From an etiopathologic viewpoint, it is useful to distinguish stenotic (or steno-incompetent) from purely incompetent TV. In fact, while stenotic TV are always structurally abnormal and few conditions can account for (mostly rheumatic valve disease), purely incompetent TV can be also functional and multiple causes are identifiable.

Ebstein Anomaly

It is a congenital malformation of the right ventricle characterized by a downward displacement into the right ventricular cavity of the insertion of the septal and/or posterior leaflet, so that a portion of the ventricular myocardium becomes atrialized and atrophic (Figs. 19.6 and 19.7) (Bharucha et al. 2010; Thiene and Frescura 2010; Ho et al. 2000; Schreiber et al. 1999; Zuberbuhler et al. 1984; Anderson et al. 1979; Frescura et al. 2000; Stellin et al. 1993). Regarding embryology, the leaflets and tensile apparatus of the TV are believed to be formed mostly by a process of delamination of the inner layers of the inlet zone of the right ventricle. The downward displacement of the leaflets in Ebstein's anomaly suggests that delamination from the inlet portion failed to occur. A wide variability of leaflet displacement towards the apex and of degree of leaflet malformation is described, from almost normal leaflets displaced less than 1 cm apically to severely malformed ones with almost apical position. It may be isolated or associated with severe malformations, like pulmonary atresia and intact septum. Ebstein anomaly accounts usually for pure TV incompetence, although rarely it has been associated with some degree of stenosis. In this condition, if the foramen ovale is patent, a right-to-left shunt occurs accounting for cyanosis. The clinical picture of these patients is also characterized by ventricular arrhythmias and pre-excitation syndrome.

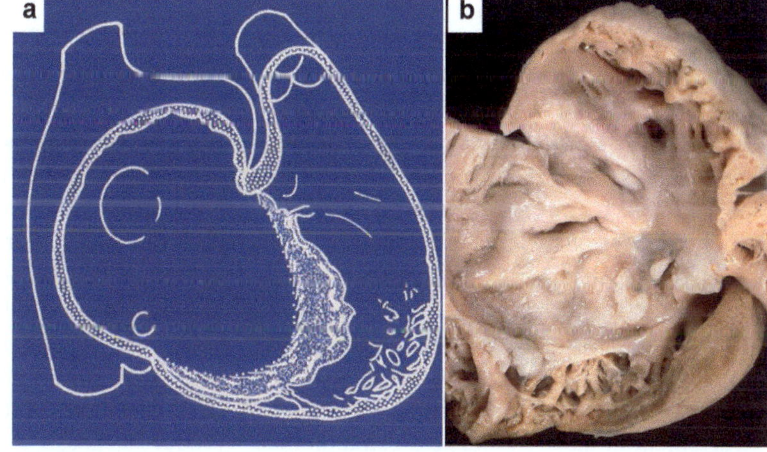

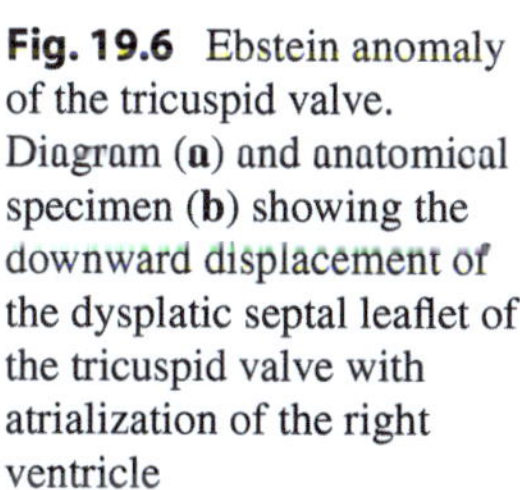
Fig. 19.6 Ebstein anomaly of the tricuspid valve. Diagram (**a**) and anatomical specimen (**b**) showing the downward displacement of the dysplatic septal leaflet of the tricuspid valve with atrialization of the right ventricle

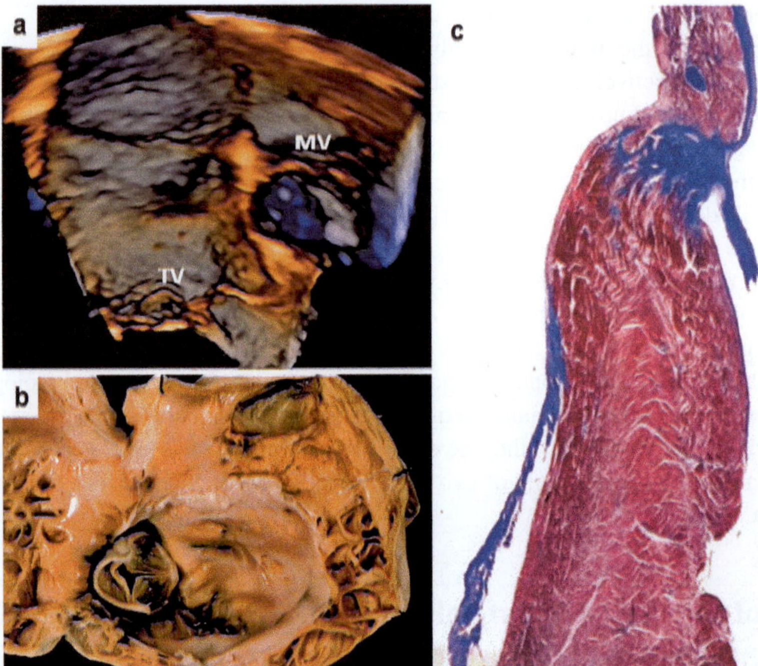

Fig. 19.7 Ebstein anomaly of the tricuspid valve. (**a**) Volume rendering display by transthoracic 3D echocardiography, illustrating the downward displacement of the tricuspid valve (*TV*) leaflet as compared to the mitral valve (*MV*) and the atrialized portion of the right ventricle. (**b**) macroscopic view of the heart of a patient who has bioprosthesis tricuspid valve replacement due to massive regurgitation in the setting of Ebstein malformation: note the septal leaflet displaced towards the apex with atrialization of the right ventricular chamber; (**c**) histology of the AV septal junction: note the apically shifted insertion of the tricuspid valve leaflet as compared to the mitral one, so that a portion of the ventricular myocardium becomes atrialized (Heidenhain trichrome stain)

Rheumatic Valve Disease

The morphologic features of rheumatic valve disease of the TV are similar to those observed in the mitral valve. Rheumatic involvement is characterized by diffuse fibrous thickening of the leaflets with fusion of the commissures, being the antero-septal the most commonly targeted (Fig. 19.8) (Waller et al. 1995a, b, c). Calcification is usually absent, at difference from rheumatic mitral valve disease. The chordae tendineae may be thickened and shortened, but chordal fusion is less frequent than in the mitral valve. All these features explain a dysfunction in terms of TV stenosis. However, when the fibrous retraction prevails with absent or mild commissural fusion, the TV dysfunction consists mostly of incompetence. Rheumatic involvement of the TV is far less common than the mitral and the aortic valves. Isolated rheumatic TV disease is rare and it is always associated with mitral valve disease (mostly stenosis), alone or in combination with aortic valve disease.

Infective Endocarditis

Acute infective endocarditis of the TV is rare and is usually associated with intravenous self-administration of drugs or with intracardiac catheter devices (pacemaker, implantable cardioverter defibrillator) (Fig. 19.9) (Waller et al. 1995a, b, c; Thiene and Basso 2006). Although it is usually accounting for TV regurgitation, due to leaflet perforation and/or chordal rupture, large infective vegetations obstructing the TV orifice may produce stenosis.

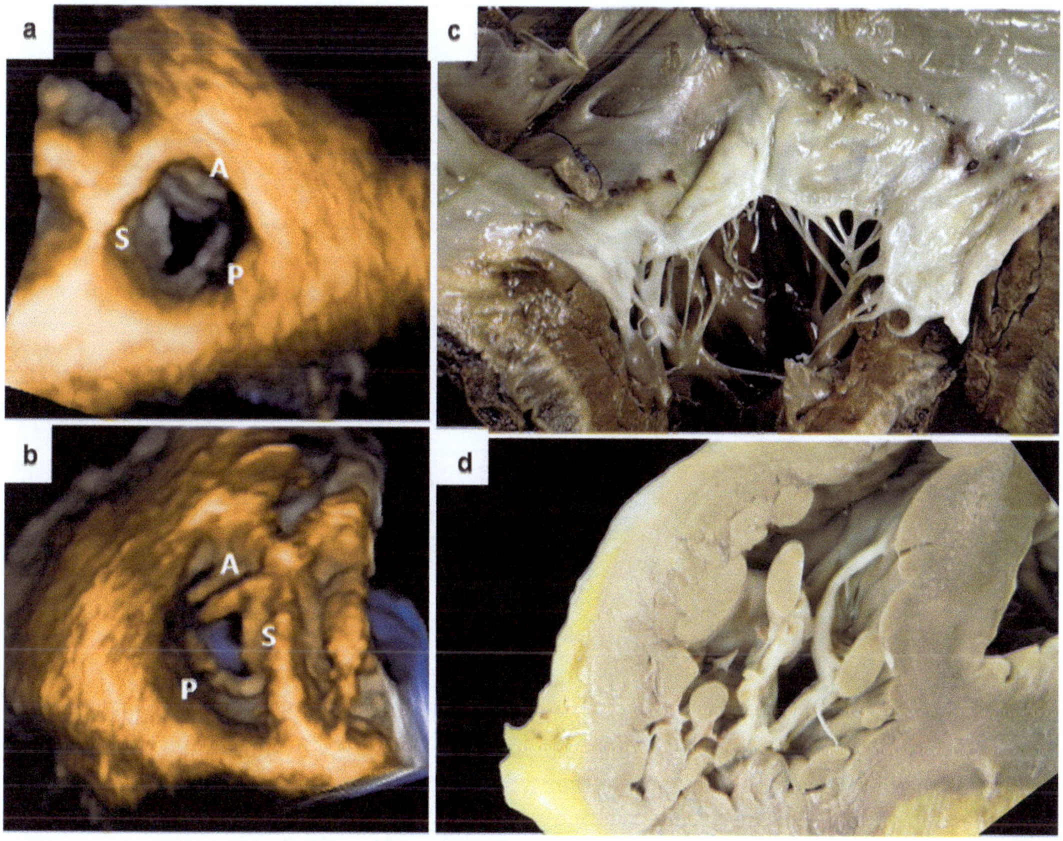

Fig. 19.8 Rheumatic tricuspid valve disease: 3D transthoracic echocardiography vs. anatomy. 3D volume rendering display, atrial view (**a**) and ventricular view (**b**) showing leaflet thickening and retraction, and commissural fusion leading to tricuspid valve steno-incompetence. Heart specimens of rheumatic tricuspid valve disease showing: (**c**) leaflet fibrous thickening, commissural fusion and surgical anulo-plasty; and (**d**) leaflet fibrous thickening with chordal thickening, fusion and retraction (same view as **b**). *P* posterior leaflet, *S* septal leaflet, *A* anterior leaflet

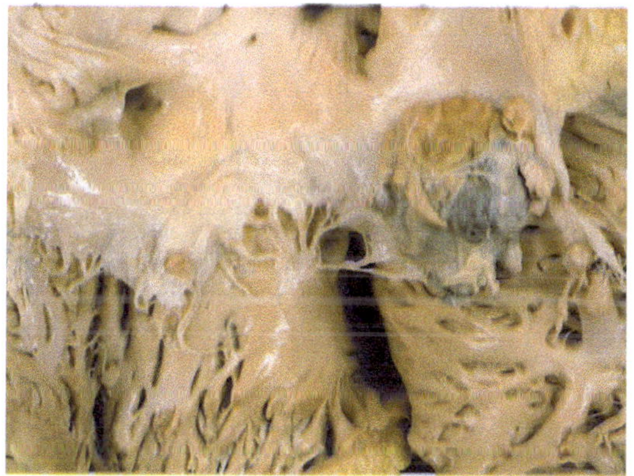

Fig. 19.9 Tricuspid valve infective endocarditis. Vegetant polypous infective endocarditis of the tricuspid valve in a drug addict

Carcinoid Valve Disease

This entity is due to carcinoid tumors that metastatize to the liver producing serotonin (5-hydroxytryptamine), then reaching the pulmonary and, to a lesser extent, the systemic circulation (due to lung inactivation). In some patients, besides the classical clinical symptoms/signs (bronchospasm, diarrhea, nausea, malabsorption, flushing, and teleangiectasia), TV and pulmonary valve disease may develop (carcinoid valve disease) (Waller et al. 1995a, b, c); Muraru et al. 2011b). Valve disease associated with Fen-phen and methysergide presents lesions which are similar to carcinoid valve disease.

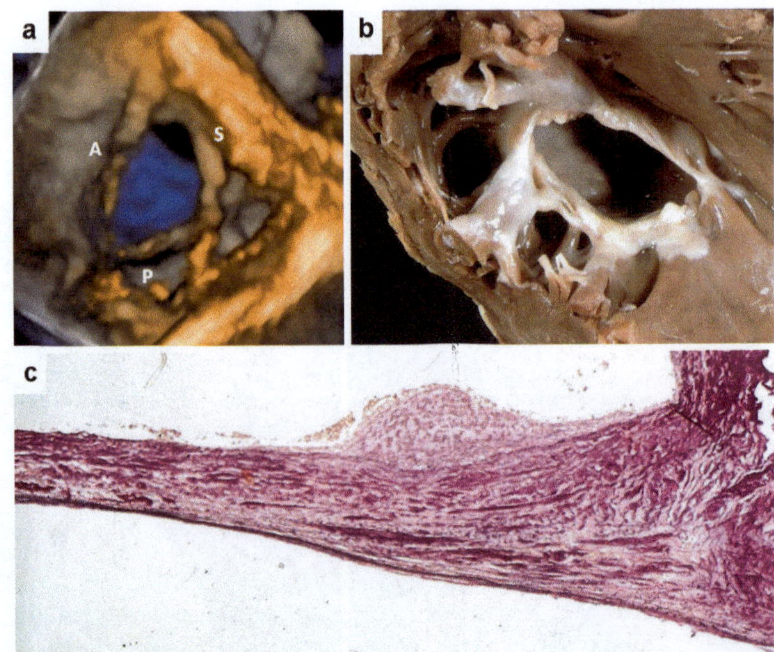

Fig. 19.10 Tricuspid valve incompetence due to carcinoid valve disease. 3D echocardiography, with volume rendering display of the valve from the right ventricle showing leaflet thickening and retraction (**a**) and corresponding anatomical view (**b**): note the leaflets thickening and whitish endocardial plaques; at histology (**c**) note the fibrous plaque superimposed upon a chorda tendinea (elastic van Gieson stain)

Macroscopically, white fibrous plaques form on the ventricular aspects of the TV and the mural endocardium (carcinoid plaques), thus accounting for leaflets' adhesion to the ventricular wall and preventing systolic closure and coaptation (Fig. 19.10). This explains why carcinoid valve disease usually account for TV incompetence or steno-incompetence. Histologic examination shows proliferation of fibrous tissue superimposed to the normal layered structure of the leaflets, at difference from rheumatic valve disease where the scarring involves the leaflet itself.

Floppy (Prolapse)

Myxoid degeneration with redundancy of the TV leaflets has been described in association with a floppy mitral valve (Waller et al. 1995a, b, c). Histologic features are similar to those reported at the mitral valve level, with expanding spongiosa and deposition of proteoglycans also in the fibrosa extending into the chordae tendinae.

Pure TV incompetence has been reported in Marfan's syndrome, usually associated with dysfunction of mitral and aortic valves (Waller et al. 1995a, b, c). Myxoid degeneration (floppy leaflets) as well as TV annulus dilatation can account for the TV dysfunction.

Papillary Muscle Dysfunction

As in the mitral valve, PM dysfunction can account for AV valve incompetence. TV PM dysfunction may result from necrosis (myocardial infarction, myocarditis), fibrosis (healed myocardial infarction, endomyocardiofibrosis) or infiltrative processes (abscess, granuloma, amyloid, iron) (Waller et al. 1995a, b, c).

Trauma/Iatrogenic

Acute TV regurgitation due to rupture of one or more papillary muscles or chordae tendinae has been described as a consequence of a severe, non penetrating, blunt chest injury (Fig. 19.11). Usually, the flail involves the anterior leaflet of the TV (Waller et al. 1995a, b, c). Rare iatrogenic variants of TV regurgitation include also trauma from pacemaker/implantable cardioverter defibrillator lead, stiff guidewire, bioptome for endomyocardial biopsy, radiofrequency ablation with damage of leaflets or subvalvular apparatus.

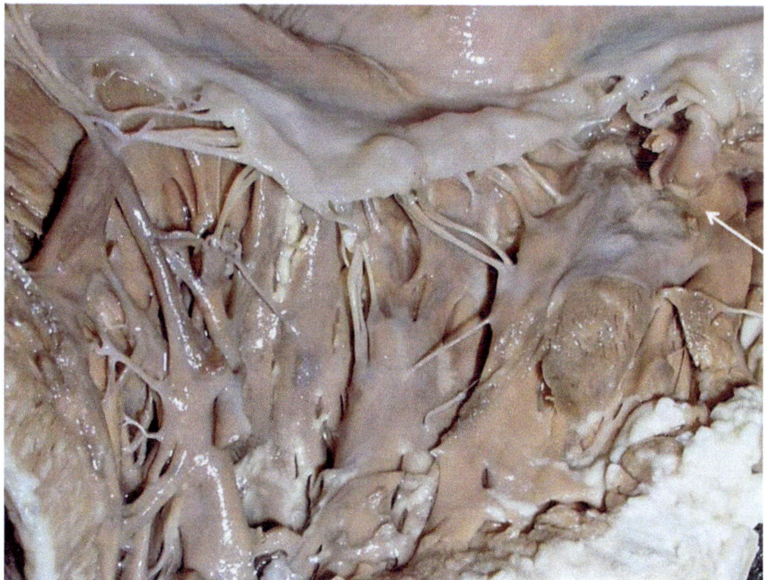

Fig. 19.11 Traumatic tricuspid valve incompetence. Acute tricuspid valve incompetence due to blunt chest trauma with rupture of the conal Lancisi's papillary muscle (*arrow*)

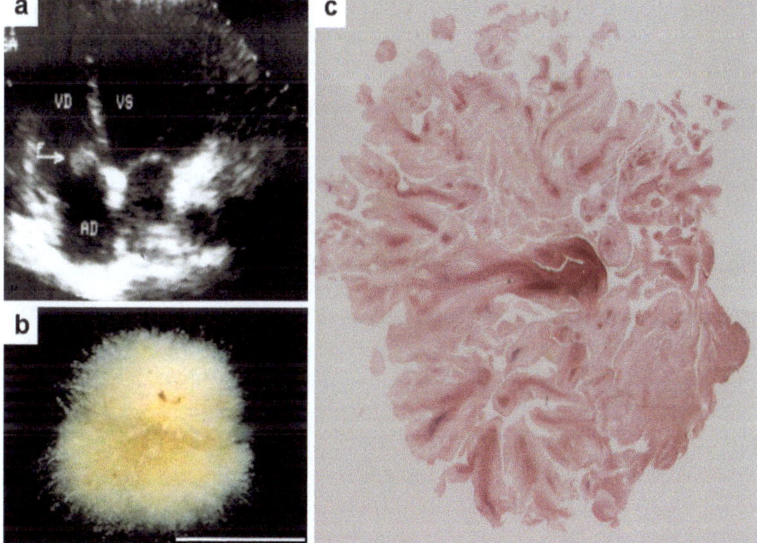

Fig. 19.12 Papillary fibroelastoma of the tricuspid valve. (**a**) Round shaped irregular mass mobile attached to the septal leaflet of the tricuspid valve; (**b**) At gross examination, the surgically resected mass appears as a sea anemone with multiple fronds; (**c**) At histology, multiple fibro-elastic fronds are branching out (elastic van Gieson stain)

Heart Valve Tumors

The right-sided valves can be affected by typical endocardial tumors such as papillary fibroelastoma (also known as endocardial papilloma) (Fig. 19.12) or hematic cyst (Fig. 19.13), the latter typically occurring in infancy (Basso et al. 2003; Valente et al. 1992; Gallucci et al. 1976; Scalia et al. 1997). While in the past these valve tumors were mostly an incidental autoptic observation, an exponential increase of clinically diagnosed fibroelastomas occurred in the last 20 years due to the widespread use of two-dimensional echocardiography, even in asymptomatic patients. At difference from left-sided fibroelastomas, the casual finding of right-sided one does not justify surgery, due to the trivial consequences of micro-embolization into the pulmonary circulation (Scalia et al. 1997), while antiplatelet therapy must be considered.

Functional TV Incompetence

Functional TV incompetence is far more frequent than the structural one. Dilatation of the right ventricular cavity and TV annulus, with consequent PM malalignement, can be due to any cause of right ventricular systolic hypertension (mitral valve stenosis, pulmonic stenosis, pulmonary hypertension as Eisenmenger's syndrome, primary pulmonary hypertension, cor pulmonale) or diastolic hypertension (dilated cardiomyopahy, right ventricular failure) (Waller et al. 1995a, b, c).

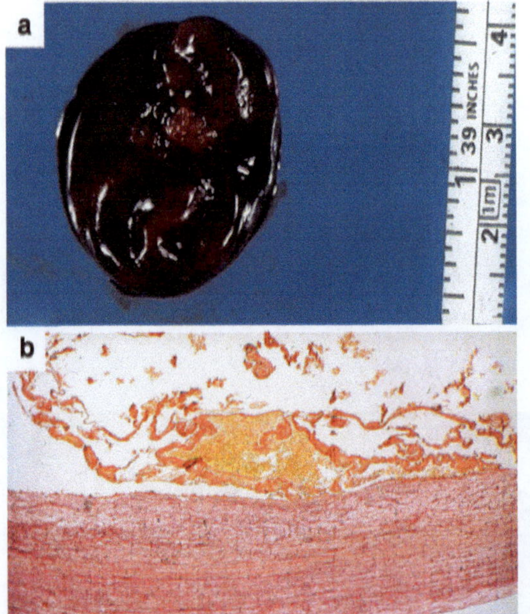

Fig. 19.13 Hematic cyst of the tricuspid valve. (**a**) Gross view of the surgically resected tricuspid valve cyst full of blood; (**b**) Histology of the previous (elastic van Gieson stain)

Pulmonary Valve Pathology

The pulmonary valve is exceptionally affected by acquired valvular diseases, such as rheumatic valve disease, infective endocarditis, carcinoid disease (Fig. 19.14) and tumors (see above), whereas congenital malformations are relatively more frequent (Stamm et al. 1998; Thiene and Frescura 2010).

The pulmonary valve may be bicuspid, much less frequently than the aortic valve, or even quadricuspid, with normally functioning valve. Bicuspid pulmonary valve is a frequent finding in tetralogy of Fallot and may be stenotic. Pulmonary valve stenosis with intact ventricular septum is one of the most frequent congenital heart diseases, accounting for up to 5–10%. The substrate of stenosis consists usually of a dome-shaped valve with central restricted orifice and three discrete raphae. When the valve stenosis is severe and associated with patent foramen ovale or fossa ovalis type atrial septal defect, an inter-atrial right-to-left shunt occurs accounting for

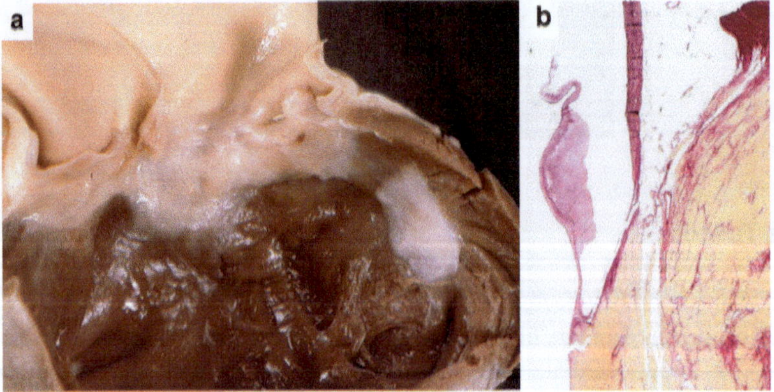

Fig. 19.14 Pulmonary valve incompetence due to carcinoid valve disease. (**a**) Right ventricular outflow tract showing the cusp fusion with the pulmonary root wall and the white fibrous carcinoid plaque superimposed to the outflow tract endocardium; (**b**) At histology, the carcinoid plaque consists of fibrous tissue proliferation on the pulmonary side, upon an underlying almost preserved semilunar cusp (elastic van Gieson stain)

cyanosis (so-called trilogy of Fallot, namely pulmonary stenosis with intact ventricular septum and atrial septal defect). More rarely, the stenotic valve shows three discrete commissures and cusps, which appear dysplastic with cauliflower excrescences. Subpulmonary valve stenosis can be due to a huge moderator band or anomalous septo-parietal band obstructing the right ventricular outflow tract.

References

Anderson KR, Zuberbuhler JR, Anderson RH, Becker AE, Lie JT. Morphologic spectrum of Ebstein's anomaly of the heart: a review. Mayo Clin Proc. 1979;5:174–80.

Badano LP, Agricola E, de Perez Isla L, Gianfagna P, Zamorano JL. Evaluation of the tricuspid valve morphology and function by transthoracic real-time three-dimensional echocardiography. Eur J Echocardiogr. 2009;10:477–84.

Basso C, Bottio T, Valente M, Bonato R, Casarotto D, Thiene G. Primary cardiac valve tumours. Heart. 2003;89:1259–60.

Bharucha T, Anderson RH, Lim ZS, Vettukattil JJ. Multiplanar review of three-dimensional echocardiography gives new insights into the morphology of Ebstein's malformation. Cardiol Young. 2010;20:49–53.

Cosío FG, Anderson RH, Kuck KH, Becker A, Borggrefe M, Campbell RW, Gaita F, Guiraudon GM, Haïssaguerre M, Rufilanchas JJ, Thiene G, Wellens HJ, Langberg J, Benditt DG, Bharati S, Klein G, Marchlinski F, Saksena S. Living anatomy of the atrioventricular junctions. A guide to electrophysiologic mapping. A Consensus Statement from the Cardiac Nomenclature Study Group, Working Group of Arrhythmias, European Society of Cardiology, and the Task Force on Cardiac Nomenclature from NASPE. Circulation. 1999;100:e31–7.

Frescura C, Angelini A, Daliento L, Thiene G. Morphological aspects of Ebstein's anomaly in adults. Thorac Cardiovasc Surg. 2000;48:203–8.

Gallucci V, Stritoni P, Fasoli G, Thiene G. Giant blood cyst of tricuspid valve. Successful excision in an infant. Br Heart J. 1976;38:990–2.

Ho SY, Goltz D, McCarthy K, Cook AC, Connell MG, Smith A, Anderson RH. The atrioventricular junctions in Ebstein malformation. Heart. 2000;83:444–9.

Lamers WH, Virágh S, Wessels A, Moorman AF, Anderson RH. Formation of the tricuspid valve in the human heart. Circulation. 1995;91:111–21.

Martinez RM, O'Leary PW, Anderson RH. Anatomy and echocardiography of the normal and abnormal tricuspid valve. Cardiol Young. 2006;16 Suppl 3:4–11.

Muraru D, Badano LP, Sarais C, Soldà E, Iliceto S. Evaluation of tricuspid valve morphology and function by transthoracic three-dimensional echocardiography. Curr Cardiol Rep. 2011a;13:242–9.

Muraru D, Tuveri MF, Marra MP, Badano LP, Iliceto S. Carcinoid tricuspid valve disease: incremental value of three-dimensional echocardiography. Eur J Echocardiogr. 2012;13:329.

Scalia D, Basso C, Rizzoli G, Lupia M, Budano S, Thiene G, Venturini A. Should right-sided fibroelastomas be operated upon? J Heart Valve Dis. 1997;6:647–50.

Schreiber C, Cook A, Ho SY, Augustin N, Anderson RH. Morphologic spectrum of Ebstein's malformation: revisitation relative to surgical repair. J Thorac Cardiovasc Surg. 1999;117:148–55.

Silver MM, Silver MD. Examination of the heart and of cardiovascular specimens in surgical pathology. In: Silver MD, Gotlieb AI, Schoen FJ, editors. Cardiovascular pathology. New York: Churchill Livingstone; 2001. p. 1–29.

Stamm C, Anderson RH, Ho SY. Clinical anatomy of the normal pulmonary root compared with that in isolated pulmonary valvular stenosis. J Am Coll Cardiol. 1998;31:1420–5.

Stellin G, Santini F, Thiene G, Bortolotti U, Daliento L, Milanesi O, Sorbara C, Mazzucco A, Casarotto D. Pulmonary atresia, intact ventricular septum, and Ebstein anomaly of the tricuspid valve. Anatomic and surgical considerations. J Thorac Cardiovasc Surg. 1993;106:255–61.

Sutton 3rd JP, Ho SY, Vogel M, Anderson RH. Is the morphologically right atrioventricular valve tricuspid? J Heart Valve Dis. 1995;4:571–5.

Thiene G, Basso C. Pathology and pathogenesis of infective endocarditis in native heart valves. Cardiovasc Pathol. 2006;15:256–63.

Thiene G, Frescura C. Anatomical and pathophysiological classification of congenital heart disease. Cardiovasc Pathol. 2010;19:259–74.

Valente M, Basso C, Thiene G, Bressan M, Stritoni P, Cocco P, Fasoli G. Fibroelastic papilloma: a not so benign cardiac tumor. Cardiovasc Pathol. 1992;1:161–6.

Veinot JP, Ghadially FN, Walley VM. Light microscopy and ultrastructure of the blood vessels and heart. In: Silver MD, Gotlieb AI, Schoen FJ, editors. Cardiovascular pathology. New York: Churchill Livingstone; 2001. p. 30–53.

Waller BF, Howard J, Fess S. Pathology of tricuspid valve stenosis and pure tricuspid regurgitation–part I. Clin Cardiol. 1995a;18:97–102.

Waller BF, Howard J, Fess S. Pathology of tricuspid valve stenosis and pure tricuspid regurgitation–part II. Clin Cardiol. 1995b;18:167–74.

Waller BF, Howard J, Fess S. Pathology of tricuspid valve stenosis and pure tricuspid regurgitation–part III. Clin Cardiol. 1995c;18:225–30.

Xanthos T, Dalivigkas I, Ekmektzoglou KA. Anatomic variations of the cardiac valves and papillary muscles of the right heart. Ital J Anat Embryol. 2011;116:111–26.

Zuberbuhler JR, Becker AE, Anderson RH, Lenox CC. Ebstein's malformation and the embryological development of the tricuspid valve. With a note on the nature of "clefts" in the atrioventricular valves. Pediatr Cardiol. 1984;5:289–95.

Mechanisms, Evaluation and Management of Tricuspid Regurgitation

20

Luigi P. Badano and Denisa Muraru

Introduction

With respect to heart valve diseases, until recently tricuspid valve regurgitation has not received as much attention as the aortic or mitral valve lesions and therefore it has been often referred as the "forgotten valve" (Mascherbauer and Maurer 2010). While trivial or mild tricuspid regurgitation may be detected in 80–90% of normal subjects undergoing modern echocardiography (Singh et al. 1999; Klein et al. 1990) and it is usually benign, hemodynamically significant tricuspid regurgitation can lead to debilitating symptoms and it is associated with poor prognosis in a number of cardiovascular diseases (Nath et al. 2004).

Today, diagnostic techniques and appropriate management strategies for patients with tricuspid regurgitation are established and continually refined. Therefore, it is important that clinicians consider assessing the severity of tricuspid regurgitation, understand its pathophysiology, choose appropriate imaging techniques and refer patients for timely intervention to prevent clinical deterioration and subsequent adverse consequences.

L.P. Badano (✉) • D. Muraru
Department of Cardiac, Thoracic and Vascular Sciences, University of Padua, Padua, Italy
e-mail: lpbadano@gmail.com

Epidemiology

Using echocardiography, the Framingham Heart study investigators found a prevalence of moderate or severe tricuspid regurgitation of 0.8% and an increased prevalence with ageing (Singh et al. 1999). Overall, the prevalence of significant tricuspid regurgitation was 4.3 times greater in females than in males.

Tricuspid regurgitation is frequently present in patients with mitral valve disease and more than one-third of patients with mitral stenosis have at least moderate tricuspid regurgitation (Sagie et al. 1997; Boyaci et al. 2007). Severe tricuspid regurgitation has been reported in 23–37% of patients after mitral valve replacement for rheumatic valve disease (Izumi et al. 2002; Porter et al. 1999). In the majority of patients, tricuspid regurgitation is not related to any primary valve pathology and it is defined "functional". Functional tricuspid regurgitation is frequently observed in the advanced stage of left-sided valvular heart disease or myocardial disease (Bruce and Connolly 2009).

In 14% of patients, tricuspid regurgitation may occur in the absence of structural tricuspid valve alterations, pulmonary hypertension or left heart dysfunction (Izumi et al. 2002).

Finally, the development of hemodynamically significant tricuspid regurgitation has been reported in 27% of patients who had only mild tricuspid regurgitation at the time of left-sided valve surgery (Dreyfus et al. 2005). In most cases, tricuspid regurgitation is diagnosed late after

N.M. Rajamannan (ed.), *Cardiac Valvular Medicine*,
DOI 10.1007/978-1-4471-4132-7_20, © Springer-Verlag London 2013

mitral valve replacement, 10 years on average, but can appear as late as 24 years after the initial surgery (Izumi et al. 2002; Porter et al. 1999). Matsunaga and Duran (2005) reported moderate or severe tricuspid regurgitation in 74% of patients who underwent surgical repair of ischemic mitral regurgitation 3 years before.

Aetiology and Mechanisms of Tricuspid Regurgitation

The aetiology of tricuspid regurgitation is generally divided into primary (or intrinsic) valve disease and secondary (or functional) valve dysfunction (Table 20.1). Primary tricuspid regurgitation results from structural abnormalities of valve apparatus, may be congenital or acquired and accounts for only 8–10% of all severe tricuspid regurgitations (Nath et al. 2004; Mutlak et al. 2007). Secondary or functional tricuspid regurgitation is usually due to tricuspid annulus dilatation caused by right ventricular dilatation and dysfunction, that may be primary or secondary to left heart diseases resulting in pulmonary hypertension (Fig. 20.1). However, despite the fact that pulmonary arterial hypertension from any cause is known to be associated with the occurrence of secondary or functional tricuspid regurgitation, not all patients with pulmonary hypertension develop significant tricuspid regurgitation, since its mechanisms are multifactorial. Mutlak et al. (2009) assessed the determinants of tricuspid regurgitation severity in a large cohort (2,139 patients) with either mild (<50 mmHg), moderate (50–70 mmHg) or severe (>70 mmHg) elevation of pulmonary artery systolic pressure. In this population, elevated pulmonary artery systolic pressure was associated with more severe tricuspid regurgitation (odds ratio 2.26 per 10 mmHg increase). However, a large number of patients with elevated pulmonary artery systolic pressure showed only mild tricuspid regurgitation (65.4% of patients with moderate and 45.6% of patients with severe pulmonary hypertension, respectively). Authors showed that other factors such as atrial fibrillation, pacemaker leads and right ventricular remodeling were also significant determinants of the severity of tricuspid regurgitation. Among them, remodeling of the right heart in response to the increase in pulmonary artery systolic pressure was the most powerful predictor of tricuspid regurgitation. This data confirms earlier observations that annular dilatation, right ventricular dilatation or tricuspid valve tenting and not pulmonary hypertension itself are the main determinants of functional tricuspid regurgitation (Sagie et al. 1994).

Even in the absence of pulmonary hypertension, tricuspid annular dilatation may cause significant regurgitation. In patients with chronic pulmonary thromboembolic hypertension and in patients with mitral stenosis in whom tricuspid regurgitation resolved after successful pulmonary

Table 20.1 Aetiology of tricuspid regurgitation

Functional (morphological normal leaflets with annular dilatation) (**75%**)
Left heart diseases (LV dysfunction or valve diseases) resulting in pulmonary hypertension
Primary pulmonary hypertension
Secondary pulmonary hypertension (e.g. chronic lung disease, pulmonary thromboembolism, left-to-right shunt)
Right ventricular dysfunction from any cause (e.g. myocardial diseases, ischemic heart disease)
Atrial fibrillation
Cardiac tumors (particularly right atrial myxomas)
Structural abnormality of the tricuspid valve (**25%**)
Rheumatic
Prolapse
Congenital Ebstein anomaly Tricuspid valve dysplasia Tricuspid valve hypoplasia Tricuspid valve cleft Double orifice tricuspid valve Unguarded tricuspid valve orifice
Endocarditis
Endomyocardial fibrosis
Carcinoid disease
Traumatic (blunt chest injury, laceration)
Iatrogenic Pace-maker/defibrillator lead interference Right ventricular biopsy Drugs (e.g. exposure to fenfluramine-phentermine, or methysergide) Radiation

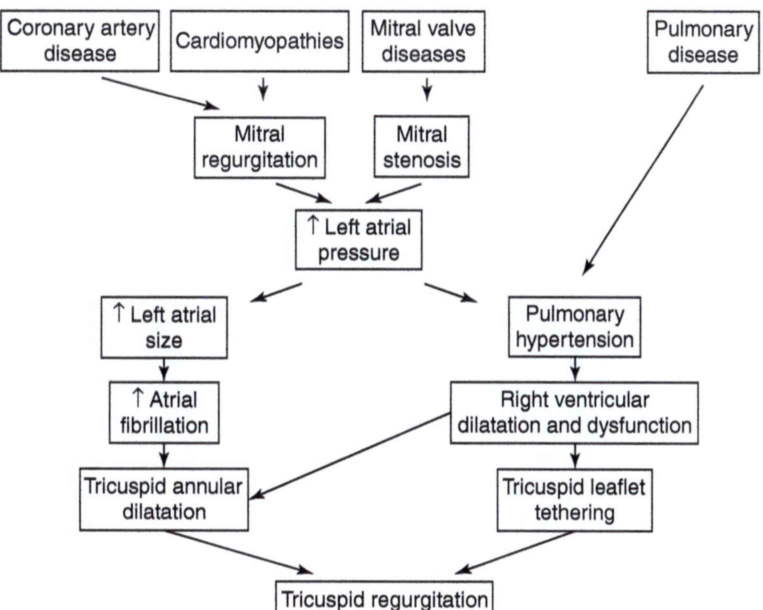

Fig. 20.1 Mechanisms of secondary or functional tricuspid regurgitation

thromboandoarterectomy or mitral balloon valvuloplasty, there was no change in tricuspid annulus diameter after the resolution of pulmonary hypertension (Sagie et al. 1997; Sadeghi et al. 2004; Song et al. 2007). These observations suggest that tricuspid annulus dilatation could be irreversible and might be the mechanism of late tricuspid regurgitation encountered in mitral valve diseases. Once tricuspid regurgitation has become significant, progressive right ventricular remodeling and dysfunction due to chronic volume overload result in papillary muscle displacement and leaflet tethering, which worsen tricuspid regurgitation and lead to further right ventricular dilatation (Fukuda et al. 2005). On the other hand, the dilated right ventricle may also compress the left ventricle via chamber interdependence, leading to an increase of pulmonary pressure which, in turn, will worsen tricuspid regurgitation.

Particular cases of tricuspid regurgitation are those developing after blunt chest trauma or as a consequence of pacemaker or defibrillator leads, which may directly interfere with leaflet coaptation while crossing the valve from the right atrium to the right ventricle. Tricuspid regurgitation is a rare complication of blunt chest trauma, most frequently of high energy road traffic accidents. If the acute rise in right intraventricular cavity pressure happens when the valve is closed, it may result in chordal rupture, however both anterior papillary muscle rupture or leaflet tears (primarily the anterior leaflet) have also been reported (van Son et al. 1994; Dounis et al. 2002). In the acute phase of the injury, the traumatic lesion can go undetected. In the chronic phase, many patients remain asymptomatic, while others exhibit symptoms and signs of right heart failure (van Son et al. 1994).

Tricuspid regurgitation due to endocardial lead implantation or removal of permanent pacemakers or implantable cardioverter defibrillators is a known complication of these procedures (Lin et al. 2005; Seo et al. 2008; Kim et al. 2008; Franceschi et al. 2009). Conflicting data have been reported about the incidence of tricuspid regurgitation related to endocardial lead implantation (Lin et al. 2005; Kim et al. 2008). The reported incidence of at least moderate tricuspid regurgitation ranged between 7% and 39% (Seo et al. 2008; Kim et al. 2008; Alizadeh et al. 2011; Klutstein et al. 2009; Kucukarslan et al. 2006; Liebowitz et al. 2000; Paniagua et al. 1998; Rubio and al-Bassam 1991; Sakai et al. 1987; Vaturi et al. 2010). However, there are significant limitations in these reports: most of them were retrospective, the number of enrolled patients was limited, the length of follow-up was not predefined, the methods used to assess the severity of tricuspid regurgitation were quite different and mainly qualitative. The mechanisms by which a right ventricular lead may induce tricuspid regurgitation remains to be clarified. Several investigators have documented a mechanical interference of the lead with the valve leaflets leading to impaired valve closure (Seo et al. 2008; Kim et al. 2008; Klutstein et al. 2009; Nucifora et al. 2007). Others have found that delayed right ventricular activation and/or alteration in right ventricular geometry and/or right ventricular dyssynchrony induced by active right ventricular pacing may cause tricuspid valve malfunction and regurgitation (Vaturi et al. 2010). The mechanical (lead interference) and functional (valve malfunction induced by active right ventricular pacing) mechanisms may also coexist, but the relative contribution of the two remains to be defined. Sakai et al. (1987) studied 26 paced hearts at autopsy and reported an interference of the pacemaker lead with the valve leaflets in 42% of cases (interference with leaflet motion in two patients, entanglement of valve chordae in four patients, and coexistence of the two in five patients). Lin et al. (2005) in a retrospective study of 41 patients identified 4 mechanisms by which right ventricular lead led to severe tricuspid regurgitation: perforation of valve leaflets, entanglement of the lead with subvalvular apparatus, impingement of the tricuspid valve leaflets, and lead adherence to the tricuspid valve.

The time course for tricuspid regurgitation development/progression after pacemaker implantation also remains to be defined. Pathological studies have detected major inflammatory changes within the heart only few days after lead implantation (Becker et al. 1972). It has been postulated that progression of inflammation over weeks to months may lead to the formation of fibrous tissue involving the pacemaker lead and resulting in lead fusion and adherence to the various components of the tricuspid valve apparatus, causing regurgitation. This has important implications on management, since an early detection of catheter-related tricuspid regurgitation may be solved by lead repositioning only if it is performed shortly after lead implantation, but the procedure can be difficult, if not impossible, during the chronic stage.

Finally, tricuspid regurgitation may be iatrogenic. Franceschi et al. (2009) performed a prospective study during which they removed 237 catheters in 208 patients implanted 46 months before. New tricuspid regurgitation occurred in 19 patients (9.1%) and it was severe in 14. Three independent risk factors of traumatic tricuspid regurgitation were identified: use of laser sheath, use of both laser sheath and lasso, and female sex. However, the strongest risk factor appears to be related to the use of specific extraction tools, due to the failure of simple traction. The anatomic substrate is related to the fibrous growth around the whole length of the lead, with attachments to surrounding structures including the tricuspid valve (Candinas et al. 1999; Robboy et al. 1969).

Another cause of iatrogenic, traumatic tricuspid regurgitation is represented by repeated endomyocardial biopsies. Tricuspid regurgitation is the most frequent valvular abnormality that occurs after cardiac transplantation (Aziz et al. 1999; Nguyen et al. 2005). Mielniczuk et al. (2005) found histologic findings of chordal tissue in 47% of endomyocardial biopsy specimens from heart transplant patients in whom a significant tricuspid regurgitation was detected. These findings suggest that chordal damage at the time of endomyocardial biopsy leading to tricuspid valve prolapse is the cause of tricuspid regurgitation in these patients. In 101 patients who underwent orthotopic cardiac transplantation and survived more than 1 year, Nguyen et al. (2005) reported that 25% developed a severe tricuspid regurgitation (4% required valve replacement for refractory right-sided heart failure). In their series, there was no case of severe tricuspid regurgitation in those patients who underwent less than 18 biopsies, conversely the incidence of severe tricuspid regurgitation was 60% in those who underwent more than 31 endomyocardial biopsies.

Tricuspid regurgitation is also a dynamic phenomenon which shows respiratory changes of large magnitude and complex pathophysiology that are independent on severity and pathogenesis of the regurgitation and degree of associated pulmonary hypertension (Topilsky et al. 2010). Topilsky et al. (2010) performed a quantitative echo-Doppler study to elucidate the mechanics of respiratory variations of tricuspid regurgitation. They observed marked right ventricular (and not right atrial) changes in size and shape during inspiration, particularly right ventricular widening. Right ventricular widening was associated with inspiratory annular enlargement, leading to less systolic annular coverage by tricuspid leaflets and increased valvular tenting, both of which contribute to coaptation loss and increase in effective regurgitant orifice. Therefore, despite a decline in regurgitant gradient, a large increase in effective regurgitant orifice occurs during inspiration causing a notable increase in regurgitant volume.

Natural History

Some patients with isolated chronic severe tricuspid regurgitation may remain asymptomatic for some time, while others may experience fatigue and decreased exercise tolerance as a result of a reduced cardiac output. As the right atrial pressure increases, patients may experience the classic symptoms caused by right-sided heart failure: peripheral oedema, abdominal fullness, ascites, hepatomegaly and decreased appetite. As the right atrium enlarges, the incidence of atrial fibrillation increases, leading itself to further right atrial and tricuspid annulus dilatation and clinical deterioration. If left untreated, severe tricuspid regurgitation will determine right ventricular failure which will result in severe peripheral oedema, ascites and severe functional limitation. It has been reported that increasing severity of tricuspid regurgitation is associated with worsening prognosis, independently from left ventricular function or pulmonary pressure (Nath et al. 2004; Messika-Zeitoun et al. 2004).

Clinical Evaluation

The most prominent features during physical examination of patients with tricuspid regurgitation are those related to the characteristics of the murmur and to the development of right-sided congestive heart failure. With severe right-sided failure, at inspection patients with severe tricuspid regurgitation show evidence of weight loss and cachexia, cyanosis and jaundice (reflecting hepatic insufficiency). Ascites and peripheral edema of variable entity may occur, and anasarca is present in severe disease.

Distended and prominent jugular veins are apparent and reflect the elevation in right atrial pressure. The normal x and x′ descents disappear, and a prominent systolic wave, i.e., a c–v wave (or s wave), due to systolic regurgitation in the right atrium becomes apparent. The descent of this wave, the y descent, is sharp and becomes the most prominent feature of the venous pulse. Jugular venous distension may be more prominent during inspiration, as a result of increased venous return. However, this finding may be difficult to detect when the venous distension is marked. A venous systolic thrill and murmur in the neck may be present in patients with severe tricuspid regurgitation.

Palpation of the chest often reveals a hyperdynamic right ventricular impulse which is thrusting in quality. The liver is often enlarged and tender and its systolic pulsations are commonly present initially. However, in patients with longstanding chronic tricuspid regurgitation the liver evolves to congestive cirrhosis and may become firm and nontender.

Auscultation usually reveals an S3 which varies in intensity and with inspiration (usually accentuated by inspiration), and originates from the right ventricle when it is extremely dilated. Intensity of P2 is usually accentuated, and splitting of S2 may be marked when tricuspid regurgitation is associated with pulmonary hypertension. The systolic murmur of tricuspid regurgitation may vary in intensity, duration, timing and location. With mild regurgitation, the murmur may be soft, short in duration, or absent.

With increasing regurgitation, the systolic murmur is usually high-pitched, holosystolic and loudest in the 4th intercostal space in the parasternal region, but occasionally is loudest in the subxyphoid area. When the right ventricle is greatly dilated and occupies the anterior surface of the heart, the murmur may be best appreciated at the apex and difficult to distinguish from that produced by mitral regurgitation.

Maneuvers which result in an increase in venous return (inspiration, leg raising, hepatic compression, exercise) characteristically increase the intensity of the murmur of tricuspid regurgitation. The murmur is characteristically augmented in intensity and duration during inspiration (Rivero-Carvallo's sign) in patients with mild to moderate tricuspid regurgitation. Respiratory variation may become difficult to appreciate in patients with severe regurgitation or marked right ventricular enlargement and dysfunction. In these cases, the inspiratory augmentation may be elicited by standing. The murmur also increases during the Mueller maneuver (forced inspiration against a closed glottis). It demonstrates an immediate overshoot after release of the Valsalva strain, but is reduced in intensity and duration in the standing position and during the strain of the Valsalva maneuver. Tricuspid valve prolapse, like mitral valve prolapse, causes nonejection systolic clicks and late systolic murmurs. However, in tricuspid valve prolapse, these findings are more prominent at the lower left sternal border. With inspiration, the clicks occur later, the murmurs intensify and become shorter in duration.

Role of Imaging Techniques

Cardiac Catheterization

Before the introduction of two-dimensional and Doppler echocardiography, cardiac catheterization was used to confirm the presence and severity of tricuspid regurgitation. The diagnosis of tricuspid regurgitation posed a greater challenge, as selective angiography into the right ventricle would often distort the tricuspid valve. In addition, right ventriculography is particularly difficult when tricuspid regurgitation is present, since it is difficult to maintain catheter position in the right ventricle. The pressure waveform in the right atrium shows the characteristic prominent systolic V wave with rapid descent only in the most severe cases. At present, diagnostic cardiac catheterization should rarely, if ever, be undertaken for the diagnosis or quantitation of tricuspid valve disease alone.

Chest X-Ray

Chest radiograph is also of limited utility. Cardiomegaly associated with prominent right-heart borders may be noted, but there are no specific findings which suggest a diagnosis of tricuspid valve disease. A prominent cardiac silhouette is observed on the right with the postero-anterior view, and the enlarged right ventricle fills in the retrosternal space on the lateral view.

Echocardiography

Two-dimensional echocardiography combined with spectral and color flow Doppler evaluation provides the most accurate laboratory test in detection and quantitation of tricuspid valve regurgitation (Lancellotti et al. 2010). "Physiological" tricuspid regurgitation is associated with normal valve leaflet morphology and normal right ventricular and atrial size. The color jet is localized in a small region adjacent to valve closure (less than 1 cm), is thin, central and often does not extend throughout systole. Peak systolic velocities are between 1.7 and 2.3 m/s.

When a "pathologic" tricuspid regurgitation is detected at color Doppler, a complete understanding of leaflet morphology and of the pathophysiological mechanisms underlying tricuspid regurgitation is mandatory. In these cases, a more comprehensive assessment of the morphology of tricuspid valve apparatus using transthoracic three-dimensional echocardiography (Figs. 20.2 and 20.3) provides important clues on the underlying aetiology and mechanisms of valve dysfunction (Badano et al. 2009; Muraru and Badano 2011).

Ebstein's anomaly is characterized by apical displacement of the septal tricuspid leaflet into the right ventricle by more than 8 mm/m² from the insertion point of the anterior mitral leaflet from the crux (Fig. 20.4). The right atrium is enlarged, composed of anatomic right atrium and atrialized proximal inflow right ventricle. The residual right ventricle is reduced in size.

The carcinoid syndrome leads to focal or diffuse deposits of fibrous tissue on the endocardium of the valvular cusps and cardiac chambers and on the intima of the great veins and coronary sinus. The white, fibrous carcinoid plaques are most extensive on the right side of the heart, where they are usually deposited on the ventricular surfaces of the tricuspid valve and cause the cusps to adhere to the underlying right ventricular wall. As a consequence, the tricuspid valve in carcinoid heart disease is characterized by thickened immobile valve leaflets held in half-open position resulting in valvular stenosis, as well as in free-flowing regurgitation at color Doppler (Fig. 20.5) (Muraru et al. 2012).

Tricuspid regurgitation associated with the use of fenfluramine-phentermine or methysergide is characterized by thickened, fibrotic and hypomobile leaflets. However, these characteristics are quite aspecific and the correct diagnosis is usually reached after confirmation of drug use.

Rheumatic tricuspid valve disease is nearly always associated with rheumatic mitral and/or aortic valve disease. However, rheumatic involvement of the tricuspid valve is less common than that of left-sided valves. Regurgitation is a consequence of deformity, shortening and retraction of one or more leaflets of the tricuspid valve (Fig. 20.6), as well as of shortening and fusion of the chordae tendinee and papillary muscles. Two-dimensional echo usually detects the thickening and the distortion of the leaflets, but cannot provide a comprehensive assessment of the extension of valve apparatus involvement, which is usually better appreciated with three-dimensional echocardiography.

Tricuspid prolapse (Fig. 20.7) is generally associated with mitral valve prolapse and is defined as a 2-mm atrial displacement of the leaflet(s) in mid-systole. The coaptation line is behind the annular plane. Tricuspid prolapse most often involves the septal and the anterior leaflet. The most common phenotype of tricuspid prolapse is diffuse myxomatous degeneration (Barlow's disease). The characteristic appearance of tricuspid valve prolapse includes dilated annulus, billowing prolapse, less commonly chordae rupture with flail leaflet, unless it is consequence of endomyocardial biopsies, trauma or endocarditis.

Pacemaker /defibrillator lead impingement of the tricuspid valve leaflet can be identified as an interference of the lead with leaflet closure. Leaflet adherence can be diagnosed by visualizing the leaflet tethering by the endocardial lead throughout the cardiac cycle (Fig. 20.8).

Functional or secondary tricuspid regurgitation is characterized by annular dilatation (greater than 40 mm) and tethering of the leaflets, with a tenting distance greater than 8 mm. In most severe cases, the leaflets fail to coapt, resulting in a wide-open regurgitation (Fig. 20.9).

Color flow Doppler and spectral Doppler are sensitive for the detection of valve regurgitation and generally accurate for a semi-quantitative assessment of its severity (Lancellotti et al. 2010).

Tricuspid regurgitation using color flow imaging can be detected using both the parasternal (tricuspid inflow view and short-axis view at great vessels level), and apical or subcostal (4- chamber view) approaches. Regurgitant jet area correlates roughly with the severity of regurgitation, being less than 5 cm² in mild, 6–10 cm² in moderate and greater than 10 cm² in severe cases. In clinical practice, a visual estimate rather than actual planimetry is utilized. Detection of a large eccentric jet adhering, swirling and reaching the posterior wall of the right atrium is in favor of significant tricuspid regurgitation. Conversely, small thin central jets usually indicate mild tricuspid regurgitation. However, color Doppler method is a source of many errors, is limited by several technical and haemodynamic factors and therefore it is not recommended to assess tricuspid regurgitation severity (Lancellotti et al. 2010). A more accurate estimate may be obtained by utilizing jet vena contracta width and PISA (Proximal Isovelocity Surface Area) measurements.

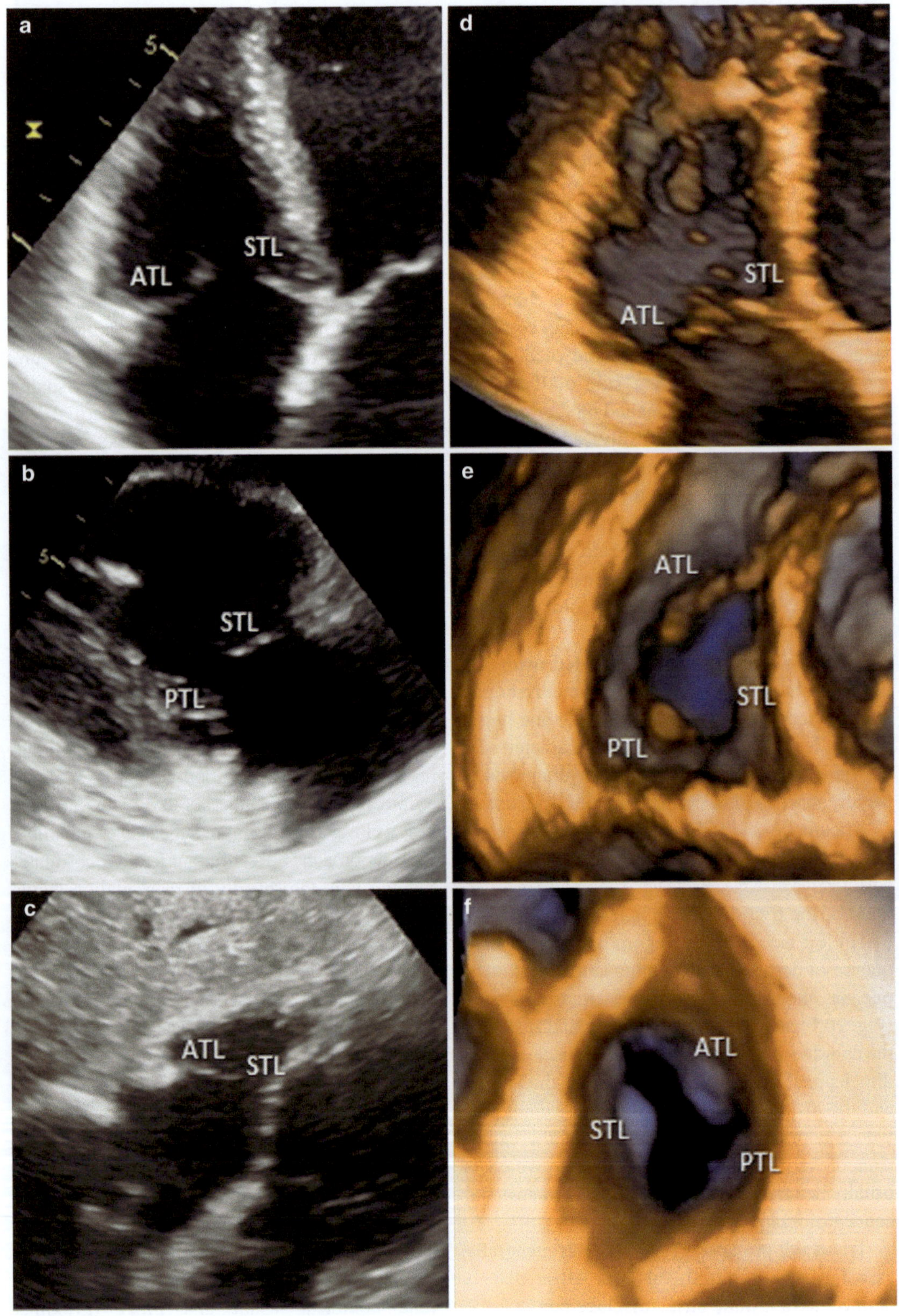
a
ATL
STL
b
STL
PTL
c
ATL
STL
d
STL
ATL
e
ATL
STL
PTL
f
ATL
STL
PTL

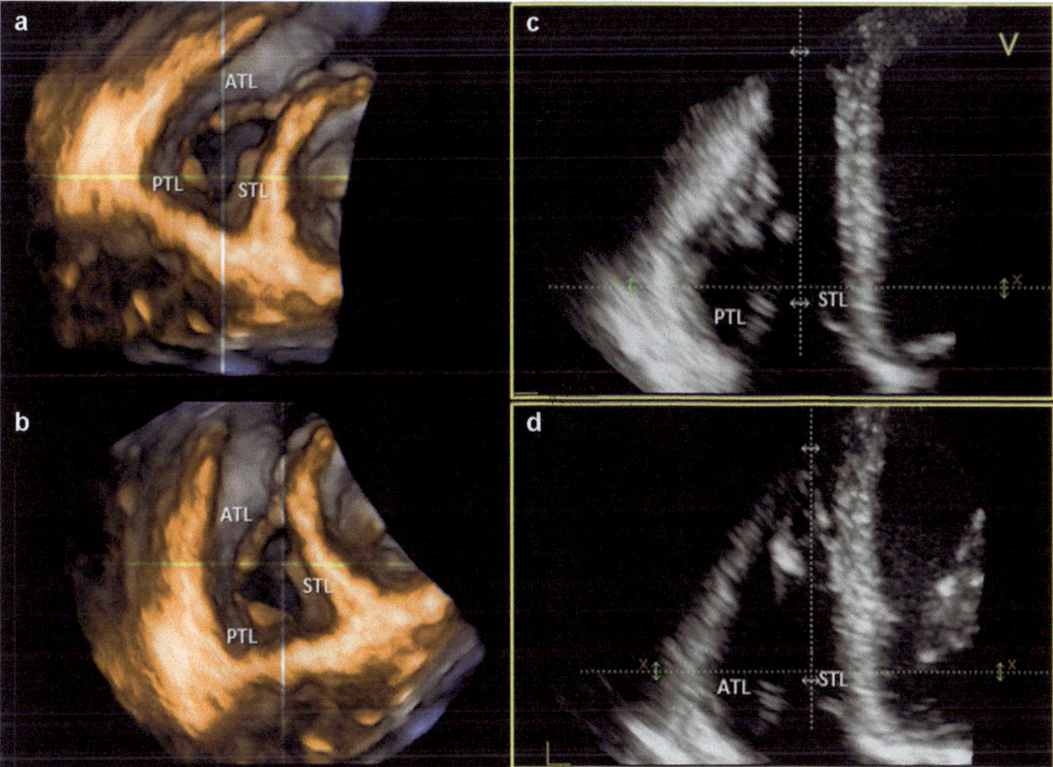

Fig. 20.3 Illustration of the variable visualization of tricuspid leaflets with 2D echocardiography (either septal and posterior, or septal and anterior), depending on the position of 4-chamber plane relative to the spatial configuration of tricuspid leaflets (*yellow horizontal line* on 3D valve rendering in (**a**) and (**c**), in correspondence with 2D views of the valve in panels (**b**) and (**d**), respectively). In contrast with 2D echocardiography which displays usually only 2 of the 3 leaflets and therefore leaves room to ambiguity, 3D echocardiography enables a precise morphologic evaluation of all three leaflets in a single view and a reliable identification of each one. Abbreviations: *ATL* anterior tricuspid leaflet, *PTL* posterior tricuspid leaflet, *STL* septal tricuspid leaflet

Vena contracta represents the cross-sectional area of the blood column as it leaves the regurgitant orifice; it reflects thus the regurgitant orifice area. The vena contracta of the tricuspid regurgitant jet is typically imaged in the apical 4-chamber view using a careful probe angulation to optimize the flow image, an adapted Nyquist limit (color Doppler scale, 40–70 cm/s) to perfectly identify the neck of the jet and a narrow sector scan coupled with the zoom mode to maximize temporal resolution and measurement accuracy (Fig. 20.10) (Tribouilloy et al. 2000). Averaging measurements over at least two-three beats is recommended. A vena contracta diameter

Fig. 20.2 Visualization of tricuspid valve apparatus by two-dimensional (**a**–**c**) and three-dimensional (**d**–**f**) echocardiography. (**a**) apical 4-chamber view; (**b**) right ventricular inflow; (**c**) subcostal view; (**d**) volume rendering of tricuspid valve apparatus with the cropping plane corresponding to apical 4-chamber view, allowing a comprehensive visualization of tricuspid leaflets, as well as of subvalvular apparatus, papillary muscles and moderator band; (**e**) volume rendering of tricuspid valve, seen en face from the right ventricle; (**f**) volume rendering of tricuspid valve, seen en face from the right atrium. Abbreviations: *ATL* anterior tricuspid leaflet, *PTL* posterior tricuspid leaflet, *STL* septal tricuspid leaflet

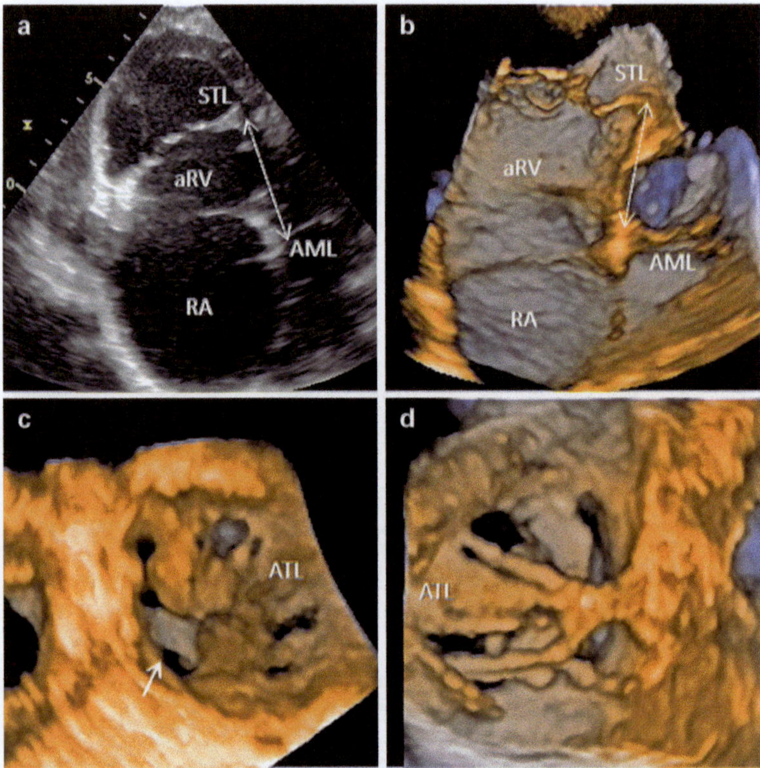

Fig. 20.4 Right heart involvement in a case with Ebstein disease. (**a**) Apical 4-chamber view, showing a severe enlargement of right heart cavities, with marked apical displacement of tricuspid septal leaflet relative to the mitral valve plane. (**b**) Similar view by 3D echocardiography, allowing a better perception of the dimensions of the atrialized portion of right ventricle. (**c**) Tricuspid valve viewed from the right atrium, depicting a large fenestrated anterior leaflet and a wide regurgitant orifice (*arrow*), while the septal and posterior leaflets are not apparent from this perspective. (**d**) Tricuspid valve viewed from the right ventricle, showing the insertion of the large anterior leaflet on the interventricular septum. Insertions of septal and posterior leaflets lay beyond the level of the cropping plane. Abbreviations: *AML* anterior mitral leaflet, *ATL* anterior tricuspid leaflet, *aRV* atrialized portion of the right ventricle, *RA* right atrium, *STL* septal tricuspid leaflet

larger than 6.5 mm is usually associated to severe tricuspid regurgitation. Intermediate values are not accurate for distinguishing moderate from mild tricuspid regurgitation. However, when measuring the vena contracta, it should be taken into account the fact that the regurgitant orifice geometry is complex and not necessarily circular (Fig. 20.10). This may explain the poor correlation found between the vena contracta width at two-dimensional color Doppler and the three-dimensional echo assessment of the effective regurgitant orifice area. Particular caution should be used in assessing eccentric jets. With three-dimensional color Doppler echo, an effective regurgitant orifice area larger than 75 mm² has been associated to severe tricuspid regurgitation (Velayudhan et al. 2006).

PISA radius measurement is by itself a good guide to severity of regurgitation, but the method should be properly performed. The apical 4-chamber view and the parasternal long- and short-axis views are classically recommended for an optimal visualization of the PISA. The area of interest is optimized by reducing imaging depth and Nyquist limit to approximately 15–40 cm/s. The PISA radius is measured at mid-systole using the first aliasing (Fig. 20.11). Qualitatively, a tricuspid regurgitation PISA radius >9 mm at a Nyquist limit of 28 cm/s has been associated with the presence of significant tricuspid regurgitation (corresponding

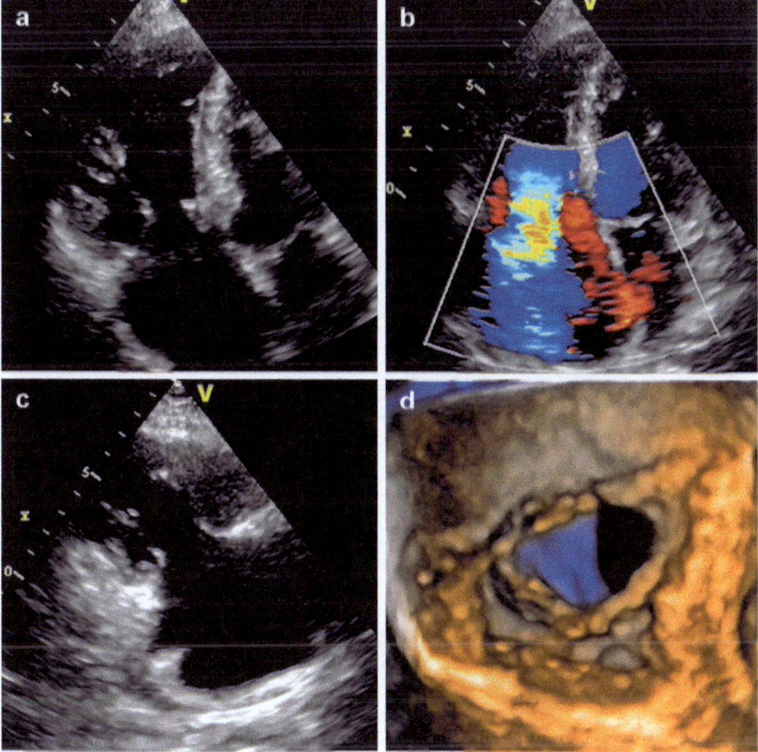

Fig. 20.5 Tricuspid valve involvement in carcinoid disease. (**a** and **c**) 4-chamber and right ventricular inflow view of tricuspid valve, showing the thickened and retracted leaflets, fixed in open position in systole and diastole, leading to massive tricuspid regurgitation (**b**); (**d**) 3D rendering of tricuspid valve seen en face from ventricular perspective, depicting the thickened fibrotic leaflets and a large central orifice resulting in tricuspid steno-insufficiency

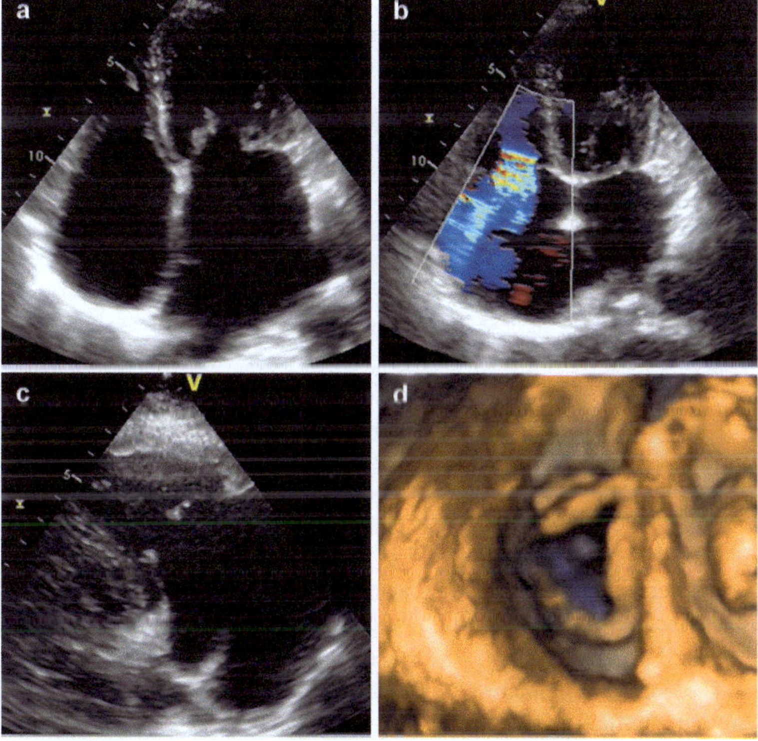

Fig. 20.6 Rheumatic tricuspid valve lesion with severe regurgitation and mild stenosis. (**a**) 4-chamber view showing severely enlarged atria and thickened leaflets of both atrio-ventricular valves; note that the opening of tricuspid valve does not seem to be reduced from this perspective. (**b**) Severe tricuspid regurgitation at color Doppler. (**c**) Tricuspid valve leaflets from right ventricular inflow view, which appear thickened and with diastolic doming. (**d**) 3D volume rendering of the tricuspid valve from ventricular perspective, showing thickened leaflets with fused commissures and restricted opening, which can be also planimetered

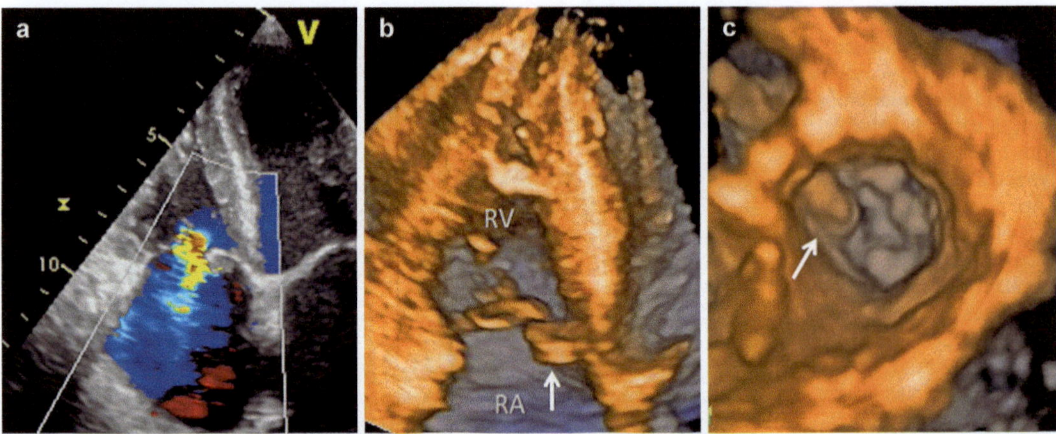

Fig. 20.7 Echocardiographic evaluation of the mechanism of tricuspid regurgitation in a heart transplant recipient. (**a**) Color Doppler showing an eccentric regurgitant jet with a large vena contracta, suggestive of severe organic tricuspid regurgitation. (**b**, **c**) 3D rendering of tricuspid valve, showing a flail of the septal leaflet (*arrow*). *RA* right atrium, *RV* right ventricle

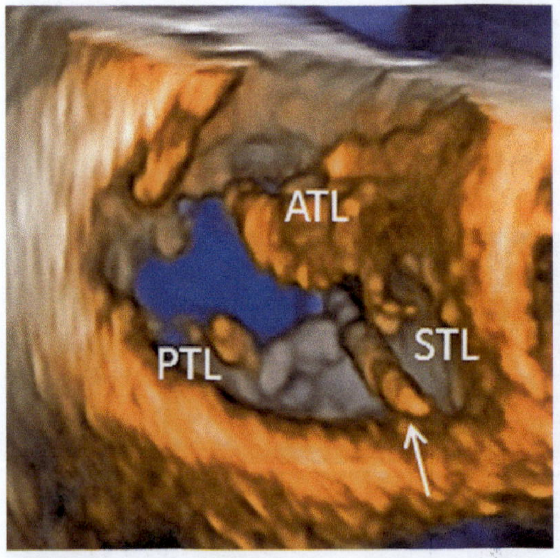

Fig. 20.8 3D volume rendering of tricuspid valve from ventricular view, demonstrating the interference of pacemaker lead (*arrow*) with the closure of septal leaflet

to an effective regurgitant orifice area larger than 40 mm² and a regurgitant volume greater than 45 ml), whereas a radius less than 5 mm suggests mild regurgitation. However, the PISA method also faces several limitations (Mascherbauer and Maurer 2010). It could underestimate the severity of TR by 30% and is less accurate in eccentric jets.

The spectral Doppler velocity tracing of tricuspid regurgitation reflects the pressure gradient between the right ventricle and the right atrium throughout systole. The shape of tricuspid regurgitation velocity profile using continuous wave Doppler provides a clue to this relationship. The regurgitation profile is generally parabolic except in severe cases, where high right atrial "C–V" waves result in a rapid equalization with right ventricular pressure, resulting in a rapid deceleration of the Doppler tracing, also described as the 'V' wave cut-off sign (Fig. 20.12).

Additional indirect clues of regurgitation severity are the density of continuous wave Doppler profile, the size of right ventricle and atrium, the paradoxical interventricular septal motion and the systolic bulge of interatrial septum toward left atrium. The hepatic vein flow may exhibit systolic reversal of flow in severe cases.

In clinical practice, echocardiographic assessment of tricuspid regurgitation includes integration of data from two- and three-dimensional imaging of the valve, right heart chambers, septal motion and inferior vena cava, as well as Doppler parameters of regurgitation severity (Table 20.2). Color flow Doppler extension of the jet should be assessed in multiple windows, and the grading of the severity of tricuspid regurgitation should be performed by measuring the vena contracta width and the PISA radius, except in the presence of mild or trivial tricuspid regurgitation (Lancellotti et al. 2010).

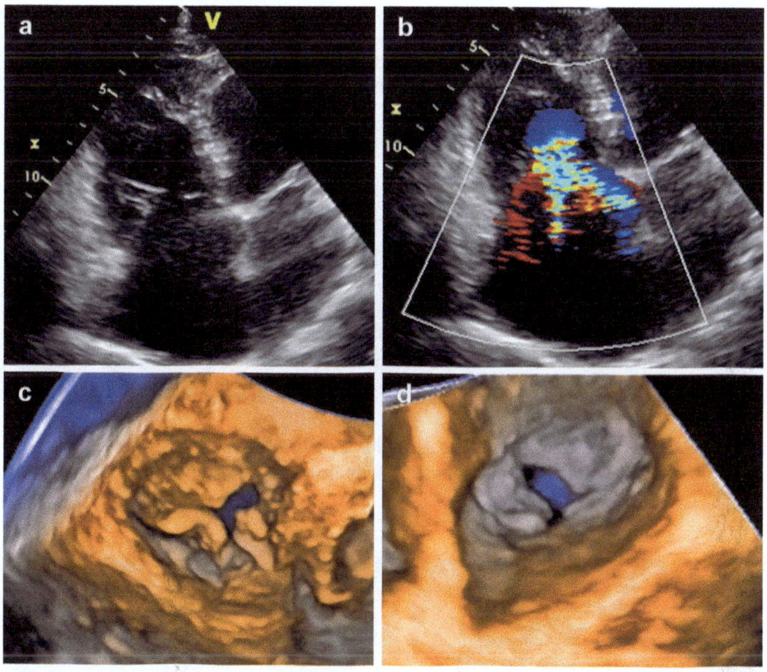

Fig. 20.9 Functional tricuspid regurgitation in a patient with sclerodermia and pulmonary arterial hypertension. (**a**) Apical 4-chamber view, showing right heart chamber enlargement with dilation of tricuspid annulus and leaflet tethering; (**b**) Color Doppler visualization of a moderate tricuspid regurgitation jet; (**c**) 3D volume rendering of tricuspid valve from the right ventricular perspective at end-systole, demonstrating tenting of tricuspid leaflets, being tethered by the attached cordae, the dilation and increased sphericity of the annulus and interventricular septal flattening as a consequence of elevated right ventricular systolic pressures; (**d**) 3D volume rendering of tricuspid leaflets during diastole

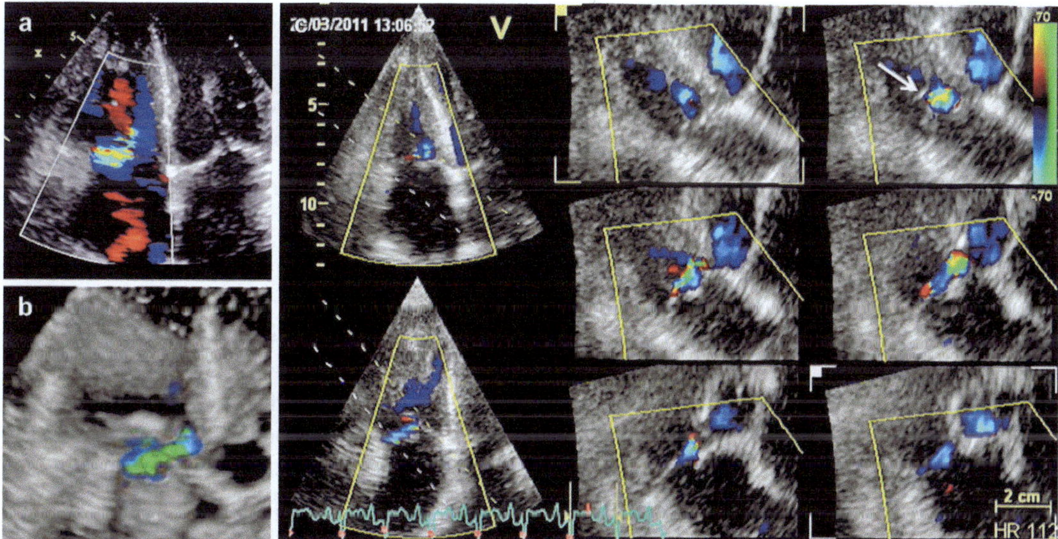

Fig. 20.10 3D color assessment of tricuspid regurgitation severity in a highly eccentric jet. (**a**) 2D color in 4-chamber view, showing a highly eccentric jet, difficult to quantify; (**b**) 3D color rendering of regurgitant jet, with a cropping plane oriented for a precise identification of jet origin and direction; (**c**) Multislice display of 3D color: 6 cross-sectional equidistant planes oriented perpendicular to the jet orientation, for the identification of vena contracta area (*arrow*)

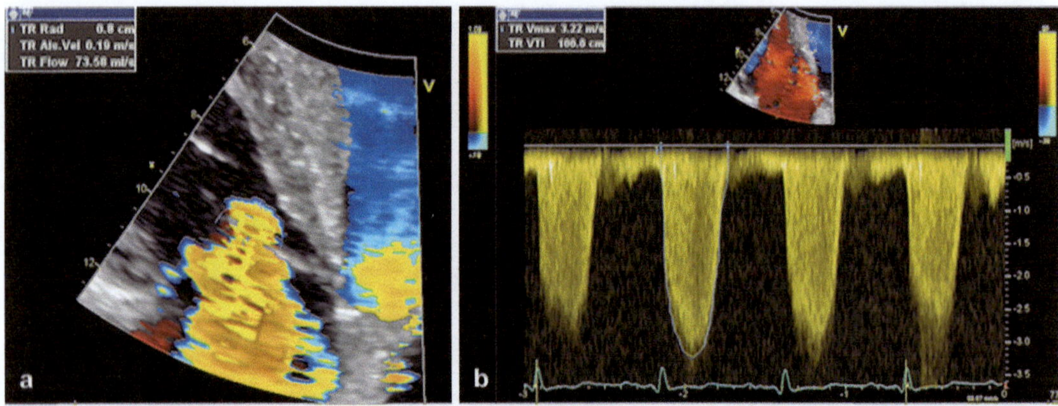

Fig. 20.11 Quantification of tricuspid regurgitation severity by PISA method. (**a**) Measurement of PISA radius. (**b**) Tracing of velocity-time integral on the continuous-wave Doppler signal of tricuspid regurgitation

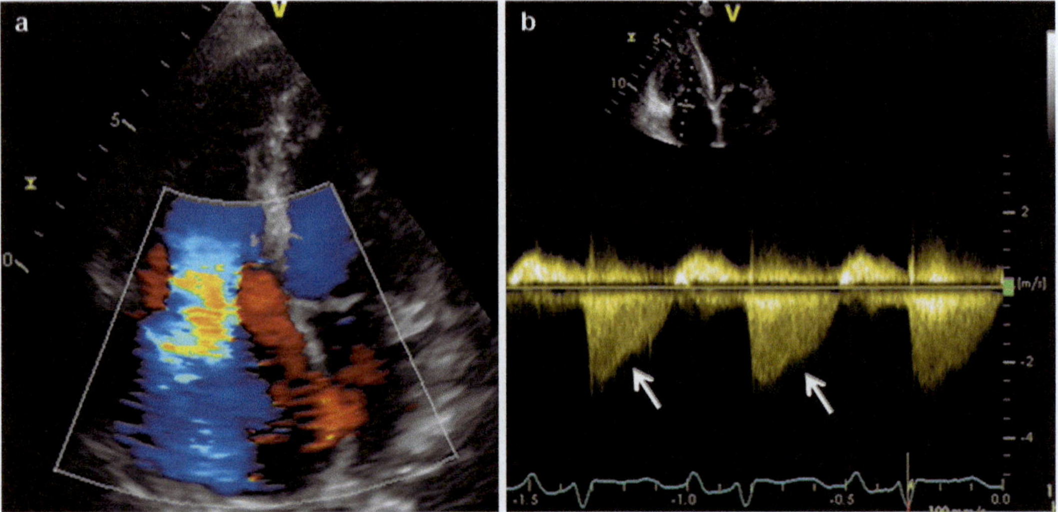

Fig. 20.12 Severe "free" tricuspid regurgitation (**a**) with the corresponding continuous Doppler signals of relatively low-amplitude, with "cut-off" sign (*arrow*, **b**)

Cardiac Magnetic Resonance

In the absence of specific contraindications, when echocardiographic imaging is limited by a suboptimal acoustic window, in patients with equivocal echocardiographic findings and when three-dimensional echocardiography is not available for assessing right ventricular volumes and function, cardiac magnetic resonance is the technique of choice to assess patients with significant tricuspid regurgitation. Cardiac magnetic resonance is not limited by acoustic window and can image the whole heart in any plane providing excellent myocardial definition. Cardiac magnetic resonance is presently the gold standard for the assessment of right ventricular morphology and function, and accurate assessment of the right ventricle is crucial to understand the underlying mechanisms and address management in patients with tricuspid regurgitation. Anwar et al. (2007) have also used cardiac magnetic resonance to assess the configuration of tricuspid valve annulus.

Table 20.2 Echocardiographic assessment of tricuspid regurgitation severity(Lancellotti et al. 2010)

Parameters	Mild	Moderate	Severe
Qualitative			
Tricuspid valve morphology	Normal/abnormal	Normal/abnormal	Abnormal/flail/large coaptation defect
Color flow TR jet (Mascherbauer and Maurer 2010)	Small, central	Intermediate	Very large central jet or eccentric wall impinging jet
CW signal of TR jet	Faint/parabolic	Dense/parabolic	Dense/triangular with early peaking (peak <2 m/s in massive TR)
Semi-quantitative			
VC width (mm)[a]	Not defined	<6.5	>6.5
PISA radius (mm)[b]	≤5	6–9	>9
Hepatic vein flow[c]	Systolic dominance	Systolic blunting	Systolic flow reversal
Tricuspid inflow	Normal	Normal	E wave dominant (≥1 cm/s)[d]
Quantitative			
EROA (mm²)	Not defined	Not defined	≥40
R Vol (ml)	Not defined	Not defined	≥ 45
+ RA/RV/IVC dimension[e]			

Modified from Lancellotti et al. (2010)

Normal 2D measurements from the apical 4-chamber view: Mid RV diameter ≤3.3 cm, RV end-diastolic area ≤28 cm², RV end-systolic area ≤16 cm², RV fractional area change >32%, maximal RA volume ≤33 ml/m², IVC diameter <1.5 cm

Abbreviations: *CW* continuous-wave Doppler, *EROA* effective regurgitant orifice area, *PISA* proximal isovelocity surface area, *RA* right atrium, *RV* right ventricle, *R Vol* regurgitant volume, *TR* tricuspid regurgitation, *VC* vena contracta

[a]At a Nyquist limit of 50–60 cm/s

[b]Baseline Nyquist limit shift of 28 cm/s

[c]Unless other reasons of systolic blunting (atrial fibrillation, elevated RA pressure)

[d]In the absence of other causes of elevated RA pressure

[e]Unless for other reasons, the RA and RV size and IVC diameter are usually normal in patients with mild TR. An end-systolic RV eccentricity index >2 is in favour of severe TR. In acute severe TR, the RV size is often normal

Management

Physicians in charge of patients with significant tricuspid regurgitation have to answer two key questions to properly address management: (1) when to treat? and (2) how to treat?.

When to Treat?

Table 20.3 summarizes the indications for the management of significant tricuspid regurgitation from the American College of Cardiology/ American Heart Association (Bonow et al. 2008) and the European Society of Cardiology (ESC) (2012). Patient's clinical status, concomitant left-sided valve surgery and the aetiology of tricuspid regurgitation usually determine the appropriate therapeutic strategy in each individual case. (McCarthy and Sales, 2010).

It is interesting to notice that, although the two documents generally share similarities, there are also some discrepancies. Both documents list a class I indication to perform tricuspid valve repair for severe tricuspid regurgitation in patients who are undergoing mitral valve surgery. However, the ESC document extends it also to the patients undergoing aortic valve surgery, as "left-sided valve surgery". Neither of the two documents provides any indication for patients with severe tricuspid regurgitation undergoing coronary artery bypass surgery.

ESC guidelines also list a class I indication for tricuspid valve repair in patients with severe primary tricuspid regurgitation and symptoms despite medical therapy without severe right ventricular dysfunction. Conversely, the ACC/AHA guidelines list it as a class IIa indication and defines it "reasonable". This is strange, since medical treatment (i.e. diuretics), even if may

Table 20.3 Comparison of American College of Cardiology/European Society of Cardiology clinical guidelines for managing patients with tricuspid regurgitation

	ACC/AHA guidelines Bonow et al. (2008)	ESC guidelines (2012)
Class IB	TV repair is beneficial for severe TR in patients with MV disease requiring MV surgery	
Class IC		Severe TR in a patient undergoing left-sided valve surgery Severe primary TR and symptoms despite medical therapy without severe right ventricular dysfunction
Class IIaC	TV replacement or annuloplasty is reasonable for severe primary TR when symptomatic. TV replacement is reasonable for severe TR secondary to diseased/abnormal TV leaflets not amenable to annuloplasty or repair.	Moderate organic TR in a patient undergoing left-sided valve surgery Moderate secondary TR with dilated annulus (>40 mm or 21 mm/m^2) in a patient undergoing left-sided valve surgery Severe TR and symptoms, after left-sided valve surgery, in the absence of left-sided myocardial, valve, or right ventricular dysfunction and without severe pulmonary hypertension (systolic pulmonary artery pressure >60 mmHg) Severe isolated TR with mild or no symptoms and progressive dilatation or deterioration of right ventricular function
Class IIbC	Tricuspid annuloplasty may be considered for less than severe TR in patients undergoing MV surgery when there is pulmonary hypertension or tricuspid annular dilatation.	
Class III	TV replacement or annuloplasty is not indicated in asymptomatic patients with TR whose pulmonary artery systolic pressure is 60 mmHg in the presence of normal MV TV replacement or annuloplasty is not indicated in patients with mild primary TR	

Abbreviations: *MV* mitral valve, *TR* tricuspid regurgitation, *TV* tricuspid valve

improve symptoms and signs of congestion, does not improve prognosis (Messika-Zeitoun et al. 2004). Moreover, this is actually an exception to the general rule stating that symptomatic heart valve disease is a Class I indication for surgery.

However, most of the discrepancies between the two documents can be found in the class II recommendations. The ESC guidelines list a IIa recommendation for severe symptomatic tricuspid regurgitation occurring after left-sided valve surgery (without left-sided valve dysfunction, right ventricular dysfunction, or pulmonary hypertension), whereas the ACC/AHA guidelines make no reference about this clinical scenario. Although the repair rate for tricuspid valve has constantly increased in the United States during the last decade (compound annual growth rate of 16.4%) according to the Society of Thoracic Surgeons data (Messika-Zeitoun et al. 2004), the above clinical situation is not uncommon. Of course, the best strategy would be to avoid this situation by being more liberal in using tricuspid valve annuloplasty at the time of initial mitral valve surgery, and this is reflected in the ESC guidelines. Conversely, the ACC/AHA guidelines are again more conservative. The ESC guidelines give a class IIa indication for moderate secondary tricuspid regurgitation with a dilated annulus (>40 mm or >21 mm/m^2) in patients undergoing left-sided valve surgery. The ACC/AHA guidelines state that tricuspid valve annuloplasty "*may be considered*" (class IIb) when there is evidence of tricuspid valve annular dilatation or pulmonary hypertension.

Finally, one of the most striking differences between ACC/AHA and ESC guidelines regards the class III indications. ACC/AHA guidelines define as class III (not indicated) tricuspid annuloplasty or replacement in asymptomatic patients with tricuspid regurgitation whose pulmonary artery systolic pressure is <60 mmHg in the presence of normal mitral valve (Bonow et al. 2008). This seems to be in contradiction with the recommendations regarding mitral regurgitation. ACC/AHA guidelines have raised mitral valve repair indication to class IIa in asymptomatic patients if a >90% success rate can be predicted in an experienced center. Since the vast majority of tricuspid valve surgeries are repair (with the exception of few organic tricuspid regurgitations), even in the less experienced centers, and knowing the insidious natural history and impact on right ventricular function of tricuspid regurgitation, it is difficult to understand the rationale behind this recommendation. The ESC guidelines for patients with severe tricuspid regurgitation and mild or no symptoms, yet with documentation of progressive dilatation or deterioration of right ventricular function, give a IIb ("*may be considered*") recommendation. This is in agreement with the rationale behind the recommendation about an earlier intervention to be performed in asymptomatic patients with severe mitral regurgitation, in order to prevent the evolution to progressive left ventricular dysfunction.

In the guidelines, it is stated that the timing of surgical intervention for tricuspid regurgitation, as well as the recommended surgical techniques remain controversial, due to the paucity of long-term data and lack of reliable quantitative parameters to assess the severity of tricuspid regurgitation. Therefore, recommendations are mostly derived from a consensus of experts, retrospective studies or registries. However, given the adverse consequences of allowing tricuspid regurgitation to progress to severe degrees (i.e. worsening symptoms of right heart failure), the fact that adding a tricuspid repair, if indicated during left-sided surgery, does not significantly increase the operative risk (Dreyfus et al. 2005; Singh et al. 2006; Tang et al. 2006), and that redo surgery to operate tricuspid valve carries a high risk and may have poor long-term results due to right ventricular irreversible dysfunction prior to operation (Mangoni et al. 2001; King et al. 1984; Hornick et al. 1996), it would seem logical that earlier intervention, especially in the presence of progressive right atrial and right ventricular enlargement, would be beneficial. However, there is currently no data that specifically addresses this important question.

A proposed algorithm for the management of tricuspid regurgitation in patients who have not previously undergone left-sided valve surgery is shown in Fig. 20.13.

How to Treat?

Medical Management

If feasible, functional tricuspid regurgitation secondary to pulmonary hypertension should be first treated by tailored medical management. In patients with pulmonary hypertension of an identifiable etiology (e.g. due to left heart diseases, lung diseases causing chronic hypoxaemia, collagen vascular diseases, left-to-right shunts, portal hypertension, HIV infection, drugs or toxins etc.), the underlying disease should be treated with specific drugs. Congenital shunt defects should be surgically corrected and accessible chronic thromboembolic disease could benefit from pulmonary thromboendarterectomy (Jamieson et al. 2003).

Moreover, it should be emphasized that functional tricuspid regurgitation is a dynamic phenomenon, its severity assessment by echocardiography being highly load dependent. Therefore, intensive management of left heart failure may dramatically decrease the perceived severity of tricuspid regurgitation. This aspect is particularly relevant in patients who are candidates to surgery for left heart disease (e.g. aortic or mitral valve diseases), while being on intensive medical treatment for heart failure. In these patients, tricuspid regurgitation requires a surgi-

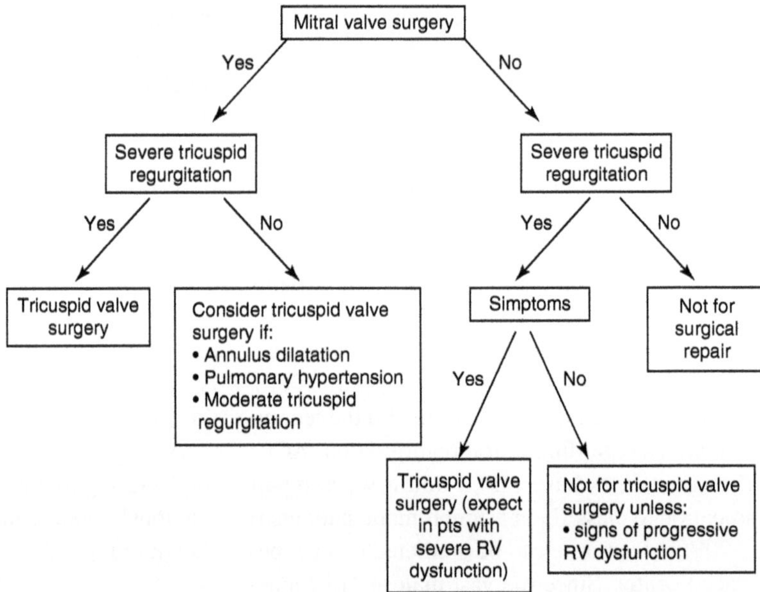

Fig. 20.13 ACC/AHA Bonow et al. (2008) and ESC (2012) guideline based algorithm for the management of tricuspid regurgitation. *MV* mitral valve, *RV* right ventricular, *TR* tricuspid regurgitation

cal correction, even if the severity is only mild or moderate at pre-operative echo.

Surgical Management

A variety of operative techniques have been developed to address the regurgitant tricuspid valve. These fall broadly into two categories: repair techniques and valve replacement.

Patients with Secondary or Functional Tricuspid Regurgitation

The goal of repair techniques is to reduce both tricuspid annulus dilatation and leaflet tethering in order to stabilize the annulus and increase leaflet coaptation. A number of surgical techniques have been developed to reach this goal. One of the oldest techniques (but still used) is the tricuspidalization of the tricuspid valve, whereby the posterior leaflet is obliterated by placation of the fibrous annulus (Kay et al. 1965; Ghanta et al. 2007). Another technique that is still used by some surgeons is the so-called De Vega purse string repair, where a double layer of a nonabsorbable suture is weaved in and out of the fibrous annulus of the anterior and posterior leaflet, and so the tricuspid valve orifice is reduced (De Vega 1972). Early results (up to 6 months) are quite good, but late follow-up studies report a significantly higher recurrence rate of tricuspid regurgitation as compared with annuloplasty techniques (McCarthy et al. 2004). However, since it is a very practical and low cost procedure, it may be the preferred approach in developing countries with high incidence of rheumatic mitral valve diseases, when a rapid and sustained fall in pulmonary artery pressure is expected following mitral valve surgery.

Peri-Guard annuloplasty consists of customized semicircular annuloplasty using bovine pericardium. However, this technique is not used anymore because of the high rate of early and late recurrence of tricuspid regurgitation.

In 1974, Carpentier and coworkers (1974) described tricuspid annuloplasty using a rigid ring with the aim to restore the tricuspid annulus to its triangular systolic shape. Flexible Dacron bands or strips of pericardium have also been used to stabilize and reduce the area of tricuspid annulus and obtain leaflet coaptation (McCarthy et al. 2004; Chang et al. 2008).

Duran flexible rings has been introduced to preserve the normal annular area change throughout the cardiac cycle. Good early and late outcome has been reported using close rigid and flexible rings, however particular care should be taken to avoid injuring the atrio-ventricular node which may lead to complete atrioventricular block.

Annuloplasty bands or incomplete rings have been used to avoid the risk of atrio-ventricular node injury. Using the data coming from three-dimensional echo, an incomplete ring, specifically designed on the three-dimensional shape of the tricuspid (ring) has been introduced with good early and mid-term outcome data (Jeong and Kim 2010).

When the tricuspid valve repair and annuloplasty techniques have been compared, tricuspid valve repair with annuloplasty ring resulted in significantly better long-term survival (46±5% vs. 36±8%, at 15 years), event free survival (34±5 vs. 17±6%, at 15 years) and survivalfree of recurrent tricuspid regurgitation compared with De Vega suture annuloplasty (Tang et al. 2006). Multivariable analysis demonstrated that the use of an annuloplasty ring was an independent predictor of long-term survival (hazard ratio [HR], 0.7; 95% confidence interval [CI], 0.5–1.0; P=0.03) and event-free survival (HR, 0.8; CI, 0.6–1.0; P=0.04). An immediate failure rate (grade 3 tricuspid regurgitation or more) around 14% of tricuspid valve repair procedures (irrespective of the technique used) has been reported (McCarthy et al. 2004). However, while patients who received a semi-rigid Carpentier-Edwards ring had no progression of tricuspid regurgitation, more than 30% of the patients who had a De Vega suture showed significant tricuspid regurgitation after 8 years (McCarthy et al. 2004).

If the dilatation of the tricuspid annulus is the only reason for functional tricuspid regurgitation, a properly performed tricuspid annuloplasty will fix the problem. However, if the right ventricle is dilated and severe tethering of the leaflets is present, annuloplasty alone may not resolve the functional tricuspid regurgitation. Despite the fact that surgeons have introduced newer techniques to circumvent this problem (such as anterior tricuspid leaflet augmentation to increase leaflet coaptation and relief the tethering leaflets (Dreyfus et al. 2008), right ventricular wall plication by placement of two strips of felts on the epicardial surface in order to reduce the right ventricular cavity size and approximate the papillary muscles (Dreyfus et al. 2008), and edge-to-edge techniques by suturing the free margins of the tricuspid leaflets to obtain a clover shaped valve in conjunction with ring annuloplasty (Lapenna et al. 2010)), this problem remains largely unresolved, also because leaflet tethering has been described only recently (Ton-Nu et al. 2006; Fukuda et al. 2006; Sukmawan et al. 2007; Park et al. 2008) (Fig. 20.14). It has been reported that the height and the area of tricuspid valve tethering are powerful predictors of the severity of early residual tricuspid regurgitation after tricuspid valve repair. Fukuda et al. (2007) reported a 55% tricuspid valve repair failure immediately after surgery in patients with preoperative tethering height larger than 10 mm. Roshanali et al. (2010) recently reported a low rate (2% at 1 month, and 8% at 1 year) of tricuspid regurgitation recurrence when a tethering height larger than 8 mm or a tethering area larger than 16 mm^2 were used as thresholds for performing an adjunctive procedure (anterior tricuspid leaflet augmentation) to reduce leaflet tethering and improve their coaptation.

In cases in whom valve leaflets are severely diseased or destroyed, the tricuspid annulus is markedly distorted and/or a severe tethering is present together with relatively small valve leaflets, a valve replacement could be necessary (Moraca et al. 2009). Despite most studies have reported superior early and long term outcome with valve repair, in some cases it is safer to replace the tricuspid valve. In primary (organic) tricuspid valve disease, valve repair has been found to be associated with better early and mid-term event free survival (90% vs. 63% at 5 years; 76% vs. 55% at 10 years; $p<0.0001$) (Singh et al. 2006). Moreover, postoperative moderate to severe right ventricular dysfunction was significantly lower in the tricuspid valve repair group (9% vs. 28%, respectively).

Despite the fact that several studies have shown no significant differences in the long-term outcome between bioprostheses and mechanical valves (Ratnatunga et al. 1998; Rizzoli et al. 2004), except in Ebstein anomaly (Brown et al. 2009), bioprostheses are generally preferred since valve thrombosis and infections following valve

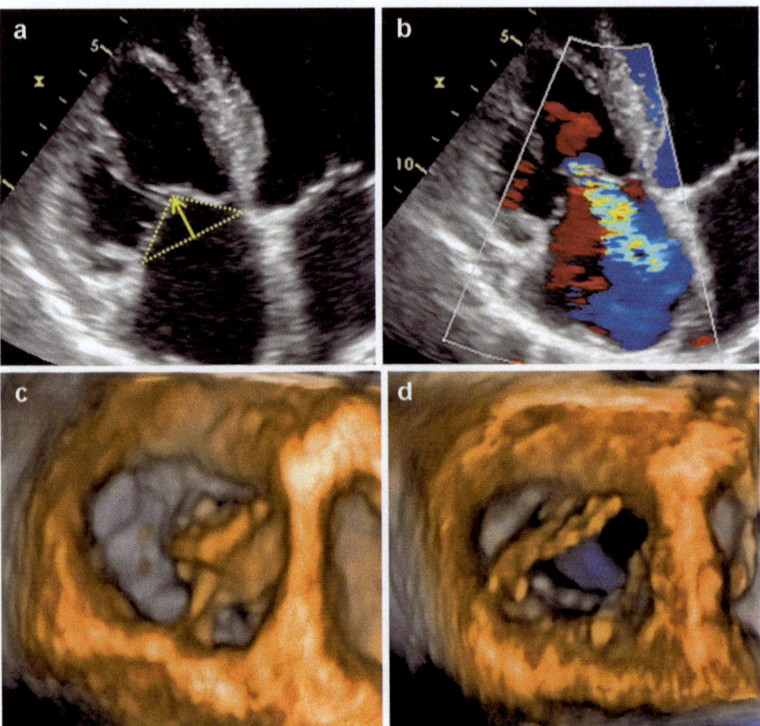

Fig. 20.14 Functional tricuspid regurgitation in a patient with sclerodermia and pulmonary arterial hypertension. (**a**) Apical 4-chamber view, showing right heart chamber enlargement with dilation of tricuspid annulus and leaflet tethering. The tenting area (*yellow dashed line*) and coaptation height (*yellow arrow*) are indicated; (**b**) Color Doppler visualization of a moderate tricuspid regurgitation jet; (**c**) 3D volume rendering of tricuspid valve from the right ventricular perspective at end-systole, demonstrating tenting of tricuspid leaflets, being tethered by the attached cordae, the dilation and increased sphericity of the annulus and interventricular septal flattening as a consequence of elevated right ventricular systolic pressures; (**d**) 3D volume rendering of tricuspid leaflets during diastole

replacement with a mechanical valve are not negligible (Sanfelippo et al. 1976). Thrombosis with mechanical valves in tricuspid position is around 1% per year. Thrombolysis is considered first-line therapy for tricuspid valve thrombosis, as opposed to left-sided valve thrombosis, for which the risks of systemic and cerebral embolism are increased.

In patients undergoing sternotomy with underlying conduction abnormalities, placement of a pacemaker lead outside prosthetic annulus or of an epicardial lead can avoid the subsequent need to pass a transvenous lead across the prosthetic valve. This technique is particularly indicated in patients who will receive a bioprosthetic tricuspid valve, in whom the placement of a trans-tricuspid pacing lead may cause prosthetic regurgitation. The major limitation of an epicardial lead is related to the increased pacing threshold which will significantly shorten the generator life.

A particularly challenging group of patients with functional tricuspid regurgitation are those who develop tricuspid regurgitation late after left-sided heart valve surgery, particularly mitral valve replacement for rheumatic disease (Matsuyama et al. 2003). Late occurrence of tricuspid regurgitation is rather uncommon after mitral valve surgery for degenerative mitral valve disease, ischemic mitral regurgitation, and functional mitral regurgitation in dilated cardiomyopathy, but it is quite common in rheumatic mitral disease (Matsunaga and Duran 2005; De Bonis et al. 2008). Aggressive management with loop diuretics and spironolactone is the mainstay of therapy and might retard tricuspid regurgitation progression. Surgery is only recommended in those with severe tricuspid regurgitation, pulmonary artery systolic pressure less than 60 mmHg and preserved right ventricular function. Operative mortality in these patients is particularly high, ranging from 10% to 20% (Mangoni et al. 2001; Hornick et al. 1996; Antunes and Barlow 2007; Kwon et al. 2006). Therefore, recommending a reoperation in these patients requires a careful consideration of the patient's functional status, comorbidities and motivation.

Established pulmonary hypertension and right ventricular failure are the most important adverse prognostic factors in these patients. In some patients in whom surgery is no longer an option, chronic dialysis may prove useful in treating volume overload and improving life quality.

Percutaneous Interventional Treatment of Tricuspid Regurgitation

The recent advent of transcatheter therapy for heart valve disease has expanded the treatment options for patients with aortic and mitral valve disease. However, no percutaneous approach is yet clinically available to treat significant tricuspid regurgitation in high-risk or nonsurgical patients. Several innovative approaches have been suggested but, to date, transcatheter treatment of tricuspid regurgitation has been performed only as compassionate treatment in isolated human cases and is still investigational. No transcatheter device specifically designed for tricuspid valve disease is commercially available and experimental data on percutaneous treatment of tricuspid valve disease is limited (Boudjemline et al. 2005; Lauten et al. 2010; Bai et al. 2012). This is partially due to the fact that transcatheter tricuspid valve replacement is associated with major challenges related to the anchorage of the percutaneous device in the highly dynamic tricuspid annulus, as well as the predominantly secondary nature of tricuspid regurgitation. In addition, the right coronary artery (which runs along the anterior portion of the tricuspid annulus) and the atrioventricular node (which is adjacent to the septal portion of the tricuspid annulus) are located close to the tricuspid valve and are exposed at risk during interventional procedures. Further, tricuspid regurgitation has traditionally assumed a lower priority than other valve diseases resulting in less commercial interest in such developments.

Compared to the mitral annulus, the tricuspid annulus offers a greater variability and less resistance for device fixation because of its larger diameter and lower proportion of fibrous tissue. Size and flexibility of the tricuspid valve and of the surrounding myocardium hamper the positioning and long-term fixation of transcatheter devices and there are no adjacent structures to facilitate implantation. Nonetheless, some of the percutaneous approaches suggested for mitral valve repair could also prove suitable for treatment of tricuspid valve disease and several new concepts of percutaneous tricuspid valve repair or replacement have been suggested.

Percutaneous Repair of the Tricuspid Valve

Thermal remodeling for annular plication has been suggested as repair concept for atrioventricular valves (Rahman et al. 2010). Catheter-based application of radiofrequency results in thermal contraction of collagen fibers which restores annulus size and dimension and reduces insufficiency. This concept is attractive, since a repeated step-wise radio frequency application could be performed until a sufficient reduction of tricuspid regurgitation is achieved. Moreover, no material is implanted, which may later allow the implantation of further devices if necessary. Thermal remodeling has been experimentally applied in the animal model for mitral annular plication (Goel et al. 2009; Heuser et al. 2008). The challenge for applying this technique to the tricuspid annulus is that it contains less collagen, possibly reducing efficacy of radiofrequency application.

Annuloplasty might also be performed by means of percutaneous ring implantation. One device under development specifically for tricuspid valve repair is the Millipede annular ring (Millipede, LLC, Ann Arbor, MI). The device mimics surgical tricuspid annuloplasty by transcatheter implantation of a flexible ring that uses a novel attachment technique to reduce annular dimensions and tricuspid regurgitation. Prior to ring fixation, the annulus is expanded to a circular shape by a dilator introduced into the right ventricle to facilitate ring placement and fixation. Although conceptually appealing, the effectiveness of tricuspid valve repair will depend on sufficient long-term fixation of this sutureless device.

Another promising technique focuses on valve repair by leaflet approximation. By way of implanting a 2-branched clip emulating the surgical Alfieri-technique used for mitral repair (Alfieri et al. 2001), the regurgitant orifice area may be reduced. Surgical edge-to-edge repair has been demonstrated to be effective in tricuspid regurgitation, however tricuspid valve has three leaflets and concomitant annular plication is considered to be a necessary adjunct and it would also be required for percutaneous tricuspid valve edge-to-edge repair. Performing interventional tricuspid edge-to-edge repair is technically challenging and is probably beyond the reach of a transcatheter approach within the near future.

Percutaneous Replacement of the Tricuspid Valve

Although percutaneous tricuspid valve repair is conceptually attractive, it is technically challenging and it is difficult to predict whether the above techniques can be adapted to the tricuspid valve and transferred to clinical practice with effective long-term results. In the presence of an unmet need for effective treatment of severe tricuspid regurgitation in non-surgical patients, transcatheter valve implantation may offer an alternative treatment option.

From the interventional perspective, there are two basic concepts regarding the percutaneous replacement of the tricuspid valve depending on the site of valve implantation – an orthotopic versus heterotopic valve replacement.

In orthotopic valve replacement, the prosthetic valve is implanted in anatomically correct position in the TV annulus, thus restoring the functional separation of the right ventricle and right atrium. Boudjemline et al. (2005) implanted a novel percutaneous tricuspid valve consisting of a bovine jugular valve mounted to a self-expanding double-disc nitinol stent into the tricuspid valve annulus of 7 sheeps using a 18F sheath. Although the technical feasibility of this approach was demonstrated to some extent, several issues related to anchorage of the self-expanding valve in the highly dynamic tricuspid annulus were observed. Due to the anatomic structure and the flexibility of the surrounding myocardium, this site of implantation offers little resistance for orthotopic long-term fixation of stent-based valves with the current technique. No further work has been done with this device.

Annulus dilatation may reach >70 mm in functional tricuspid regurgitation and is associated with the loss of anatomical landmarks between right ventricle and right atrium. A device intended for orthotopic tricuspid valve replacement would require unique solutions for stent- and catheter design as well as tissue valve engineering (e.g. a 70-mm size bioprosthesis would require a leaflet height of >40 mm to avoid prolapsing into the right atrium). Therefore, it is unlikely that the various difficulties associated with orthotopic valve replacement will be resolved within the near future.

However, orthotopic percutaneous tricuspid valve implantation has been performed as a valve-in-valve-procedure using balloon-expandable stent valves designed for either aortic (Edwards Sapien, Edwards Lifescience, Irvine, CA, US) or pulmonary (Melody® valve, Medtronic, Minneapolis, MN, US) valve implantation after failure of surgically implanted bioprosthetic valves or conduits (Van Garsse et al. 2011; Zegdi et al. 2006; Tanous et al. 2009; Straver et al. 2011). In these reports, percutaneous valve replacement has been performed with a high rate of technical and functional success. Although long-term results are not available yet, this concept may be considered as potential treatment option for degenerated bioprosthetic tricuspid valves in selected patients.

An alternative percutaneous option is heterotopic tricuspid valve implant involving implantation of stent valves into the inferior (and superior) vena cava. This procedure has recently been performed for the first time for compassionate treatment in a human patient (Lauten et al. 2010). In this patient, the authors implanted a self-expanding valve at the cavoatrial junction to reduce regurgitant backflow into the inferior vena cava. In this experience, excellent valve function was observed after resulting deployment in a marked reduction of caval pressure and an abolition of backflow to the inferior vena cava. Compared to the orthotopic approach, this procedure benefits from the advantage of a straightforward implantation procedure due to the distance to vulnerable cardiac structures. The introduction of foreign material in the right ventricular inflow tract is avoided, permitting a potentially lower risk of injury to ventricular structures and making this an attractive approach to the interventional cardiologist.

However, although caval valve implantation is a rather simple procedure this approach has significant limitations, restricting its use to severely ill patients with significant tricuspid regurgitation, in end-stage heart disease. Although venous regurgitation is prevented by heterotopic valves, right ventricular and right atrial overload persist, resulting in ventricularization of the right atrium with potential deleterious effects on cardiac function and atrial rhythm during long-term follow-up. Furthermore, caval valve implantation addresses the regurgitation of blood in the caval veins, a condition not found in every patient with severe tricuspid regurgitation. In severe tricuspid regurgitation, the atrium functions as a compliant reservoir by retaining part of the regurgitant volume and limiting the systolic flow reversal in the caval veins. However, since pulsatile blood flow and systolic flow reversal in the caval veins are prerequisites for the proper function of the caval valves, proof of regurgitation into the inferior vena cava and preserved right ventricular function are required prior to heterotopic valve implantation. A preserved right ventricular function is already known to affect the outcome after tricuspid valve surgery, and must also be taken into account to a larger extent in any potential percutaneous tricuspid valve intervention.

In conclusion, although transcatheter tricuspid valve repair or replacement is desirable as it would avoid the trauma and risks of conventional surgery and has the potential to improve outcome, this treatment modality currently remains at an investigational level.

Conclusions

Hemodynamically significant tricuspid regurgitation cannot be ignored when performing corrective surgical procedures for left-sided valve disease. Particularly in patients undergoing mitral valve surgery, since tricuspid regurgitation does not disappear in most of patients despite successful operation, and reoperation for recurrent tricuspid regurgitation carries high mortality rates, preventive tricuspid valve annuloplasty should be considered in patients with enlarged tricuspid valve annulus and at least moderate tricuspid regurgitation. Challenges to emerging minimally invasive or percutaneous approaches are numerous, but should be surmountable with evolving surgical, imaging and interventional techniques.

References

Alfieri O, Maisano F, De Bonis M, et al. The double-orifice technique in mitral valve repair: a simple solution for complex problems. J Thorac Cardiovasc Surg. 2001;122:674–81.

Alizadeh A, Sanati HR, Haji-Karimi M, et al. Induction and aggravation of atrioventricular valve regurgitation in the course of chronic right ventricular apical pacing. Europace. 2011;13(11):1587–90.

Antunes MJ, Barlow JB. Management of tricuspid valve regurgitation. Heart. 2007;93:271–6.

Anwar AM, Soliman OI, Nemes A, van Geuns RJ, Geleijnse MI, ten Cate FJ. Value of assessment of tricuspid annulus: real-time three-dimensional echocardiography and magnetic resonance imaging. Int J Cardiovasc Imaging. 2007;23:701–5.

Aziz T, Burgess MI, Rahman AN, Campbell CS, Deiraniya AK, Yonan NA. Risk factors for tricuspid valve regurgitation after orthotopic heart transplantation. Ann Thorac Surg. 1999;68:1247–51.

Badano LP, Agricola E, de Perez Isla L, Gianfagna P, Zamorano JL. Evaluation of the tricuspid valve morphology and function by transthoracic real-time three-dimensional echocardiography. Eur J Echocardiogr. 2009;10:477–84.

Bai Y, Zong GJ, Wang HR, et al. An integrated pericardial valved stent special for percutaneous tricuspid implantation: an animal feasibility study. J Surg Res. 2012;160:215–21.

Becker AE, Becker MJ, Claudon DG, Edwards JE. Surface thrombosis and fibrous encapsulation of intravenous pacemaker catheter electrode. Circulation. 1972;46:409–12.

Bonow RO, Carabello BA, Chatterjee K, et al. 2008 focused update incorporated into the ACC/AHA 2006 guidelines for the management of patients with valvular heart disease: a report of the American College of Cardiology/American Heart Association Task Force on Practice Guidelines (Writing Committee to revise the 1998 guidelines for the management of patients with valvular heart disease). Endorsed by the Society of Cardiovascular Anesthesiologists, Society for Cardiovascular Angiography and Interventions, and Society of Thoracic Surgeons. J Am Coll Cardiol. 2008;52:e1–142.

Boudjemline Y, Agnoletti G, Bonnet D, et al. Steps toward the percutaneous replacement of atrioventricular valves an experimental study. J Am Coll Cardiol. 2005;46:360–5.

Boyaci A, Gokce V, Topaloglu S, Korkmaz S, Goksel S. Outcome of significant functional tricuspid regurgitation late after mitral valve replacement for predominant rheumatic mitral stenosis. Angiology. 2007;58:336–42.

Brown ML, Dearani JA, Danielson GK, et al. Comparison of the outcome of porcine bioprosthetic versus mechanical prosthetic replacement of the tricuspid valve in the Ebstein anomaly. Am J Cardiol. 2009;103:555–61.

Bruce CJ, Connolly HM. Right-sided valve diseases deserves a little more respect. Circulation. 2009;119:2726–34.

Candinas R, Duru F, Schneider J, et al. Postmortem analysis of encapsulation around long-term ventricular endocardial pacing leads. Mayo Clin Proc. 1999;74:120–5.

Carpentier A, Deloche A, Hanania G, et al. Surgical management of acquired tricuspid valve diseases. J Thorac Cardiovasc Surg. 1974;67:53–65.

Chang BC, Song SW, Lee S, Yoo KJK, Kang MS, Chung N. Eight-year outcome of tricuspid annuloplasty using autologus pericardial strip for functional tricuspid regurgitation. Ann Thorac Surg. 2008;86:1485–92.

De Bonis M, Lapenna E, Sorrentino F, et al. Evolution of tricuspid regurgitation after mitral valve repair for functional mitral regurgitation in dilated cardiomyopathy. Eur J Cardiothorac Surg. 2008;33:600–6.

De Vega NG. Selective, adjustable and permanent annuloplasty. An original technique for the treatment of tricuspid regurgitation. Rev Esp Cardiol. 1972;25:555–6.

Dounis G, Matsakas E, Poularas J, Papakostantinou K, Kalogeromitros A, Karabinis A. Traumatic tricuspid insufficiency: a case report with a review of the literature. Eur J Emerg Med. 2002;9:258–61.

Dreyfus GD, Corbi PJ, Chan KM, Bahrami T. Secondary tricuspid regurgitation or dilatation: which should be the criteria for surgical repair? Ann Thorac Surg. 2005;79:127–32.

Dreyfus GD, Raja SG, John Chan KM. Tricuspid leaflet augmentation to address severe tethering in functional tricuspid regurgitation. Eur J Cardiothorac Surg. 2008;34:908–10.

Vahanian A, Alfieri O, Andreotti F, et al. ESC Guidelines on the management of valvular heart diseases (Version 2012). Eur Heart J 2012; in press.

Franceschi F, Thuny F, Giorgi R, et al. Incidence, risk factors, and outcome of traumatic tricuspid regurgitation after percutaneous ventricular lead removal. J Am Coll Cardiol. 2009;53:2168–74.

Fukuda S, Song JM, Gillinov AM, et al. Tricuspid valve tethering predicts residual tricuspid regurgitation after tricuspid annuloplasty. Circulation. 2005;111:975–9.

Fukuda S, Saracino G, Matsumara Y, et al. Three-dimensional geometry of the tricuspid annulus in healthy subjects and in patients with functional tricuspid regurgitation: a real-time, 3-dimensional echocardiographic study. Circulation. 2006;I-114:I-492–8.

Fukuda S, Gillinov AM, McCarthy PM, et al. Echocardiographic follow-up of tricuspid annuloplasty with a new three-dimensional ring in patients with functional tricuspid regurgitation. J Am Soc Echocardiogr. 2007;20:1236–12242.

Ghanta RV, Chen R, Narayanasamy N, et al. Suture bicuspidalization of the tricuspid valve versus ring annuloplasty for repair of functional tricuspid regurgitation: midterm results in 237 consecutive patients. J Thorac Cardiovasc Surg. 2007;133:117–26.

Goel R, Witzel T, Dickens D, Takeda PA, Heuser RR. The QuantumCor device for treating mitral regurgitation: an animal study. Catheter Cardiovasc Interv. 2009;74:43–8.

Heuser RR, Witzel T, Dickens D, Takeda PA. Percutaneous treatment for mitral regurgitation: the QuantumCor system. J Interv Cardiol. 2008;21:178–82.

Hornick P, Harris PA, Taylor KM. Tricuspid valve replacement subsequent to previous open heart surgery. J Heart Valve Dis. 1996;5:20–5.

Izumi C, Iga K, Konishi T. Progression of isolated tricuspid regurgitation late after mitral valve surgery for rheumatic mitral valve disease. J Heart Valve Dis. 2002;11:353–6.

Jamieson SW, Kapelanski DP, Sakakibara N, et al. Pulmonary endarterectomy: experience and lessons learned in 1,500 cases. Ann Thorac Surg. 2003;76:1457–62.

Jeong DS, Kim KH. Tricuspid annuloplasty using the MC3 ring for functional tricuspid regurgitation. Circ J. 2010;74:278–83.

Kay JH, Maselli-Campagna G, Tsuji KK. Surgical treatment of tricuspid insufficiency. Ann Surg. 1965;162:53–8.

Kim JB, Spevack DM, Tunick PA, et al. The effect of transvenous pacemaker and implantable cardioverter defibrillator lead placement on tricuspid valve function: an observational study. J Am Soc Echocardiogr. 2008;21:284–7.

King RM, Schaff HV, Danielson GK, et al. Surgery for tricuspid regurgitation late after mitral valve replacement. Circulation. 1984;70:I193–7.

Klein A, Burstow D, Tajik A, et al. Age-related prevalence of valvular regurgitation in normal subjects: a comprehensive color-flow examination in 118 volunteers. J Am Soc Echocardiogr. 1990;3:54–63.

Klutstein M, Balkin J, Butnaru A, Ilan M, Lahad A, Rosenmann D. Tricuspid incompetence following permanent pacemaker implantation. Pacing Clin Eletrophysiol. 2009;32 suppl 1:S135–7.

Kucukarslan N, Kirilmaz A, Ulusoy E, et al. Tricuspid insufficiency does not increase early after permanent implantation of pacemaker leads. J Card Surg. 2006;21:391–4.

Kwon DA, Park JS, Chang HJ, et al. Prediction of outcome in patients undergoing surgery for severe tricuspid regurgitation following mitral valve surgery. Am J Cardiol. 2006;98:659–61.

Lancellotti P, Moura L, Pierard LA, et al. European Association of Echocardiography recommendations for the assessment of valvular regurgitation. Part 2:mitral and tricuspid regurgitation (native valve diseases). Eur J Echocardiogr. 2010;11:307–32.

Lapenna E, De Bonis M, Verzini A, et al. The clover technique for the treatment of complex tricuspid valve insufficiency: midterm clinical and echocardiographic results in 66 patients. Eur J Cardiothorac Surg. 2010;37:1297–303.

Lauten A, Figulla HR, Willich C, et al. Heterotopic valve replacement as an interventional approach to tricuspid regurgitation. J Am Coll Cardiol. 2010;55:499–500.

Liebowitz DW, Rosenheck S, Pollak A, Geist M, Gilon D. Transvenous pacemaker leads do not worsen tricuspid regurgitation: a prospective echocardiographc study. Cardiology. 2000;93:74–7.

Lin G, Nishimura RA, Connolly HM, Dearani JA, Sundt 3rd TM, Hayes DL. Severe symptomatic tricuspid valve regurgitation due to permanent pacemaker or implantable cardioverter-defibrillator leads. J Am Coll Cardiol. 2005;45:1672–5.

Mangoni AA, DiSalvo TG, Vlahakes GJ, Polanczyk CA, Fifer MA. Outcome following isolated tricuspid valve replacement. Eur J Cardiothorac Surg. 2001;19:68–73.

Mascherbauer J, Maurer G. The forgotten valve: lessons to be learned in tricuspid regurgitation. Eur Heart J. 2010;31:2841–3.

Matsunaga A, Duran CM. Progression of TR after repaired functional ischemic mitral regurgitation. Circulation. 2005;112(suppl):I-453–7.

Matsuyama K, Matsumoto M, Sugita T, Nishizawa J, Tokuda Y, Matsuo T. Predictors of residual tricuspid regurgitation after mitral valve surgery. Ann Thorac Surg. 2003;75:1826–8.

McCarthy PM, Sales VL. Evolving indications for tricuspid valve surgery. Curr Treat Options Cardiovasc Med. 2010;12:587–97.

McCarthy PM, Bhudia SK, Rajeswaran J, et al. Tricuspid valve repair:durability and risk factors for failure. J Thorac Cardiovasc Surg. 2004;127:674–85.

Messika-Zeitoun D, Thomson H, et al. Medical and surgical outcome of tricuspid regurgitation caused by flail leaflets. J Thorac Cardiovasc Surg. 2004;128: 296–302.

Mielniczuk L, Haddad H, Davies RA, Veinot JP. Tricuspid valve chordal tissue in endomyocardial biopsy specimens of patients with significant tricuspid regurgitation. J Heart Lung Transplant. 2005;24:1586–90.

Moraca RJ, Moon MR, Guthrie TJ, et al. Outcomes of tricuspid valve repair and replacement: a propensity analysis. Ann Thorac Surg. 2009;87:83–8.

Muraru D, Badano LP. Assessment of tricuspid valve morphology and function. In: Badano LP, Lang RM, Zamorano JL, editors. Textbook of real-time three dimensional echocardiography. London: Springer; 2011. p. 173–82.

Muraru D, Tuveri MF, Peazzolo-Marra M, Badano LP, Iliceto S. Carcinoid tricuspid valve disease: incremental value of three-dimensional echocardiography. Eur Heart J Cardiovasc Imaging. 2012;13:329.

Mutlak D, Lessick J, Reisner SA, et al. Echocardiography-based spectrum of sever tricuspid regurgitation: the frequency of apparently idiopathic tricuspid regurgitation. J Am Soc Echocardiogr. 2007;20:405–8.

Mutlak D, Aronson D, Lessick J, Reisner SA, Dabbah S, Agmon Y. Functional tricuspid regurgitation in patients with pulmonary hypertension: is pulmonary artery pressure the only determinant of regurgitation severity? Chest. 2009;135:115–21.

Nath J, Foster E, Heidenreich PA. Impact of tricuspid regurgitation on long-term survival. J Am Coll Cardiol. 2004;43:405–9.

Nguyen V, Cantarovich M, Cecere R, Giannetti N. Tricuspid regurgitation after cardiac transplantation: how many biopsies arc too many? J Ilcart Lung Transplant. 2005;24:S227–31.

Nucifora G, Badano LP, Allocca G, et al. Severe tricuspid regurgitation due to entrapment of the anterior leaflet of the valve by a permanent pacemaker lead: role of real-time three-dimensional echocardiography. Echocardiography. 2007;24:649–52.

Paniagua D, Aldrich HR, Lieberman EH, Lamas GA, Agatston AS. Increased prevalence of significant tricuspid regurgitation in patients with transvenous pacemaker leads. Am J Cardiol. 1998;82:1130–2.

Park YH, Song JM, Lee EY, Kim YJ, Kang DH, Song JK. Geometric and hemodynamic determinants of functional tricuspid regurgitation secondary to pulmonary hypertension: a real-time three dimensional echocardiographic study. Int J Cardiol. 2008;124: 160–5.

Porter A, Shapira Y, Wurzel M, et al. Tricuspid regurgitation late after mitral valve replacement: clinical and echocardiographic evaluation. J Heart Valve Dis. 1999;8:57–62.

Rahman S, Eid N, Murarka S, Heuser RR. Remodeling of the mitral valve using radiofrequency energy: review of a new treatment modality for mitral regurgitation. Cardiovasc Revasc Med. 2010;11:249–59.

Ratnatunga CP, Edwards MB, Dore CJ, Taylor KM. Tricuspid valve replacement: UK heart valve registry mid-term results comparing mechanical and biological prostheses. Ann Thorac Surg. 1998;66: 1940–7.

Rizzoli G, Vendramin I, Nesseris G, Bottio T, Guglielmi CSL. Biological and mechanical prostheses in tricuspid position? A meta-analysis of intra-institutional results. Ann Thorac Surg. 2004;77:1607–14.

Robboy SJ, Harthorne JW, Leinbach RC, et al. Autopsy findings with permanent pervenous pacemakers. Circulation. 1969;39:495–501.

Roshanali F, Saidi B, Mandegar MH. Echocardiographic approach to the decision-making process for tricuspid valve repair. J Thorac Cardiovasc Surg. 2010;139: 1483–7.

Rubio PA, al-Bassam MS. Pacemaker-lead puncture of the tricuspid valve. Successful diagnosis and treatment. Chest. 1991;99:1519–20.

Sadeghi HM, Kimura BJ, Raisinghani A, et al. Does lowering pulmonary arterial pressure eliminate severe functional tricuspid regurgitation? Insights from pulmonary thromboendoarterectomy. J Am Coll Cardiol. 2004;44:126–32.

Sagie A, Schwammenthal E, Padial LR, de Vazquez Prada JA, Weyman AE, Levine RA. Determinants of functional tricuspid regurgitation in incomplete tricuspid valve closure: Doppler color flow study of 109 patients. J Am Coll Cardiol. 1994;24:446–53.

Sagie A, Freitas N, Chen MH, Marshall JE, Weyman AE, Levine RA. Echocardiographic assessment of mitral stenosis and its associated valvular lesions in 205 patients and lack of association with mitral valve prolapse. J Am Soc Echocardiogr. 1997;10:141–8.

Sakai M, Ohkawa S, Ueda K, et al. Tricuspid regurgitation induced by transvenous right ventricular pacing: echocardiographic and pathological observations. J Cardiol. 1987;17:311–20.

Sanfelippo PM, Giuliani ER, Danielson GK, Wallace RB, Pluth JR, McGoon DC. Tricuspid valve prosthetic replacement. Early and late results with the Starr-Edwards prosthesis. J Thorac Cardiovasc Surg. 1976;71: 441–5.

Seo Y, Ishizu T, Nakajima H, Sekiguchi Y, Watanabe S, Aonuma K. Clinical utility of 3-dimensional echocardiography in the evaluation of tricuspid regurgitation caused by pace-maker leads. Circ J. 2008;72:1465–70.

Singh JP, Evans JC, Levy D, et al. Prevalence and clinical determinants of mitral, tricuspid, and aortic regurgitation (the Framingham Heart Study). Am J Cardiol. 1999;83:897–902.

Singh SK, Tang GH, Maganti MD, et al. Midterm outcomes of tricuspid valve repair versus replacement for organic tricuspid disease. Ann Thorac Surg. 2006;82:1735–41.

Song H, Kang DH, Kim JH, et al. Percutaneous mitral valvuloplasty versus surgical treatment in mitral stenosis with severe tricuspid regurgitation. Circulation. 2007;116:1246–50.

Straver B, Wagenaar LJ, Blom NA, et al. Percutaneous tricuspid valve implantation in a Fontan patient with congestive heart failure and protein-losing enteropathy. Circ Cardiovasc Interv. 2011;4:112–3.

Sukmawan R, Watanabe N, Ogasawara Y, et al. Geometric changes of tricuspid valve tenting in tricuspid regurgitation secondary to pulmonary hypertension quantified by novel system with transthoracic real-time 3-dimensional echocardiography. J Am Soc Echocardiogr. 2007;20:470–6.

Tang GH, David TE, Singh SK, Maganti MD, Armstrong S, Borger MA. Tricuspid valve repair with an annuloplasty ring results in improved long-term outcomes. Circulation. 2006;114:1735–41.

Tanous D, Nadeem SN, Mason X, Colman JM, Benson LN, Horlick EM. Creation of a functional tricuspid valve: novel use of percutaneously implanted valve in right atrial to right ventricular conduit in a patient with tricuspid atresia. Int J Cardiol. 2009;144:e8–10.

Ton-Nu TT, Levine RA, Handschumacher MD, et al. Geometric determinants of functional tricuspid regurgitation:insights from 3-dimensional echocardiography. Circulation. 2006;114:143–9.

Topilsky Y, Tribouilloy C, Michelena HI, Pislaru S, Mahoney DW, Enriquez-Sarano M. Pathophysiology of tricuspid regurgitation. Quantitative Doppler echocardiographic assessment of respiratory dependence. Circulation. 2010;122:1505–13.

Tribouilloy C, Enriquez-Sarano M, Bailey K, Tajik A, Seward J. Quantification of tricuspid regurgitation by measuring the width of the vena contracta with Doppler color flow imaging: a clinical study. J Am Coll Cardiol. 2000;36:472–8.

Van Garsse LA, Ter Bekke RM, van Ommen VG. Percutaneous transcatheter valve-in-valve implantation in stenosed tricuspid valve bioprosthesis. Circulation. 2011;123:e219–21.

van Son JA, Danielson GK, Schaff HV, Miller FA. Traumatic tricuspid valve insufficiency. Experience in thirteen patients. J Thorac Cardiovasc Surg. 1994;108:893–8.

Vaturi M, Kusniec J, Shapira Y, et al. Right ventricular pacing increases tricuspid regurgitation grade regardless of the mechanical interference to the valve by the electrode. Eur J Echocardiogr. 2010;11(6):550–3.

Velayudhan DE, Brown TM, Nanda NC, et al. Quantification of tricuspid regurgitation by live three-dimensional transthoracic echocardiographic measurements of vena contracta area. Echocardiography. 2006;23:793–800.

Zegdi R, Khabbaz Z, Borenstein N, Fabiani JN. A repositionable valved stent for endovascular treatment of deteriorated bioprostheses. J Am Coll Cardiol. 2006;48:1365–8.

Index

N.M. Rajamannan (ed.), *Cardiac Valvular Medicine*,
DOI 10.1007/978-1-4471-4132-7, © Springer-Verlag London 2013

V

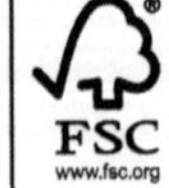

MIX
Papier aus verantwortungsvollen Quellen
Paper from responsible sources
FSC® C105338

If you have any concerns about our products,
you can contact us on
ProductSafety@springernature.com

In case Publisher is established outside the EU,
the EU authorized representative is:
Springer Nature Customer Service Center GmbH
Europaplatz 3, 69115 Heidelberg, Germany

Printed by Libri Plureos GmbH
in Hamburg, Germany